The National Collaborating Centre

for Chronic Conditions

Funded to produce guidelines for the NHS by NICE

OSTEOARTHRITIS

National clinical guideline for care and management in adults

Published by

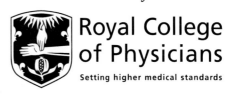

Royal College
of Physicians
Setting higher medical standards

Mission statement

The Royal College of Physicians plays a leading role in the delivery of high quality patient care by setting standards of medical practice and promoting clinical excellence. We provide physicians in the United Kingdom and overseas with education, training and support throughout their careers. As an independent body representing over 20,000 Fellows and Members worldwide, we advise and work with government, the public, patients and other professions to improve health and healthcare.

The National Collaborating Centre for Chronic Conditions

The National Collaborating Centre for Chronic Conditions (NCC-CC) is a collaborative, multiprofessional centre undertaking commissions to develop clinical guidance for the NHS in England and Wales. The NCC-CC was established in 2001. It is an independent body, housed within the Clinical Standards Department at the Royal College of Physicians of London. The NCC-CC is funded by the National Institute for Health and Clinical Excellence (NICE) to undertake commissions for national clinical guidelines on an annual rolling programme.

Citation for this document

National Collaborating Centre for Chronic Conditions. *Osteoarthritis: national clinical guideline for care and management in adults.* London: Royal College of Physicians, 2008.

Contents

DEVELOPMENT OF THE GUIDELINE

1   Introduction

2   Methodology

3   Key messages of the guideline

THE GUIDELINE

4   Holistic approach to osteoarthritis assessment and management

Members of the Guideline Development Group

Professor Philip Conaghan *(Chair)*
Professor of Musculoskeletal Medicine, University of Leeds; Consultant Rheumatologist, Leeds Teaching Hospitals Trust

Dr Fraser Birrell
Consultant Rheumatologist, Northumbria Healthcare NHS Trust;
Honorary Clinical Senior Lecturer, University of Newcastle upon Tyne

Dr Michael Burke
General Practitioner, Merseyside

Ms Jo Cumming
Patient and Carer Representative, London

Dr John Dickson
Clinical Adviser to the GDG; Clinical Lead for Musculoskeletal Services,
Redcar and Cleveland Primary Care Trust

Professor Paul Dieppe
Professor of Health Services Research, University of Bristol

Dr Mike Doherty
Head of Academic Rheumatology, University of Nottingham,
and Honorary Consultant Rheumatologist, Nottingham University Hospitals NHS Trust

Dr Krysia Dziedzic
Senior Lecturer in Physiotherapy, Primary Care Musculoskeletal Research Centre,
Keele University

Professor Roger Francis
Professor of Geriatric Medicine, University of Newcastle upon Tyne

Mr Rob Grant
Senior Project Manager, NCC-CC and Medical Statistician, Royal College of Physicians of London

Mrs Christine Kell
Patient and Carer Representative, County Durham

Mr Nick Latimer
Health Economist, NCC-CC; Research Fellow, Queen Mary University of London

Dr Alex MacGregor
Professor of Chronic Diseases Epidemiology, University of East Anglia;
Consultant Rheumatologist, Norfolk and Norwich University Hospital NHS Trust

Ms Carolyn Naisby
Consultant Physiotherapist, City Hospitals Sunderland NHS Foundation Trust

Dr Rachel O'Mahony
Health Services Research Fellow in Guideline Development, NCC-CC

Mrs Susan Oliver
Nurse Consultant in Rheumatology, Litchdon Medical Centre, Barnstaple, Devon

Mrs Alison Richards
Information Scientist, NCC-CC

Dr Martin Underwood
Vice-dean, Warwick Medical School

The following experts were invited to attend specific meetings and to advise the Guideline Development Group:

Dr Marta Buszewicz
Senior Lecturer in Community-based Teaching and Research, University College London

Dr Alison Carr
Lecturer in Musculoskeletal Epidemiology, University of Nottingham

Mr Mark Emerton
Consultant Orthopaedic Surgeon, Leeds Teaching Hospitals NHS Trust

Professor Edzard Ernst
Laing Professor of Complementary Medicine, Peninsula Medical School

Dr Alison Hammond
Arthritis Research Campaign Senior Lecturer, Brighton University

Dr Mike Hurley
Reader in Physiotherapy; ARC Research Fellow, King's College London

Professor Andrew McCaskie
Professor of Orthopaedics, University of Newcastle upon Tyne

Dr Mark Porcheret
General Practitioner Research Fellow, Keele University

Dr Tony Redmond
Arthritis Research Campaign Lecturer in Podiatric Rheumatology, University of Leeds

Dr Adrian White
Clinical Research Fellow, Peninsula Medical School

Ms Rahana Mohammed of Arthritis Care attended one meeting as a deputy for Ms Jo Cumming

Acknowledgements

The Guideline Development Group (GDG) are grateful to Bernard Higgins, Jane Ingham, Ian Lockhart, Jill Parnham, Nicole Stack, Susan Tann and Claire Turner of the NCC-CC for their support throughout the development of the guideline.

The GDG would especially like to record their gratitude for the great amount of work voluntarily given to the refinement of the economic model of non-steroidal anti-inflammatory drugs by Dr Joanne Lord of the National Institute for Health and Clinical Excellence (NICE).

The GDG would also like to thank the following people for giving their time to advise us on the design and interpretation of the economic model:

- Dr Phil Alderson, NICE
- Mr Garry Barton, School of Economics, University of Nottingham
- Professor Chris Hawkey, Institute of Clinical Research, University of Nottingham
- Professor Tom MacDonald, Hypertension Research Centre and Medicines Monitoring Unit, University of Dundee
- Dr Jayne Spink, NICE
- Dr Rafe Suvarna, Medicines and Healthcare Regulatory Agency
- Professor Richard Thomson, Professor of Epidemiology and Public Health, University of Newcastle upon Tyne
- Dr Weiya Zhang, Associate Professor, Centre for Population Sciences, University of Nottingham.

Preface

Osteoarthritis is the most common disease of the joints, and one of the most widespread of all chronic diseases. Frequently described as 'wear and tear', its prevalence increases steadily with age and by retirement age the associated radiological changes can be observed in over half the population. Symptoms can vary from minimal to severe pain and stiffness, but overall the disease is responsible for considerable morbidity and is a common reason for GP consultation. Unfortunately, it is also difficult to treat and inevitably a wide range of potential therapies have been advocated, both by conventional and complementary practitioners, and not necessarily with strong supporting evidence.

The high prevalence of osteoarthritis, the numerous forms of potential treatment and the uncertainty around these all make the disorder an excellent topic for a clinical guideline. The lack of evidence in some areas is a less favourable feature, and although this has presented something of a challenge, the GDG has risen to this admirably. As with all NICE guidelines, an exhaustive literature search has been performed and the papers identified in this process have been rigorously assessed. Where it is possible to make recommendations based on good evidence, the GDG have done so; where evidence is not available or is weak, they have either made recommendations on the basis of strong clinical consensus, or have advocated appropriate research.

The guideline contains a number of recommendations which are not currently routine practice for many clinicians. While the place of paracetamol in early pain management is confirmed, the guideline also suggests early consideration of topical non-steroidal anti-inflammatory drugs (NSAIDs) for knee and hand arthritis, and suggests that wherever systemic NSAIDs or cyclooxygenase-2 (COX-2) inhibitors are used, they should be coprescribed with cover from a proton pump inhibitor (PPI). This latter recommendation will surprise many, but with PPIs now coming off patent, it is clearly backed up by our health economic analysis. The positive role of exercise is emphasised in contrast to the natural inclination some might have to rest when a joint is affected by osteoarthritis. The GDG has also not shied away from negative recommendations. They suggest that arthroscopic lavage and debridement is not suitable therapy for osteoarthritis except in clear instances where this is associated with mechanical locking; and they do not recommend the use of intra-articular hyaluronans. Elsewhere, there is only restricted support for the use of acupuncture.

The process of producing a guideline is rarely straightforward and there have been occasional difficulties along the way. The GDG have navigated all these with good humour and a consistent desire to evaluate all evidence as thoroughly as they possibly could in order to improve the management of this difficult condition. We at the NCC-CC are grateful to them for all of their work. The guideline is a tribute to their efforts and we hope and expect that it can be used both to practical benefit and to raise the profile of this sometimes neglected condition.

Dr Bernard Higgins MD FRCP
Director, National Collaborating Centre for Chronic Conditions

Abbreviations

ADL	Activities of daily living
AE	Adverse event
AHI	Arthritis Helplessness Index
AIMS	Arthritis Impact Measurement Scale
AL-TENS	Acupuncture-like transcutaneous electrical nerve stimulation
AQoL	Assessment of quality of life instrument
ARC	Arthritis Research Campaign
AT	Assistive technology
BDI	Beck Depression Inventory
BMI	Body mass index
CES-D Scale	Center for Epidemiologic Studies Depression Scale
CI	Confidence interval (95% unless stated otherwise)
COX-2	Cyclooxegenase-2
CV	Cardio-vascular
DASS21	Depression, Anxiety and Stress Scale
EQ-5D	EuroQol 5-dimensional outcomes questionnaire
FABER	Flexion, abduction, external rotation test
GDG	Guideline Development Group
GI	Gastrointestinal
HAD	Hospital Anxiety and Depression Scale
HAQ score	Stanford health assessment questionnaire score
HR	Hazard ratio
HRG	Healthcare resource groups
HS	Harris hip score
HSS	Hospital for special surgery knee score
IRGL Pain Scale	Impact of Rheumatic Diseases on General Health and Lifestyle Pain Scale
ITT	Intention to treat analysis
KOOS	Knee injury and osteoarthritis outcome score
KSPS	Knee-specific Pain Scale
LASER	Light amplification by stimulated emission of radiation
LI	Lequesne index
MA	Meta-analysis
MACTAR	McMaster Toronto Arthritis patient preference questionnaire
MHRA	Medicines and Healthcare products Regulatory Agency
MI	Myocardial infarction
NCC-CC	National Collaborating Centre for Chronic Conditions
NHP Pain Scale	Nottingham Health Profile Pain Scale

NHS	National Health Service; this guideline is intended for use in the NHS in England and Wales
NICE	National Institute for Health and Clinical Excellence
NNT	Number needed to treat
NPRS	Numerical Pain Rating Scale
NRS-101	Numerical Rating Scale
NS	Not significant (at the 5% level unless stated otherwise)
NSAID	Non-steroidal anti-inflammatory drugs
OARSI	Osteoarthritis Research Society international assessment questionnaire
OR	Odds ratio
PASE	Physical Activity Scale for the Elderly
PEMF	Pulsed electromagnetic field
PEME	Pulsed electromagnetic energy
PPI	Proton pump inhibitor, **also** Present pain intensity score
PPT	Pressure pain tolerance
PSFS	Patient-specific Functional Scale
PUB	Perforation (gastric), ulceration, or bleed
QALY	Quality of life-adjusted year
QoLS	Quality of life score
QWB	Quality of Well-being Scale
RAOS	Rheumatoid and arthritis outcome score
RCT	Randomised clinical trial
ROM	Range of motion
RR	Relative risk
SDS Pain Scale	Simple Descriptive Scale
SF-12	Short Form (12 point) questionnaire
SF-36	Short Form (36 point) questionnaire
SIP	Sickness impact profile
SMD	Standardised mean difference
SNRI	Serotonin and noradrenalin reuptake inhibitor
SR	Systematic review
SSRI	Selective serotonin reuptake inhibitor
SWD	Short wave diathermy
TEFR	Therapeutic education and functional re-adaptation programme
TENS	Transcutaneous electrical nerve stimulation
TJA	Total joint arthroplasty (joint replacement surgery)
TSK	Tampa scale of kinesiophobia
TTU	Transfer to utility
VAS	Visual analogue scale
WOMAC	Western Ontario and McMaster Osteoarthritis Index
WMD	Weighted mean differences

Glossary

Clinically significant improvement	Some trials define a dichotomous outcome of clinically significant pain relief as having been achieved above a specific threshold on a pain score, for example, WOMAC pain VAS. However, there is no standard threshold and each such trial should be considered individually.
Cohort study	A retrospective or prospective follow-up study. Groups of individuals to be followed up are defined on the basis of presence or absence of exposure to a suspected risk factor or intervention. A cohort study can be comparative, in which case two or more groups are selected on the basis of differences in their exposure to the agent of interest.
Confidence interval (CI)	A range of values which provide a measure of certainty in a statistic. The interval is calculated from sample data, and generally straddles the sample estimate. The 95% confidence value means that if the study is repeated many times, then 95% of the estimates of the statistic in question will lie within the confidence interval.
Cochrane library	The Cochrane Library consists of a regularly updated collection of evidence-based medicine databases including the Cochrane Database of Systematic Reviews (reviews of randomised controlled trials prepared by the Cochrane Collaboration).
Concordance	A concept reflecting the extent to which a course of action agreed between clinicians and a patient is actually carried out, often but not solely used in the sense of therapeutic interventions or behavioural changes.
Cost–consequence analysis	A type of economic evaluation where, for each intervention, various health outcomes are reported in addition to cost, but there is no overall measure of health gain.
Cost–effectiveness analysis	An economic study design in which consequences of different interventions are measured using a single outcome, usually in natural units (for example, life-years gained, deaths avoided, heart attacks avoided, cases detected). Alternative interventions are then compared in terms of cost per unit of effectiveness.
Cost–utility analysis	A form of cost–effectiveness analysis in which the units of effectiveness are quality adjusted life-years (QALYs).
Electrotherapy	In this guideline, electrotherapy is used to describe any intervention suggested to be useful in controlling pain in osteoarthritis through applying local electrical or electromagnetic stimulation.
Escape medication	See rescue medication
Implementation study	A pragmatic approach to assess the real-life effectiveness of a programme of healthcare interventions as a complete package, typically around information and communication. Measurements are made before and after the implementation of the new programme. The study design suffers from contemporaneous confounding changes in the healthcare system, lack of blinding, primacy/recency effects and a historical control group.
Incremental cost	The cost of one alternative less the cost of another.
Incremental cost–effectiveness ratio (ICER)	The ratio of the difference in costs between two alternatives to the difference in effectiveness between the same two alternatives.
Kellgren-Lawrence scale	A tool for classifying severity of osteoarthritis based on radiographic findings.
Manual therapy	A range of physiotherapy techniques where the affected joint (typically the hip) is manipulated and stretched beyond the range of motion that the person with osteoarthritis is able to use.
Meta-analysis	A statistical technique for combining (pooling) the results of a number of studies that address the same question and report on the same outcomes to produce a summary result.

Methodological limitations	Features of the design or reporting of a clinical study which are known to be associated with risk of bias or lack of validity. Where a study is reported in this guideline as having significant methodological limitations, a recommendation has not been directly derived from it.
Observational study	A retrospective or prospective study in which the investigator observes the natural course of events with or without control groups, for example cohort studies and case-control studies.
Odds ratio	A measure of treatment effectiveness: the odds of an event happening in the intervention group, divided by the odds of it happening in the control group. The 'odds' is the ratio of non-events to events.
p-values	The probability that an observed difference could have occurred by chance. A p-value of less than 0.05 is conventionally considered to be 'statistically significant'.
Quality of life	Refers to the level of comfort, enjoyment and ability to pursue daily activities.
Quality-of-life adjusted year (QALY)	A measure of health outcome which assigns to each period of time a weight, ranging from 0 to 1, corresponding to the health-related quality of life during that period, where a weight of 1 corresponds to optimal health, and a weight of 0 corresponds to a health state judged equivalent to death; these are then aggregated across time periods.
Randomised clinical trial (RCT)	A trial in which people are randomly assigned to two (or more) groups: one (the experimental group) receiving the treatment that is being tested, and the other (the comparison or control group) receiving an alternative treatment, a placebo (dummy treatment) or no treatment. The two groups are followed up to compare differences in outcomes to see how effective the experimental treatment was. Such trial designs help minimise experimental bias.
Rescue medication	In this guideline, this is an outcome recorded by some studies. The rate of rescue medication use is the rate at which participants had to use a stronger medication (typically for analgesia).
Self-management	A term used for aspects of osteoarthritis care which a person can do for themselves with advice from the primary care team, such as the GP, nurse, physiotherapist, occupational therapist and from information leaflets.
Sensitivity analysis	A measure of the extent to which small changes in parameters and variables affect a result calculated from them. In this guideline, sensitivity analysis is used in health economic modelling.
Stakeholder	Any national organisation, including patient and carers' groups, healthcare professionals and commercial companies with an interest in the guideline under development.
Statistical significance	A result is deemed statistically significant if the probability of the result occurring by chance is less than 1 in 20 (p<0.05).
Systematic review	Research that summarises the evidence on a clearly formulated question according to a pre-defined protocol using systematic and explicit methods to identify, select and appraise relevant studies, and to extract, collate and report their findings. It may or may not use statistical meta-analysis.
Technology appraisal	Formal ascertainment and review of the evidence surrounding a health technology, restricted in the current document to appraisals undertaken by NICE.
Transfer to utility	A method of deriving health utilities from clinical outcomes through finding an equation that best links the two.
Utility	A number between 0 and 1 that can be assigned to a particular state of health, assessing the holistic impact on quality of life and allowing states to be ranked in order of (average) patient preference.

DEVELOPMENT OF THE GUIDELINE

1 Introduction

1.1 What is osteoarthritis?

Osteoarthritis (OA) refers to a clinical syndrome of joint pain accompanied by varying degrees of functional limitation and reduced quality of life. It is by far the most common form of arthritis and one of the leading causes of pain and disability worldwide. Any synovial joint can develop osteoarthritis but knees, hips and small hand joints are the peripheral sites most commonly affected. Although pain, reduced function and participation restriction can be important consequences of osteoarthritis, structural changes commonly occur without accompanying symptoms. Such frequent discordance between osteoarthritis pathology, symptoms and disability means that each of these need separate consideration in epidemiological studies and clinical trials of osteoarthritis treatments.

Osteoarthritis is a metabolically active, dynamic process that involves all joint tissues (cartilage, bone, synovium/capsule, ligaments and muscle). Key pathological changes include localised loss of articular (hyaline) cartilage and remodelling of adjacent bone with new bone formation (osteophyte) at the joint margins. This combination of tissue loss and new tissue synthesis supports the view of osteoarthritis as the *repair process* of synovial joints. A variety of joint traumas may trigger the need to repair, but once initiated all the joint tissues take part, showing increased cell activity and new tissue production. In general, osteoarthritis is a slow but efficient repair process that often compensates for the initial trauma, resulting in a structurally altered but symptom-free joint. In some people, however, either because of overwhelming insult or compromised repair potential, the osteoarthritis process cannot compensate, resulting in continuing tissue damage and eventual presentation with symptomatic osteoarthritis or 'joint failure'. This explains the extreme variability in clinical presentation and outcome, both between individuals and at different joint sites. The specific targeting of osteoarthritis for certain joints remains unexplained, but one hypothesis suggests an evolutionary fault where joints that have most recently altered are biomechanically underdesigned and thus more often fail.

1.2 Risk factors for osteoarthritis

Osteoarthritis is defined not as a disease or a single condition but as a *common complex disorder* with multiple *risk factors*. These risk factors are broadly divisible into:
- *genetic* factors (heritability estimates for hand, knee and hip osteoarthritis are high at 40–60%, though the responsible genes are largely unknown)
- *constitutional* factors (for example, ageing, female sex, obesity, high bone density)
- more local, largely *biomechanical* risk factors (for example, joint injury, occupational/recreational usage, reduced muscle strength, joint laxity, joint malalignment).

Importantly, many environmental/lifestyle risk factors are reversible (for example, obesity, muscle weakness) or avoidable (for example, occupational or recreational joint trauma) which has important implications for secondary and primary prevention. However, the importance of individual risk factors varies, and even differs, between joint sites. Also, risk factors for developing osteoarthritis may differ from risk factors for progression and poor clinical outcome (eg high bone density is a risk factor for development, but low bone density is a risk factor for progression of knee and hip osteoarthritis). This means that knowledge, including treatments, for osteoarthritis at one joint site cannot necessarily be extrapolated to all joint sites.

1.3 The epidemiology of osteoarthritis pain and structural pathology

The exact incidence and prevalence of osteoarthritis is difficult to determine because the clinical syndrome of osteoarthritis (joint pain and stiffness) does not always correspond with the structural changes of osteoarthritis (usually defined as abnormal changes in the appearance of joints on radiographs). This area is becoming more complex with sensitive imaging techniques such as magnetic resonance imaging, which demonstrate more frequent structural abnormalities than detected by radiographs.

Osteoarthritis at individual joint sites (notably knee, hip and hand) demonstrates consistent age-related increases in prevalence (Arthritis and Musculoskeletal Alliance 2004). However, symptomatic osteoarthritis **is not an inevitable consequence of ageing**. Although prevalence of osteoarthritis rises in frequency with age, it does affect substantial numbers of people of working age. The number of people with osteoarthritis in the UK is increasing as the population ages, and as the prevalence of risk factors such as obesity and poor levels of physical fitness also continues to rise.

▷ Joint pain

The cause of joint pain in osteoarthritis is not well understood. Estimates suggest that up to 8.5 million people in the UK are affected by joint pain that may be attributed to osteoarthritis (Arthritis Care 2004). Population estimates of the prevalence of joint symptoms depend heavily on the specific definition used, but there is general agreement that the occurrence of symptoms is more common than radiographic osteoarthritis in any given joint among older people. This may be due to joint pain arising from causes other than osteoarthritis (for example bursitis, tendonitis) and differing radiographic protocols.

In adults 45 years old and over, the most common site of peripheral joint pain lasting for more than one week in the past month is in the knee (19%) and the highest prevalence of knee pain is among women aged 75 and over (35%) (Urwin et al. 1998). Global disability is also high among those reporting isolated knee pain. In adults aged 50 years old and over, 23% report severe pain and disability (Jinks et al. 2004). One-month period prevalence of hand pain ranges from 12% in adults 45 years and over (Urwin et al. 1998) to 30% in adults 50 years and over (Dziedzic et al. 2007) and is more common in women than men, increasing in prevalence in the oldest age groups (Dziedzic 2007).

▷ Radiographic osteoarthritis

Although joint pain is more common than radiographic osteoarthritis, much radiographic osteoarthritis occurs in the absence of symptoms. At least 4.4 million people in the UK have x-ray evidence of moderate to severe osteoarthritis of their hands, over 0.5 million have moderate to severe osteoarthritis of the knees and 210,000 have moderate to severe osteoarthritis of the hips (Arthritis Research Campaign 2002; Arthritis and Musculoskeletal Alliance 2004). The prevalence of radiographic osteoarthritis, like symptoms, is also dependent on the particular images acquired and definitions used (Duncan et al. 2006).

The prevalence of radiographic osteoarthritis is higher in women than men, especially after the age of 50 and for hand and knee osteoarthritis. Radiographic osteoarthritis of the knee affects about 25% of community populations of adults aged 50 years and over (Peat 2001).

Ethnic differences in radiographic osteoarthritis prevalence have been more difficult to distinguish, especially in studied African-American groups. However, recent reports (Peat et al. 2006) comparing Chinese and US populations have demonstrated much lower levels of hip osteoarthritis in the Chinese, although levels of knee and hand osteoarthritis generally were similar despite varying patterns.

▷ The relationship between symptomatic and radiographic osteoarthritis

Although symptoms and radiographic changes do not always overlap, radiographic osteoarthritis is still more common in persons with a longer history and more persistent symptoms. There is a consistent association at the knee, for example, between severity of pain, stiffness and physical function and the presence of radiographic osteoarthritis (Duncan et al. 2007). Concordance between symptoms and radiographic osteoarthritis seems greater with more advanced structural damage (Peat et al. 2006).

Half of adults aged 50 years and over with radiographic osteoarthritis of the knee have symptoms (Peat et al. 2006). Of the 25% of older adults with significant knee joint pain, two thirds have radiographic disease. The prevalence of painful, disabling radiographic knee osteoarthritis in the UK populations aged over 55 has been estimated at approximately 10%. The prevalence of symptomatic radiographic osteoarthritis is higher in women than men, especially after the age of 50. Within the knee joint of symptomatic individuals, the most common radiographic osteoarthritis pattern of involvement is combined tibiofemoral and patellofemoral changes (Duncan et al. 2006). Although there are few good studies, symptomatic radiographic hand osteoarthritis has been reported in less than 3% of the population, while rates of symptomatic radiographic hip osteoarthritis have varied from 5 to 9%.

Table 1.1 Prevalence of radiographic and symptomatic osteoarthritis in older adults		
	Radiographic osteoarthritis (%)	Symptomatic osteoarthritis (%)
Knee (Peat et al. 2001)	25	13
Hip (Croft;* Lau et al. 1996)	11	5
Hand (Wilder et al. 2006)	41	3

* The 5% symptomatic OA prevalence: personal communication 2007.

1.4 Prognosis and outcome

A common misconception in the UK, held by the public as well as many healthcare professionals, is that osteoarthritis is a slowly progressive disease that inevitably gets worse and results in increasing pain and disability over time. However, the osteoarthritis process is one of attempted repair, and this repair process effectively limits the damage and symptoms in the majority of cases.

The need to consider osteoarthritis of the knee, hip and hand as separate entities is apparent from their different natural histories and outcomes. *Hand osteoarthritis* has a particularly good prognosis. Most cases of interphalangeal joint osteoarthritis become asymptomatic after a few years, although patients are left with permanent swellings of the distal or proximal interphalangeal joints (called Heberden's and Bouchard's nodes respectively). Involvement of the thumb base may have a worse prognosis, as in some cases this causes continuing pain on certain activities (such as pinch grip), and thus lasting disability.

Knee osteoarthritis is very variable in its outcome. Improvement in the structure of the joint, as shown by radiographs, is rare once the condition has become established. However, improvement in pain and disability over time is common. The data on clinical outcomes, as opposed to radiographic changes, are sparse, but it would seem that over a period of several years about a third of cases improve, a third stay much the same, and the remaining third of patients develop progressive symptomatic disease. Little is known about the risk factors for progression, which may be different from those for initiation of the disease, but obesity probably makes an important contribution.

Hip osteoarthritis probably has the worst overall outcome of the three major sites considered in this guideline. As with the knee, relatively little is known about the natural history of symptomatic disease, but we do know that a significant number of people progress to a point where hip replacement is needed in 1 to 5 years. In contrast, some hips heal spontaneously, with improvement in the radiographic changes as well as the symptoms.

Osteoarthritis predominantly affects older people, and often coexists with other conditions associated with aging and obesity, such as cardiovascular disease and diabetes, as well as with common sensory (for example, poor vision) and psychosocial problems (for example, anxiety, depression and social isolation). The prognosis and outcome depends on these comorbidities as much as it does on the joint disease.

1.5 The impact on the individual

Osteoarthritis is the most common cause of disability in the UK. Pain, stiffness, joint deformity and loss of joint mobility have a substantial impact on individuals.

Pain is the most frequent reason for patients to present to their GP and over half of people with osteoarthritis say that pain is their worse problem. Many people with osteoarthritis experience persistent pain (Arthritis Research Campaign 2002). Severity of pain is also important, with the likelihood of mobility problems increasing as pain increases (Wilkie et al. 2006). It can affect every aspect of a person's daily life, and their overall quality of life (Doherty et al. 2003).

I mean, if I sit too long, that doesn't help either. But the worst part is if I'm asleep and my legs are bent and I haven't woke up, the pain, I can't tell you what it is like. I can not move it ... and what I do is I grip both hands round the knee and try to force my leg straight and I break out in a hot sweat. All I can say is that it is a bony pain. I could shout out with the pain (Jinks et al. 2007).

Osteoarthritis of the large joints reduces people's mobility. The disorder accounts for more trouble with climbing stairs and walking than any other disease (Felson et al. 2000). Furthermore, 80% of people with the condition have some degree of limitation of movement and 25% cannot perform their major activities of daily life (World Health Organization 2003). In small joints such as the hands and fingers osteoarthritis makes many ordinary tasks difficult and painful (Arthritis and Musculoskeletal Alliance 2004).

When it first happened [knee pain], I couldn't put weight on my foot. It was horrible. I can't tell you what it was like. Really really severe ... painful; absolutely painful. I used to walk a lot, that stopped me from walking, but now I'm walking again so that's better isn't it? I thought I'd be a cripple for life. I couldn't see it going. I couldn't see what would make it go, but physio helped and those tablets helped (Jinks et al. 2007).

Older adults with joint pain are more likely to have participation restriction in areas of life such as getting out and about, looking after others and work, than those without joint pain (Wilkie et al 2007). Although it is difficult to be certain from studies of elderly populations with significant comorbid medical problems, it may be that there is an increased mortality associated with multiple-joint osteoarthritis.

1.6 The impact on society

Increases in life expectancy and ageing populations are expected to make osteoarthritis the fourth leading cause of disability by the year 2020 (Woolf and Pfleger 2003).

- Osteoarthritis was estimated to be the eighth leading non-fatal burden of disease in the world in 1990, accounting for 2.8% of total years of living with disability, around the same percentage as schizophrenia and congenital anomalies (Murray and Lopez 1996; Woolf and Pfleger 2003)
- Osteoarthritis was the sixth leading cause of years living with disability at a global level, accounting for 3% of the total global years of living with disability (Woolf and Pfelger 2003).

Osteoarthritis has considerable impact on health services.

- Each year 2 million adults visit their GP because of osteoarthritis (Arthritis Research Campaign 2002).
- Consultations for osteoarthritis account for 15% of all musculoskeletal consultations in those aged 45 years old and over, peaking at 25% in those aged 75 years old and over. Of those aged over 45 years old, 5% have an osteoarthritis-recorded primary care consultation in the course of a year. This rises to 10% in those aged 75 years and over (Jordan et al. 2007).
- The incidence of a new GP consultation for knee pain in adults aged 50 and over is approximately 10% per year (Jordan et al. 2006).
- Over a 1-year period there were 114,500 hospital admissions (Arthrtis Research Campaign 2002).
- In 2000, over 44,000 hip replacements and over 35,000 knee replacements were performed at a cost of £405 million.

Although some people do consult their GP, many others do not. In a recent study, over half of people with severe and disabling knee pain had not visited their GP about this in the past 12 months. People's perception of osteoarthritis is that it is a part of normal ageing. The perception that 'nothing can be done' is a dominant feature in many accounts (Sanders et al. 2004).

Osteoarthritis has a significant negative impact on the UK economy, with its total cost estimated as equivalent of 1% of GNP per year (Arthritis and Musculoskeletal Alliance 2004; Levy et al. 1993; Doherty et al. 1995, 2003). Only a very few people who are receiving incapacity benefit – around one in 200 – later return to work (Arthritis and Musculoskeletal Alliance 2004; Arthritis Research Campaign 2002). In 1999/2000, 36 million working days were lost due to osteoarthritis alone, at an estimated cost of £3.2 billion in lost production. At the same time, £43 million was spent on community services and £215 million was spent on social services for osteoarthritis.

1.7   Features of the evidence base for osteoarthritis

The following guidelines and recommendations for osteoarthritis are based on an evidence-based appraisal of a vast amount of literature as well as on expert opinion, especially where the evidence base is particularly lacking.

Where appropriate, these guidelines have focused on *patient-centred* outcomes (often patient-reported outcomes) concerning pain, function and quality of life. We also included some performance-based outcomes measures, especially where there is some face validity that they may relate to function, for example, proprioception outcome measures which may be relevant to the potential for falls. Unfortunately, many studies do not include a quality of life measure, and often the only non-pain outcomes reported may be a generic health-related quality of life measure such as the SF-36.

There are always limitations to the evidence on which such guidelines are based, and the recommendations need to be viewed in light of these limitations.

- The majority of the published evidence relates to osteoarthritis of the knee. We have tried to highlight where the evidence pertains to an individual anatomical location, and have presented these as related to knee, hip, hand or mixed sites.
- There are very limited data on the effects of *combinations* of therapies.
- Many trials have looked at single joint involvement when many patients have *multiple* joint involvement which may alter the reported efficacy of a particular therapeutic intervention.
- There is a major problem interpreting the duration of efficacy of therapies since many studies, especially those including pharmacological therapies, are of short duration.
- Similarly, side effects may only be detected after long-term follow-up; therefore, where possible we have included toxicity data from long-term observational studies as well as randomised trials.
- When looking at studies of pharmacological therapies, there is the complexity of comparing different doses of drugs.
- Many studies do not reflect 'real-life' patient use of therapies or their compliance. Patients may not use pharmacological therapies on a daily basis or at the full recommended

dosages. Also, the use of over-the-counter medications has not been well studied in osteoarthritis populations.

- Most studies have not included patients with very severe osteoarthritis (for example, severely functional compromised patients who cannot walk, or patients with severe structural damage such as grade 4 Kellgren Lawrence radiographic damage). This may limit the extrapolation of the reported benefits of a therapy to these patients.
- Studies often include patients who are not at high risk of drug side effects. Many studies have not included very elderly patients.
- There is an inherent bias with time-related improvement in design of studies: there tends to be better designs with more recent studies, and often with pharmaceutical company funding.

1.8 The working diagnosis of osteoarthritis

This guideline applies to people with a working diagnosis of osteoarthritis who present for treatment or whose activities of daily living are significantly affected by their osteoarthritis. The management of neck or back pain related to degenerative changes in spine are not part of this guideline.

People presenting to health professionals with osteoarthritis complain of joint pain, they do not complain of radiological change. Thus, these guidelines are primarily about the management of older patients presenting for treatment of peripheral joint pain, treatment of the pain itself and of the consequences of such pain for patients who have a working diagnosis of osteoarthritis. The Guideline Development Group (GDG) recognised that many of the studies reviewed will have only included participants with symptomatic radiological osteoarthritis and that they are inferring any positive or negative treatment effects apply equally to those with or without radiological change.

The GDG considered the following to represent a clinician's working diagnosis of peripheral joint osteoarthritis:
- persistent joint pain that is worse with use
- age 45 years old and over
- morning stiffness lasting no more than half an hour.

The GDG felt that patients meeting their working diagnosis of osteoarthritis do not normally require radiological or laboratory investigations. This working diagnosis is very similar to the American College of Rheumatologists' clinical diagnostic criteria for osteoarthritis of the knee that were designed to differentiate between an inflammatory arthritis such as rheumatoid arthritis and osteoarthritis (Altman et al. 1986).

Other symptoms/findings which will, if required, add to diagnostic certainty include:
- inactivity pain and stiffness, known as 'gelling'. This is very common, for example after prolonged sitting, and should be distinguished from locking, which is a feature normally associated with prevention of limb straightening during gait, and suggests meniscal pathology
- examination findings of crepitus or bony swelling

- radiological evidence of osteoarthritis (joint space loss, osteophyte formation, subchondral bone thickening or cyst formation)
- absence of clinical/laboratory evidence of inflammation such as acutely inflamed joints or markers of inflammation (raised erythrocyte sedimentation rate/C-reactive protein/plasma viscosity).

The working diagnosis of osteoarthritis excludes the following joint disorders which are not addressed in these guidelines: inflammatory arthritis (including rheumatoid and psoriatic arthritis, ankylosing spondylitis, gout and reactive arthritis) and connective tissue disorders with associated arthritides. However, it is important to recognise that many patients with inflammatory arthritis have secondary osteoarthritis and that these guidelines could also apply to these patients.

1.9 This guideline and the previous technology appraisal on COX-2 inhibitors

This guideline replaces the osteoarthritis aspects only of the NICE technology appraisal TA27 (National Institute for Health and Clinical Excellence 2001). The guideline recommendations are based on up-to-date evidence on efficacy and adverse events, contemporary costs and an expanded health economic analysis of cost effectiveness. This has led to an increased role for COX-2 inhibitors, blanket warning of adverse events (not just gastro-intestinal) and a clear recommendation to coprescribe a proton pump inhibitor. It is important to bear in mind that technology appraisals carry a governmental obligation for implementation while guidelines do not.

2 Methodology

2.1 Aim

The aim of the National Collaborating Centre for Chronic Conditions (NCC-CC) is to provide a user-friendly, clinical, evidence-based guideline for the NHS in England and Wales that:

- offers best clinical advice for osteoarthritis
- is based on best published clinical and economic evidence, alongside expert consensus
- takes into account patient choice and informed decision-making
- defines the major components of NHS care provision for osteoarthritis
- details areas of uncertainty or controversy requiring further research
- provides a choice of guideline versions for differing audiences.

2.2 Scope

The guideline was developed in accordance with a scope, which detailed the remit of the guideline originating from the Department of Health and specified those aspects of osteoarthritis care to be included and excluded.

Prior to the commencement of the guideline development, the scope was subjected to stakeholder consultation in accordance with processes established by NICE (National Institute for Health and Clinical Excellence 2006). The full scope is shown in Appendix B, available online at www.rcplondon.ac.uk/pubs/brochure.aspx?e=242

2.3 Audience

The guideline is intended for use by the following people or organisations:

- all healthcare professionals
- people with osteoarthritis and their parents and carers
- patient support groups
- commissioning organisations
- service providers.

2.4 Involvement of people with osteoarthritis

The NCC-CC was keen to ensure the views and preferences of people with osteoarthritis and their carers informed all stages of the guideline. This was achieved by:

- having a person with osteoarthritis and a user-organisation representative on the guideline development group
- consulting the Patient and Public Involvement Programme (PPIP) housed within NICE during the predevelopment (scoping) and final validation stages of the guideline project.

2.5 Guideline limitations

Guideline limitations comprise those listed below.

- NICE clinical guidelines usually do not cover issues of **service** delivery, organisation or provision (unless specified in the remit from the Department of Health).
- NICE is primarily concerned with health services and so recommendations are not provided for social services and the voluntary sector. However, the guideline may address important issues in how NHS clinicians interface with these other sectors.
- Generally, the guideline does not cover rare, complex, complicated or unusual conditions.
- Where a meta-analysis has been used to look at a particular outcome such as pain, the individual component papers were considered to ensure that studies were not excluded that contained outcome measures relevant to function and quality of life.
- It is not possible in the development of a clinical guideline to complete extensive systematic literature review of all pharmacological toxicity, although NICE expect their guidelines to be read alongside the summaries of product characteristics.

2.6 Other work relevant to the guideline

NICE has published technology appraisal guidance on selective COX-2 inhibitors for osteo-arthritis (which is superseded by publication of this guideline) and rheumatoid arthritis. This is available from www.nice.org.uk under the number TA27 (National Institute for Health and Clinical Excellence 2001).

NICE has also published interventional procedures guidance on artificial metacarpophalangeal and interphalangeal joint replacement for end-stage arthritis. This is available from www.nice.org.uk under the number IPG110.

The NCC-CC and NICE are developing a clinical guideline on rheumatoid arthritis (publication is expected in 2009).

Other guidance referred to in this guideline:

- 'Obesity: the prevention, identification, assessment and management of overweight and obesity in adults and children', available from www.nice.org.uk (number CG43).
- 'Depression: management of depression in primary and secondary care', available from www.nice.org.uk (number CG23).
- 'Dyspepsia: managing dyspesia in adults in primary care', available from www.nice.org.uk (number CG17).

2.7 Background

The development of this evidence-based clinical guideline draws upon the methods described by NICE's 'Guidelines manual' (National Institute for Health and Clinical Excellence 2006) and the online methodology pack (National Collaborating Centre for Chronic Conditions 2006) specifically developed by the NCC-CC for each chronic condition guideline (see www.rcplondon. ac.uk/college/ceeu/ncc-cc/index.asp). The developers' role and remit is summarised in Table 2.1.

Table 2.1 Role and remit of the developers	
National Collaborating Centre for Chronic Conditions (NCC-CC)	The NCC-CC was set up in 2001 and is housed within the Royal College of Physicians (RCP). The NCC-CC undertakes commissions received from NICE. A multiprofessional partners' board inclusive of patient groups and NHS management governs the NCC-CC.
NCC-CC Technical Team	The technical team met approximately two weeks before each Guideline Development Group (GDG) meeting and comprised the following members: GDG Chair GDG Clinical Adviser Information Scientist Research Fellow Health Economist Project Manager.
Guideline Development Group	The GDG met monthly (May 2006 to May 2007) and comprised a multidisciplinary team of professionals, people with osteoarthritis and patient organisation representatives who were supported by the technical team. The GDG membership details including patient representation and professional groups are detailed in the GDG membership page (p v).
Guideline Project Executive (PE)	The PE was involved in overseeing all phases of the guideline. It also reviewed the quality of the guideline and compliance with the Department of Health remit and NICE scope. The PE comprised: NCC-CC Director NCC-CC Assistant Director NCC-CC Manager NICE Commissioning Manager Technical Team.
Formal consensus	At the end of the guideline development process the GDG met to review and agree the guideline recommendations.

Members of the GDG declared any interests in accordance with NICE's 'Guideline manual' (National Institute for Health and Clinical Excellence 2006). A register is given in Appendix E, available online at www.rcplondon.ac.uk/pubs/brochure.aspx?e=242

2.8 The process of guideline development

The basic steps in the process of producing a guideline are:
- developing clinical evidence-based questions
- systematically searching for the evidence
- critically appraising the evidence
- incorporating health economic evidence
- distilling and synthesising the evidence and writing recommendations
- grading the evidence statements
- agreeing the recommendations

- structuring and writing the guideline
- updating the guideline.

▷ Developing evidence-based questions

The technical team drafted a series of clinical questions that covered the guideline scope. The GDG and Project Executive refine and approve these questions, which are shown in Appendix A available online at www.rcplondon.ac.uk/pubs/brochure.aspx?e=242

▷ Searching for the evidence

The information scientist developed a search strategy for each question. Key words for the search were identified by the GDG. In addition, the health economist searched for additional papers providing economic evidence or to inform detailed health economic work (for example, modelling). Papers that were published or accepted for publication in peer-reviewed journals were considered as evidence by the GDG. Conference paper abstracts and non-English language papers were excluded from the searches.

Each clinical question dictated the appropriate study design that was prioritised in the search strategy but the strategy was not limited solely to these study types. The research fellow or health economist identified titles and abstracts from the search results that appeared to be relevant to the question. Exclusion lists were generated for each question together with the rationale for the exclusion. The exclusion lists were presented to the GDG. Full papers were obtained where relevant. See Appendix A for literature search details; available online at www.rcplondon.ac.uk/pubs/brochure.aspx?e=242

▷ Appraising the evidence

The research fellow or health economist, as appropriate, critically appraised the full papers. In general, no formal contact was made with authors; however, there were ad hoc occasions when this was required in order to clarify specific details. Critical appraisal checklists were compiled for each full paper. One research fellow undertook the critical appraisal and data extraction. The evidence was considered carefully by the GDG for accuracy and completeness.

All procedures are fully compliant with the:
- NICE methodology as detailed in the 'Guideline development methods – information for national collaborating centres and guideline developers manual' (National Institute for Health and Clinical Excellence 2006)
- NCC-CC quality assurance document and systematic review chart available at: www.rcplondon.ac.uk/college/ncc-cc/index.asp

▷ Health economic evidence

Areas for health economic modelling were agreed by the GDG after the formation of the clinical questions. The Health Economist reviewed the clinical questions to consider the potential application of health economic modelling, and these priorities were agreed with the GDG. In this guideline, a broad cost-consequence comparison was performed. Details are given in Appendix C available online at www.rcplondon.ac.uk/pubs/brochure.aspx?e=242 An in-depth economic model was created to compare non-steroidal anti-inflammatory drugs (NSAIDs), including the selective COX-2 inhibitors, and this is described in section 8.3 with details in Appendix D, available online at www.rcplondon.ac.uk/pubs/brochure.aspx?e=242

The health economist performed supplemental literature searches to obtain additional data for modelling. Assumptions and designs of the models were explained to and agreed by the GDG members during meetings, and they commented on subsequent revisions.

▷ Distilling and synthesising the evidence and developing recommendations

The evidence from each full paper was distilled into an evidence table and synthesised into evidence statements before being presented to the GDG. This evidence was then reviewed by the GDG and used as a basis upon which to formulate recommendations. The criteria for grading evidence are shown in Table 2.2.

Evidence tables are available online at available online at
www.rcplondon.ac.uk/pubs/brochure.aspx?e=242

▷ Grading the evidence statements

Table 2.2 Grading the evidence statements (National Institute for Health and Clinical Excellence 2006)	
Level of evidence	**Type of evidence**
1++	High-quality meta-analyses (MA), systematic reviews of RCTs, or RCTs with a very low risk of bias.
1+	Well-conducted meta-analyses, systematic reviews of RCTs, or RCTs with a low risk of bias.
1–	Meta-analyses, systematic reviews of RCTs, or RCTs with a high risk of bias.*
2++	High-quality systematic reviews of case-control or cohort studies. High-quality case-control or cohort studies with a very low risk of confounding, bias or chance and a high probability that the relationship is causal.
2+	Well-conducted case-control or cohort studies with a low risk of confounding, bias or chance and a moderate probability that the relationship is causal.
2–	Case-control or cohort studies with a high risk of confounding, bias or chance and a significant risk that the relationship is not causal.*
3	Non-analytic studies (for example case reports, case series).
4	Expert opinion, formal consensus.

*Studies with a level of evidence '–' are not used as a basis for making a recommendation.

▷ Agreeing the recommendations

The GDG employed formal consensus techniques to:
- ensure that the recommendations reflected the evidence base
- approve recommendations based on lesser evidence or extrapolations from other situations
- reach consensus recommendations where the evidence was inadequate
- debate areas of disagreement and finalise recommendations.

The GDG also reached agreement on the following:

- five to ten recommendations as key priorities for implementation
- five key research recommendations
- algorithms.

In prioritising key recommendations for implementation, the GDG took into account the following criteria:

- high clinical impact
- high impact on reducing variation
- more efficient use of NHS resources
- allowing the patient to reach critical points in the care pathway more quickly.

Audit criteria will be produced for NICE by Clinical Accountability Service Planning and Evaluation (CASPE) Research following publication in order to provide suggestions of areas for audit in line with the key recommendations for implementation.

▷ Structuring and writing the guideline

The guideline is divided into sections for ease of reading. For each section the layout is similar and contains the following parts.

- *Clinical introduction* sets a succinct background and describes the current clinical context.
- *Methodological introduction* describes any issues or limitations that were apparent when reading the evidence base.
- *Evidence statements* provide a synthesis of the evidence base and usually describe what the evidence showed in relation to the outcomes of interest.
- *Health economics* presents, where appropriate, an overview of the cost-effectiveness evidence base, or any economic modelling.
- *From evidence to recommendations* sets out the GDG decision-making rationale providing a clear and explicit audit trail from the evidence to the evolution of the recommendations.
- *Recommendations* provide stand alone, action-orientated recommendations.
- *Evidence tables* are not published as part of the full guideline but are available online at www.rcplondon.ac.uk/pubs/brochure.aspx?e=242 These describe comprehensive details of the primary evidence that was considered during the writing of each section.

▷ Writing the guideline

The first draft version of the guideline was drawn up by the technical team in accord with the decisions of the GDG, incorporating contributions from individual GDG members in their expert areas and edited for consistency of style and terminology. The guideline was then submitted for a formal public and stakeholder consultation prior to publication. The registered stakeholders for this guideline are detailed on the NICE website (www.nice.org.uk). Editorial responsibility for the full guideline rests with the GDG.

Table 2.3 Versions of this guideline	
Full version	Details the recommendations, the supporting evidence base and the expert considerations of the GDG. Published by the NCC-CC. Available at www.rcplondon.ac.uk/pubs/brochure.aspx?e=242
NICE version	Documents the recommendations without any supporting evidence. Available at www.nice.org.uk
'Quick reference guide'	An abridged version. Available at www.rcplondon.ac.uk/pubs/brochure.aspx?e=242
'Understanding NICE guidance'	A lay version of the guideline recommendations. Available at www.rcplondon.ac.uk/pubs/brochure.aspx?e=242

▷ Updating the guideline

Literature searches were repeated for all of the evidence-based questions at the end of the GDG development process, allowing any relevant papers published up until 16 April 2007 to be considered. Future guideline updates will consider evidence published after this cut-off date.

Two years after publication of the guideline, NICE will ask a national collaborating centre to determine whether the evidence base has progressed significantly to alter the guideline recommendations and warrant an early update. If not, the guideline will be considered for update approximately 4 years after publication.

2.9 Disclaimer

Healthcare providers need to use clinical judgement, knowledge and expertise when deciding whether it is appropriate to apply guidelines. The recommendations cited here are a guide and may not be appropriate for use in all situations. The decision to adopt any of the recommendations cited here must be made by the practitioner in light of individual patient circumstances, the wishes of the patient, clinical expertise and resources.

The NCC-CC disclaims any responsibility for damages arising out of the use or non-use of these guidelines and the literature used in support of these guidelines.

2.10 Funding

The NCC-CC was commissioned by the NICE to undertake the work on this guideline.

3 Key messages of the guideline

3.1 Key priorities for implementation

Exercise* should be a core treatment (see Fig 3.2) for people with osteoarthritis, irrespective of age, comorbidity, pain severity and disability. Exercise should include:

- local muscle strengthening
- general aerobic fitness.

Referral for arthroscopic lavage and debridement** should not be offered as part of treatment for osteoarthritis, unless the person has knee osteoarthritis with a clear history of mechanical locking in knee osteoarthritis (not gelling, 'giving way' or X-ray evidence of loose bodies).

Healthcare professionals should consider offering paracetamol for pain relief in addition to core treatment (see Fig 3.2); regular dosing may be required. Paracetamol and/or topical NSAIDs should be considered ahead of oral NSAIDs, COX-2 inhibitors or opioids.

Healthcare professionals should consider offering topical NSAIDs for pain relief in addition to core treatment (see Fig 3.2) for people with knee or hand osteoarthritis. Topical NSAIDs and/or paracetamol should be considered ahead of oral NSAIDs, COX-2 inhibitors or opioids.

When offering treatment with an oral NSAID/COX-2 inhibitor, the first choice should be either a COX-2 inhibitor (other than etoricoxib 60mg), or a standard NSAID. In either case these should be coprescribed with a proton pump inhibitor (PPI), choosing the one with the lowest acquisition cost.†

Referral for joint replacement surgery should be considered for people with osteoarthritis who experience joint symptoms (pain, stiffness, reduced function) that impact substantially on their quality of life and are refractory to non-surgical treatment. Referral should be made before there is prolonged and established functional limitation and severe pain.

---

* It has not been specified whether exercise should be provided by the NHS or whether the healthcare professional should provide advice and encouragement to the patient to obtain and carry out the intervention themselves. Exercise has been found to be beneficial but the clinician needs to make a judgement in each case on how effectively to ensure patient participation. This will depend on the patient's individual needs, circumstances, self-motivation and the availability of local facilities.

** This recommendation is a refinement of the indication in 'Arthroscopic knee washout, with or without debridement, for the treatment of osteoarthritis' (NICE interventional procedure guidance 230). This guideline has reviewed the clinical and cost-effectiveness evidence, which has led to this more specific recommendation on the indication for which arthroscopic lavage and debridement is judged to be clinically and cost effective.

† This guideline replaces the osteoarthritis aspects only of NICE technology appraisal guidance 27. The guideline recommendations are based on up-to-date evidence on efficacy and adverse events, current costs and an expanded health-economic analysis of cost effectiveness. This has led to an increased role for COX-2 inhibitors, an increased awareness of all potential adverse events (gastrointestinal, liver and cardio-renal) and a recommendation to coprescribe a proton pump inhibitor (PPI). This is based on health economic modelling with generic omeprazole, therefore the cheapest available PPI should be considered first.

3.2   Algorithms

3.2.1   Holistic assessment

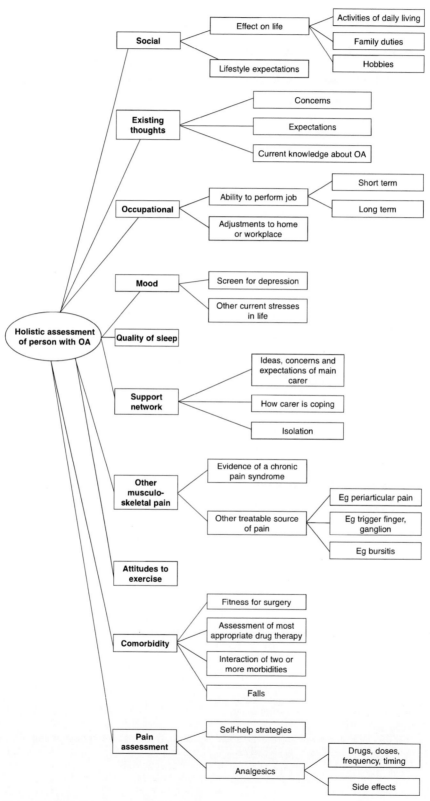

Figure 3.1 Holistic assessment algorithm

Assessing needs: how to use this algorithm

This layout is intended as an aide memoire to provide a breakdown of key topics which are of common concern when assessing people with osteoarthritis. Within each topic are a few suggested specific points worth assessing. Not every topic will be of concern for everyone with osteoarthritis, and there are other specifics which may warrant consideration for particular individuals.

3.2.2 Targeting treatment

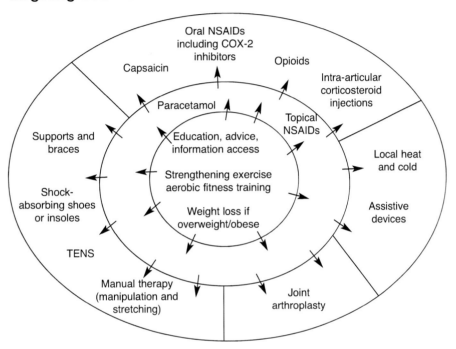

Figure 3.2 Targeting treatment algorithm. COX-2 = cyclooxegenase-2; NSAIDs = non-steroidal anti-inflammatory drugs; TENS = transcutaneous electrical nerve stimulation.

Targeting treatment: how to use this algorithm

Starting at the centre and working outward, the treatments are arranged in the order in which they should be considered for people with osteoarthritis, given that individual needs, risk factors and preferences will modulate this approach. In accordance with the recommendations in the guideline, there are three **core interventions** which should be considered for every person with osteoarthritis – these are given in the central circle. Some of these may not be relevant, depending on the individual. Where further treatment is required, consideration should be given to the second ring, which contains **relatively safe pharmaceutical options**. Again, these should be considered in light of the person's needs and preferences. A third outer circle gives **adjunctive treatments**. These treatments all meet at least one of the following criteria: less well-proven efficacy, less symptom relief or increased risk to the patient. They are presented here in four groups: pharmaceutical options, self-management techniques, surgery and other non-pharmaceutical treatments.

THE GUIDELINE

4 Holistic approach to oesteoarthritis assessment and management

4.1 Principles of good osteoarthritis care

4.1.1 General introduction

People with osteoarthritis may experience a number of challenges to their lives as a consequence of their symptoms. Some of these challenges have an effect on the individual's ability to contribute to society or enjoy a reasonable quality of life. A holistic approach to care considers the global needs of an individual, taking into account social and psychological factors that have an effect on their quality of life and the ability to carry out activities of daily living, employment-related activities, family commitments and hobbies (Salaffi et al. 1991).

A holistic assessment of the individual's medical, social and psychological needs can enable a tailored approach to treatment options encouraging positive health-seeking behaviours that are relevant to the individual's goals. A therapeutic relationship based on shared decision-making endorses the individual's ability to self-manage their condition and reduces the reliance on pharmacological therapies, hence providing a greater sense of empowerment for the individual (Sobel 1995; Corben and Rosen 2005).

These principles should also encompass a patient-centred approach to communication providing a mutual goal-sharing approach that encourages a positive approach to rehabilitation (Stewart et al. 2003).

RECOMMENDATIONS

R1   Healthcare professionals should assess the effect of osteoarthritis on the individual's function, quality of life, occupation, mood, relationships and leisure activities.

R2   People with symptomatic osteoarthritis should have periodic review tailored to their individual needs.

R3   Healthcare professionals should formulate a management plan in partnership with the person with osteoarthritis.

R4   Comorbidities that compound the effect of osteoarthritis should be taken into consideration in the management plan.

R5   Healthcare professionals should offer all people with clinically symptomatic osteoarthritis advice on the following core treatments:
   - access to appropriate information (see section 5.1)
   - activity and exercise (see section 6.1)
   - interventions to effect weight loss if overweight or obese (see section 6.2 and NICE guideline number 43 on obesity, National Institute for Health and Clinical Excellence 2006b).

R6   The risks and benefits of treatment options, taking into account comorbidities, should be communicated to the patient in ways that can be understood.

See sections 3.2.1 and 3.2.2 for the associated algorithms.

4.2 Patient experience and perceptions

4.2.1 Clinical introduction

This guideline provides practitioners with evidence-based recommendations on treatments for people with osteoarthritis. The guidance on specific treatments is necessary but not sufficient for the provision of effective, high quality healthcare: other information is required. This includes the physical, psychological and social assessment of the patient and the effect that joint pain or joint dysfunction has on their life. The skills of good history taking and clinical examination of the locomotor system are crucial, as is the knowledge of when to request further investigations and the interpretation of these tests. Effective communication skills allow the practitioner to fully understand the context of osteoarthritis in their patient's life and to provide the patient with an accurate assessment, explanation and prognosis. Management options, benefits and risks can be shared with the patient to allow an informed decision to be made. A good knowledge of the context of musculoskeletal healthcare provision and expertise in the locality as well as good communication with the providers of health and social care are also necessary.

4.2.2 Methodological introduction

We looked for studies that investigated patient experiences of osteoarthritis and its treatments and how patient perceptions influence their preference and outcome for treatments. Due to the large volume of evidence, studies were excluded if they used a mixed arthritis population of which less than 75% had osteoarthritis or if the population was not relevant to the UK.

One cohort study (Gignac et al. 2006) and 18 observational studies (Ballantyne et al. 2007; Brenes et al. 2002; Cook et al. 2007; Downe-Wamboldt 1991; Ferreira and Sherman 2007; Hampson et al. 1994, 1996; Hill and Bird 2007; Laborde and Powers 1985; Lastowiecka et al. 2006; Rejeski et al. 1996; Rejeski et al. 1998; Sanders et al. 2002; Tak and Laffrey 2003; Tallon et al. 2000; Tubach et al. 2006; Victor et al. 2004; Weinberger et al. 1989) were found on patient experiences of osteoarthritis and its treatments. One of these studies (Downe-Wamboldt 1991) was excluded due to methodological limitations.

The cohort study assessed the experiences of 90 patients, comparing those with osteoarthritis with non-osteoarthritis patients.

The 17 included observational studies were all methodologically sound and differed with respect to study design (N=11 observational-correlation; N=3 qualitative; N=1 observational; N=1 case series) and trial size.

4.3.2 Evidence statements

All evidence statements in this section are level 3.

▷ Body function and structure (symptoms)

Ten studies (Cook et al. 2007; Ferreira and Sherman 2007; Gignac et al. 2006; Hampson et al. 1994, 1996; Laborde and Powers 1985; Sanders et al. 2002; Tallon et al. 2000; Tubach et al. 2006; Victor et al. 2004)

Observational and qualitative studies found that pain, function and negative feelings were important factors affecting the lives of patients with OA. Patients found their pain was distressing and that their OA caused limitations and had a major impact on their daily life. The areas that caused major problems for patients were: pain, stiffness, fatigue, disability, depression, anxiety and sleep disturbance.

▷ Activities and participation

Nine studies (Brenes et al. 2002; Cook et al. 2007; Gignac et al. 2006; Lastowiecka et al. 2006; Rejeski et al. 1996, 1998; Sanders et al. 2002; Tallon et al. 2000; Victor et al. 2004)

Observational and qualitative studies found that poor performance of tasks was associated with female gender, BMI, pain and pessimism. Patients often felt embarrassed at not being able to do things that their peers could do and one of the things they felt most distressing was not being able to do activities that they used to be able to do. The most frequent activities affected by osteoarthritis were: leisure activities, social activities, close relationships, community mobility, employment and heavy housework. Personal care activities were rarely mentioned. OA also impacted employment status. Both middle-aged and older-age adults described the loss of valuable roles and leisure activities such as travel, and were less likely to mention employment. Loss of these activities was described as extremely upsetting.

Pre-task self-efficacy beliefs and knee pain was found to influence the speed of movement, post-task difficulty ratings and perceptions of physical ability. Work ability did not differ with gender; however, patients with hip OA had the worst work ability scores and in non-retired patients, white-collar workers had significantly higher work ability than blue-collar workers, regardless of age.

▷ Psychosocial and personal factors: feeling old

Two studies (Gignac et al. 2006; Sanders et al. 2002)

Observational and qualitative studies found that many patients viewed their OA symptoms as an inevitable part of getting old, that their older age had rendered their disabilities 'invisible' and they were not viewed as being legitimately disabled because they were old (that is, disability should be expected and accepted in old age). Many also felt that there were negative stereotypes of older age and that they were a burden on society and wanted to distance themselves from such stereotypes. Patients often minimised or normalised their condition (which was more commonly done among older patients who attributed it to age).

▷ Psychosocial and personal factors: depression, anxiety, life satisfaction

Eleven studies (Ballantyne et al. 2007; Brenes et al. 2002; Cook et al. 2007; Ferreira and Sherman 2007; Gignac et al. 2006; Hampson et al. 1994, 1996; Laborde and Powers 1985; Lastowiecka et al. 2006; Tak and Laffrey 2003; Tallon et al. 2000)

Observational and qualitative studies found that pessimism was correlated with all physical outcome measures. More joint involvement was associated with negative feelings about treatment and with negative mood. Being female was associated with less impact of osteoarthritis on Arthritis Impact Measurement Scale (AIMS)2 affective status; and stressed women reported greater use of emotion-focused coping strategies, felt their health was under external control, perceived less social support and were less satisfied with their lives. Greater perceived social support was related to higher internal health locus of control. Patients expressed that their aspirations for future life satisfaction had declined appreciably and that depression and anxiety were major problems that they experienced. Older patients with advanced OA felt that the disease threatened their self-identities and they were overwhelmed by health and activity changes and felt powerless to change their situation. Many ignored their disease and tried to carry on as normal despite experiencing exacerbated symptoms.

Patients were unable to guarantee relief from symptoms based on lifestyle changes alone and this was linked to upset feelings, helplessness and depression. Many expressed frustration, anxiety and fear about the future. Pain was correlated with greater depression and lower life satisfaction whereas support and optimism were correlated with fewer depressive symptoms and greater life satisfaction.

In non-retired patients, white-collar workers had worse mental status than blue-collar workers. Those with hip OA also had the worst mental status. Those with worse mental status had lower work ability. Mental health was worse for persons with OA compared with those not suffering from OA.

▷ Psychosocial and personal factors: relationships

Three studies (Ballantyne et al. 2007; Gignac et al. 2006; Hampson et al. 1994)

Observational and qualitative studies found that in OA patients, symptoms affected mood and made them frustrated and annoyed with others. Informal social networks (family, friends and neighbours) were critical to patient's management and coping, particularly marital relationships and the decision not to have joint replacement surgery. This was because networks helped with tasks, gave emotional support and helped keep patients socially involved and connected to others despite their physical limitations, reinforcing the idea that surgery is avoidable. Decisions were made on the marital couple's ability to cope rather than the individual's capacity and thus health professionals may need to consider the couple as the patient when considering disease-management options.

▷ Psychosocial and personal factors: knowledge of arthritis and its management

Six studies (Ballantyne et al. 2007; Hampson et al. 1994; Hill and Bird 2007; Laborde and Powers 1985; Sanders et al. 2002; Victor et al. 2004)

Observational and qualitative studies found that most patients expected to have OA permanently and did not believe that a cure for OA was likely or that there was an effective way of treating OA and thus they were reluctant to seek treatment for their OA. Beliefs about the cause and control of OA and the helpfulness of treatment showed no relationship to general health perceptions. Patients were predominantly externally controlled in terms of their health beliefs (that is, they believed that their health was the result of fate or another's actions). Most patients thought their OA was a 'normal' and 'integral' part of their life history, was an inevitable result of hardship or hard work (a common view among men and women and across different occupational groups). Some felt that younger people might be more 'deserving' of treatment than themselves. Younger respondents did not perceive their symptoms as being normal, this affected their approach to management and their determination to get formal treatment.

Many patients were unsure as to the causes and physiology of OA, were uncertain of how to manage an acute episode and unclear as to the likely 'end point' of the disease (ending up in a wheelchair). The most frequently cited causes were: accidents/injuries, occupational factors, cold or damp weather, too much acid in the joints, old age, weight and climatic factors. Many patients knew about NSAIDs and steroid injections but did not always know about their side effects and some thought that taking their drug therapy regularly would reduce the progression of their OA. Many also knew about the benefits of exercise and weight loss but did not know suitable forms of exercise. Many did not know about the benefits of lifestyle changes or using aids and devices. Arthritis was perceived as debilitating but was not the primary health concern in participants' lives.

▷ Psychosocial and personal factors: expectations desired from treatment

Three studies (Hampson et al. 1994; Sanders et al. 2002; Victor et al. 2004)

Observational and qualitative studies found that most patients felt it was 'very' or 'extremely' important to try to prevent their OA from getting worse. Areas where patients most wanted improvements were in pain management, mobility/functional ability and maintaining an independent life in the community. Pain was a major concern for most patients. However, their main goals were to maximise and increase their daily activity as a strategy to manage their pain, rather than identifying 'pain control' itself as a major or single issue.

▷ Psychosocial and personal factors: use of self-management methods

Five studies (Hampson et al. 1994; Hampson et al. 1996; Sanders et al. 2002; Tak and Laffrey 2003; Tallon et al. 2000)

Observational and qualitative studies found that patients with more education were more likely to use active pain coping methods. The more serious and symptomatic participants perceived their condition to be, the less positive they felt about the management methods they used to control it). Patients reporting use of alcohol (compared with never using alcohol) reported less control over good and bad days. Use of self-management methods was associated with symptoms and seriousness but not with age or gender. A number of patients felt embarrassed about their disabilities and felt stigma in using walking aids or wheelchairs – some disguised their needs for using walking aids. Frequent use of problem-focused coping strategies was associated with greater perceived social support. Alternative therapies (for example, ginger, cod-liver oil, acupuncture, magnets and others) were frequently used by many of the patients. Some felt they were helpful and others thought benefits were due to placebo effects. Despite lack of evidence for complementary therapies and dismissal from the medical profession, patients were prepared to try anything that others had found helpful. Patients wanted more information about the condition, self-help and available treatment options. Coping strategies used by patients included carrying on regardless, taking medication as required, exercise, use of aids to daily living, restricting movement and resting.

▷ Psychosocial and personal factors: treatment/healthcare

Seven studies (Ballantyne et al. 2007; Gignac et al. 2006; Hampson et al. 1994; Sanders et al. 2002; Tallon et al. 2000; Victor et al. 2004)

Observational and qualitative studies found that most patients found at least one aspect of their treatment made them feel better, no aspect of their treatment made them feel worse, and perceived helpfulness of treatment was inversely related to negative feelings about treatment. Older patients and women were more likely to rate their treatment as more helpful. Patients with higher occupational status were more likely to feel more negatively about their treatment. Employed younger respondents had all paid for private referrals to specialists and had all undergone or were being considered for total joint replacement surgery. Drugs were seen as helpful, surgery was perceived as the only way to 'cure' the disease (but some avoided it due to fear of risks or felt they were too old to benefit). Canes were perceived as useful but some felt embarrassed and did not use them. Physiotherapy and regular exercise were seen as beneficial treatments. Most patients were satisfied with their treatment and felt there was little more their GP could do for them.

Treatments most used by patients were: tablets, aids and adaptations, physical therapy (used very often) and treatments most patients had not tried were injections, removal of fluid/debris, aids and adaptations, physical therapy, complementary therapy, education and advice, no treatment and knee replacement. Treatments found moderately helpful by patients were tablets and top treatments found extremely helpful were tablets, physical therapy, aids and adaptations and removal of fluid/debris. The top treatment found not helpful was physical therapy. Treatments that patients felt should be made priority for researchers were knee replacement, pain relief, cure, reduced swelling, education and advice and physical therapy.

Many patients were unwilling to use medication and obtained information on activities and foods that were perceived as harmful. Treating pain with medication for these people was seen as masking rather than curing symptoms and was seen as potentially harmful due to increased risk of unwanted side effects. Long delays between experiencing symptoms and an OA diagnosis made OA symptoms more difficult to deal with. Younger respondents attributed this delay to health professionals not considering OA as a possibility because participants were 'too young' to have arthritis. Barriers to receiving support noted mainly by younger OA patients were the 'invisibility' of symptoms and their unpredictable nature. Others often exhorted them to engage in activities when they were in pain, were disappointed when plans were unexpectedly cancelled or were suspicious about the inability of participants to engage in some activities.

Patients felt that they there was a real lack of information and support given to them (from their GP and other primary care team members) about their condition, especially in the areas of managing pain and coping with daily activities. Many found difficulties in communicating with doctors and some were extremely dissatisfied with the service they had received. Many patients reported that their doctor/health professional ignored their symptoms and had re-enforced the view that their OA was normal for their age and patients were aware that they could be considered a burden on the NHS. Obtaining information and more visits to the doctor was associated with reporting more symptoms and with believing treatment to be more helpful.

Common problems reported by patients were: an inadequate supply of medications to last until their next GP appointment, gastrointestinal (GI) problems, barriers to attending clinic (for example, finances, transportation) and problems requiring rapid intervention. Women were significantly more likely to have inadequate supply of medication and GI complaints were more prevalent among persons who were Caucasian, younger and non-compliant. Persons with worse AIMS ratings or with poorer psychological health were more likely to have reported barriers to care.

Some participants mentioned that previous non-arthritis-related surgical experiences (their own or others) created fear and mistrust of surgery that contributed to the avoidance of total joint arthroplasty (TJA). Some noted that previous experience with physicians, particularly around prescribing medications, had undermined their trust in their physicians and often left them believing that their interests came second. Several noted that their family physician had never discussed surgery with them and because they were regarded as experts in treatment, participants assumed that surgery was not possible and was also not a viable option and were given the impression that surgery was something to be avoided. Where surgery had been mentioned by health professionals, it was often described as a last resort, leaving many participants wanting to try all other alternatives before TJA.

4.2.4 From evidence to recommendations

▷ Assessment of the individual

Every patient brings their thoughts, health beliefs, experiences, concerns and expectations to the consultation. It is important to acknowledge distress and assess current ability to cope.

Exploring the background to distress is fruitful as psychosocial factors are often more closely associated with health status, quality of life and functional status than measures of disease severity (such as X-rays) (Salaffi et al. 1991; Sobel 1995). Identifying psychosocial barriers to recovery and rehabilitation is important in a subgroup of patients.

There is evidence to show that patients' perception of how patient centred a consultation is strongly predicts positive health outcomes and health resource efficiency (that is, fewer referrals and investigations) (Stewart et al. 2003).

The GDG considered that there were three key areas to include in patient-centred assessment:

1 Employment and social activities

There is an association with osteoarthritis and certain occupations (for example, farmers and hip osteoarthritis, footballers with a history of knee injuries and knee osteoarthritis). Health and employment are closely intertwined and conversely unemployment can be associated with ill health and depression. Patients with osteoarthritis can have difficult choices to make with regard to continuing in work, returning to work after time away, changing the nature of their work, or deciding to stop working. Practitioners provide sickness certification and therefore often have to give guidance, discuss work options and know sources of further help, both in the short term and the long term. The Disability Discrimination Act (DDA) 1995 makes it unlawful for employers to treat a disabled person less favourably than anyone else because of their disability, in terms of recruitment, training, promotion and dismissal. It also requires employers to make reasonable adjustments to working practices or premises to overcome substantial disadvantage caused by disability. Reasonable adjustments can include, where possible: changing or modifying tasks; altering work patterns; special equipment; time off to attend appointments; or help with travel to work. Advice about workplace adjustments can be made by physiotherapists, occupational therapists or an occupational health department if available. There are government schemes and initiatives available to help patients if they wish to start, return or continue working: www.direct.gov.uk/en/DisabledPeople/Employmentsupport/index.htm

2 Comorbidity

Osteoarthritis is more common in older age groups and therefore it is more likely that other conditions will coexist: this raises several issues.

- A patient's ability to adhere with exercise, for example if angina, chronic obstructive pulmonary disease, previous stroke or obesity are present.
- Polypharmacy issues. The choice of drug treatments for osteoarthritis as outlined in this guidance can be influenced by the drugs taken for other conditions, for example patients who are taking warfarin should not take NSAIDs, and may find that other analgesics alter the levels of anticoagulation.
- Other medical conditions can influence the choice of treatments for osteoarthritis, such as a history of duodenal ulcer, chronic kidney impairment, heart failure and liver problems.
- The risk of falls increases with polypharmacy, increasing age, osteoarthritis and other medical conditions.
- The presence of severe comorbid conditions may influence the decision to perform joint replacement surgery.
- Prognosis of osteoarthritis disability is worse in the presence of two or more comorbidities.

- Quality of sleep can be adversely affected by osteoarthritis and other comorbid conditions.
- Depression can accompany any chronic and long-term condition. The NICE guideline on depression (CG23) (National Institute for Health and Clinical Excellence 2007) recommends that screening should be undertaken in primary care and general hospital settings for depression in high-risk groups, for example, those with significant physical illnesses causing disability.

3 Support network

Carers provide help and support. They also need support themselves. It is important to be aware of the health beliefs of carers and to respect their ideas, concerns and expectations as well as those of the patient. Advice is available for support for carers both nationally (www.direct.gov.uk) and locally via social services. Some patients have no social support and risk becoming isolated if their osteoarthritis is progressive. Good communication between primary care and social services is essential in this scenario.

▷ Clinical assessment

The evidence base given in other parts of this guideline tends to assess interventions in terms of patient-reported outcomes. The working diagnosis of osteoarthritis is a clinical one based on symptoms and therefore when considering which treatment options to discuss with the patient, it is also important to assess accurately and examine the locomotor system. There are several points to consider.

- It is important to assess function. For example, assessment of the lower limb should always include an assessment of gait (see section 6.5 for evidence base).
- The joints above and below the affected joint should be examined. Sometimes pain can be referred to a more distal joint, for example hip pathology can cause knee pain.
- An assessment should be made as to whether the joint pain is related to that region only, whether other joints are involved, or whether there is evidence of a widespread pain disorder.
- It is worth looking for other treatable periarticular sources of pain such as bursitis, trigger finger, ganglions, very localised ligament pain, etc, which could respond quickly to appropriate treatment (see section 7.1 for evidence base).
- An assessment should be made of the severity of joint pain and/or dysfunction to decide whether early referral to an orthopaedic surgeon is required. There is evidence that delaying joint replacement until after disability is well established reduces the likelihood of benefit from surgery (see section 8 for evidence base).

▷ Pain assessment

Pain is the most common presentation of osteoarthritis. It can be episodic, activity related or constant. It can disturb sleep. Analgesics are readily available over the counter, or prescribed, or sometimes borrowed from others. It is important to know how the analgesics are being taken – regularly, 'as required', or both, as well as timing, dose frequency and different drugs being used. Attitudes to taking painkillers and side effects (experienced or anticipated) are all relevant in understanding the impact of painful joints for the patient as well as providing valuable information for a management plan. Disturbed sleep can lead to the loss of restorative sleep which in turn can cause daytime fatigue, deconditioning of muscles and muscle pain similar to that found in chronic widespread pain syndromes. Some patients can progress to developing chronic pain which is now known to be maintained by several pathophysiological mechanisms, which currently can be dealt with only partially.

▷ Patient-centred decision-making

In order to achieve a holistic approach to care, patients must be encouraged to consider a range of factors that can enhance their self-management approaches to coping with their condition (Department of Work and Pensions 2005; King's Fund 2005).

Self-management requires a 'toolbox' approach of core treatments and adjuncts which can be tried if required. The patient is then able to deal with exacerbations confidently and quickly.

It is worth considering what part of the osteoarthritis journey the patient is on. In the early stages there is joint pain and uncertain diagnosis, later on symptomatic flares, with possible periods of quiescence of varying length. In one longitudinal study in primary care over 7 years (Peters et al. 2005), 25% of patients with symptomatic osteoarthritis improved. Some people have rapidly progressive osteoarthritis; others have progressive osteoarthritis which may benefit from surgery. Some patients will opt for and benefit from long-term palliation of their symptoms. As a rough guide, osteoarthritis of the hip joint can progress to requiring joint replacement fairly quickly over the first few years, osteoarthritis of the knee joint often has a slower progression over 5 to 10 years, and nodal hand osteoarthritis can have a good prognosis, at least in terms of pain. Within these generalisations there can be substantial variation.

To deliver these evidence-based guidelines effectively a holistic approach to the needs of the patient needs to be made by the practitioner. One focus of this should be the promotion of their health and general wellbeing. An important task of the practitioner is to reduce risk factors for osteoarthritis by promoting self-care and empowering the patient to make behavioural changes to their lifestyle. To increase the likelihood of success, any changes need to be relevant to that person, and to be specific with achievable, measurable goals in both the short term and the long term. Devising and sharing the management plan with the patient in partnership, including offering management options, allows for the patient's personality, family, daily life, economic circumstances, physical surroundings and social context to be taken into account. This patient-centred approach not only increases patient satisfaction but also adherence with the treatment plan. Rehabilitation and palliation of symptoms often requires coordination of care with other healthcare professionals and other agencies such as social services. The General Medical Council publication 'Good medical practice' (General Medical Council 2006) encourages practitioners to share with patients – in a way they can understand – the information they want or need to know about their condition, its likely progression, and the treatment options available to them, including associated risks and uncertainties. This is particularly relevant when discussing surgical options or using drugs such as NSAIDs. Risk is best presented to patients in several ways at once: for example as absolute risk, as relative risk and as 'number needed to harm'.

These guidelines give many different options for the management of a patient who has osteo-arthritis. The core recommendations can be offered to all patients and a choice can be made from the other evidence-based and cost-effective recommendations. The knowledge that osteoarthritis is a dynamic process which does include the potential for repair if adverse factors are minimised, in addition to the many different interventions, should allow practitioners to give advice and support which is positive and constructive. The power of the therapeutic effect of the practitioner–patient relationship must not be forgotten. Good communication skills imparting accurate information honestly and sensitively and in a positive way greatly enhance the ability of the patient to cope. Conversely, negative practitioner attitudes to osteoarthritis can increase the distress experienced.

▷ Joint protection

These guidelines indirectly address the concept of joint protection by looking specifically at evidence bases for single interventions. The principles are:

- resting inflamed joints by reducing loading, time in use and repetitions
- using the largest muscles and joints that can do the job. For example, standing up from a chair using hips and knees rather than pushing up with hands
- using proper movement techniques for lifting, sitting, standing, bending and reaching
- using appliances, gadgets and modifications for home equipment to minimise stress on joints. Examples include raising the height of a chair to make standing and sitting easier, using a smaller kettle with less water, boiling potatoes in a chip sieve to facilitate removal when cooked
- planning the week ahead to anticipate difficulties
- using biomechanics to best effect. This will include good posture, aligning joints correctly, and avoiding staying in one position for a long time
- balancing activity with rest and organising the day to pace activities
- simplifying tasks
- recruiting others to help
- making exercise a part of everyday life including exercises which improve joint range of movement, stamina and strength. Exercise should also be for cardiovascular fitness and to maintain or improve balance.

▷ Pain

Pain is a complex phenomenon. Effective pain relief may require using a number of analgesics or pain-relieving strategies together. The complexity of multiple pain pathways and processes often mean that two or more treatments may combine synergistically or in a complementary way to act on the different components of the pain response. This technique is known as balanced or multimodal analgesia.

By tackling pain early and effectively it is hoped that the development of chronic pain can be stopped but more work needs to be done in this area. Timing of analgesia is important. Regular analgesia will be appropriate if the pain is constant. Pain with exertion can be helped by taking the analgesia before the exercise. Some patients will need palliative care for their joint pain. For these people long-term opioids can be of benefit (see section 7.1).

5 Education and self-management

5.1 Patient information

5.1.1 Clinical introduction

There is limited disease-specific evidence on the benefits of providing information for osteoarthritis. It is essential that the consultation is one of information sharing and achieving concordance in the treatment regimes suggested (Cox et al. 2004; Elwyn et al. 1999). Recognising that the patient should be treated as an individual and not as a disease state is imperative in improving communication and outcomes (Donovan and Blake 2000).

People will vary in how they adjust to their condition or instigate changes as a result of the information and advice provided. This is likely to depend on a number of factors:

- the disease severity and levels of pain, fatigue, depression, disability or loss of mobility
- prior knowledge and beliefs about the condition
- the social and psychological context at the time
- health beliefs and learnt behaviours.

5.1.2 Methodological introduction

We looked for studies that investigated:

- the effectiveness of patient information provision/education methods compared with each other or to no information/education
- the effectiveness of patient self-management programmes compared with each other or no self-management
- both with respect to symptoms, function, quality of life.

Due to the large volume of evidence, studies were excluded if they used a mixed arthritis population of which less than 75% had osteoarthritis or if population was not relevant to the UK.

Two systematic reviews and meta-analyses (MA) (Chodosh et al. 2005; Superio-Cabuslay et al. 1996), eight RCTs (Heuts 2005; Calfas et al. 1992; Nunez et al. 2006; Victor and Triggs 2005; Buszewicz et al. 2006; Maisiak et al. 1996; Pariser et al. 2005; Keefe and Blumenthal 2004), one implementation study (De Jong et al. 2004) and one observational study (Hampson et al. 1993) were found on patient education and self-management methods. Two of these studies (Pariser et al. 2005; Keefe 2004) were excluded due to methodological limitations.

The first MA (Chodosh et al. 2005) included 14 RCTs on osteoarthritis self-management programmes compared with usual care or control programmes (attending classes which were unrelated to osteoarthritis self-management). Follow-up was between 4–6 months for all studies. The quality of the included RCTs was assessed but the results of this are not mentioned. The MA pooled together all data for the outcomes of pain and function.

The second MA (Superio-Cabuslay et al. 1996) included ten RCTs/CCTs on osteoarthritis patient education (information about arthritis and symptom management) compared with control (types of controls not mentioned). Quality of the included RCTs was not assessed. The

MA pooled together all data for the outcomes of pain and functional disability. Studies differed with respect to sample size and duration.

The six RCTs not included in the systematic reviews were all randomised, parallel group studies but differed with respect to:

- osteoarthritis site (two RCTs knee, two RCTs hip and/or knee, two RCTs not specified)
- treatment (five RCTs group sessions of self-management/education programmes, one RCT telephone intervention – treatment counselling and symptom monitoring)
- comparison (two RCTs usual care, two RCTs waiting list, one RCT education booklet, one RCT education lecture)
- trial size, blinding and length.

The implementation study (De Jong et al. 2004) was methodologically sound and compared the effects of a 6-week knee osteoarthritis self-management programme (N=204 patients) and a 9-week hip osteoarthritis self-management programme (N=169 patients) with pretreatment values in patients from urban and semi-rural communities.

The observational-correlation study was methodologically sound and consisted of giving questionnaires to, and interviewing, N=61 osteoarthritis patients in order to assess their use of self-management methods to deal with the symptoms of osteoarthritis.

5.1.3 Evidence statements

Table 5.1 Symptoms: pain

Pain outcome	Reference	Intervention	Assessment time	Outcome/effect size
Knee				
Pain severity (VAS, change from baseline)	1 implementation study (De Jong et al. 2004) (N=204)	Knee programme (pre-test vs post-test)	6 weeks, end of intervention	–5.4, p=0.002 Favours intervention
Pain tolerance (VAS, change from baseline)	1 implementation study (De Jong et al. 2004) (N=204)	Knee programme (pre-test vs post-test)	6 weeks, end of intervention	–3.9, p=0.034 Favours intervention
IRGL pain scale (scale 5-25, change from baseline)	1 implementation study (De Jong et al. 2004) (N=204)	Knee programme (pre-test vs post-test)	6 weeks, end of intervention	–0.4, p=0.015 Favours intervention
WOMAC pain	1 RCT (Nunez et al. 2006) (N=100)	Therapeutic education and functional readaptation programme (TEFR) + conventional (pharmacologic) treatment vs control (waiting list) + pharmacologic treatment	9 months, 6 months post-intervention	NS
WOMAC pain	1 RCT (Victor and Triggs 2005) (N=193)	Education programme (nurse-led) vs control (waiting list) group	1 month (end of intervention) and at 1 year (11 months post-intervention)	NS

continued

Table 5.1 Symptoms: pain – *continued*

Pain outcome	Reference	Intervention	Assessment time	Outcome/effect size
Hip				
Pain severity (VAS, change from baseline)	1 implementation study (De Jong et al. 2004) (N=169)	Hip programme (pre-test vs post-test)	9 weeks, end of intervention	–4.7, p=0.007 Favours intervention
Pain tolerance (VAS, change from baseline)	1 implementation study (De Jong et al. 2004) (N=169)	Hip programme (pre-test vs post-test)	9 weeks, end of intervention	–4.9, p=0.004 Favours intervention
IRGL pain scale (scale 5–25, change from baseline)	1 implementation study (De Jong et al. 2004) (N=169)	Hip programme (pre-test vs post-test)	9 weeks, end of intervention	–0.4, p=0.032 Favours intervention
Knee and/or hip				
WOMAC Pain	1 RCT (Buszewicz et al. 2006) (N=812)	Self-management programme + education booklet vs education booklet alone	4 months and 12 months post-intervention	NS
Unspecified site				
Pain (weighted average standardised gain difference)	1 MA (Superio-Cabuslay et al. 1996) (9 RCTs), N=9 RCTs	Patient education vs control	Study duration between 1 to 42 months	Effect size: 0.16, 95% CI –0.69 to 1.02 No p–values given
Pain (Pooled estimate)	1 MA (Chodosh et al. 2005) (14 RCTs)	Self-management programmes vs control groups (mostly usual care or programme control)	4 to 6 months follow-up	Effect size: –0.06, 95% CI –0.10 to –0.02, p<0.05. Favours intervention Effect size equivalent to improvement of <2mm on VAS pain scale
Knee pain (VAS)	1 RCT (Heuts 2005) (N=297)	Self-management programme vs usual care	3 months post-intervention and 21 months post-intervention	Mean improvement 3 months: 0.67 (self-management) and 0.01 (usual care), p=0.023 21 months: 0.39 (self-management) and –0.48 (usual care), p=0.004
Hip pain (VAS)	1 RCT (Heuts 2005) (N=297)	Self-management programme vs usual care	3 months post-intervention and 21 months post-intervention	NS

Table 5.2 Symptoms: stiffness

Stiffness outcome	Reference	Intervention	Assessment time	Outcome/effect size
Knee				
WOMAC stiffness	1 RCT (Nunez et al. 2006) (N=100)	Therapeutic education and functional readaptation programme (TEFR) + conventional (pharmacologic) treatment vs control (waiting list) + pharmacologic treatment	9 months, 6 months post-intervention	NS
WOMAC stiffness	1 RCT (Victor and Triggs 2005) (N=193)	Education programme (nurse-led) vs control (waiting list) group	1 month (end of intervention) and at 1 year (11 months post-intervention)	NS
Knee and/or hip				
WOMAC stiffness	1 RCT (Buszewicz et al. 2006) (N=812)	Self-management programme + education booklet vs education booklet alone	4 months and 12 months post-intervention	NS

Table 5.3 Function

Function outcome	Reference	Intervention	Assessment time	Outcome/effect size
Knee				
IRGL mobility scale (scale 7–28, change from baseline)	1 implementation study (De Jong et al. 2004) (N=204)	Knee programme (pre-test vs post-test)	6 weeks, end of intervention	NS
WOMAC function	1 RCT (Nunez et al. 2006) (N=100)	Therapeutic education and functional readaptation programme (TEFR) + conventional (pharmacologic) treatment vs control (waiting list) + pharmacologic treatment	9 months, 6 months post-intervention	Mean values: 35.3 (TEFR) and 40.9 (control), p=0.035 Favours intervention
WOMAC disability	1 RCT (Victor and Triggs 2005) (N=193)	Education programme (nurse-led) vs control (waiting list) group	1 month (end of intervention) and at 1 year (11 months post-intervention).	NS
Hip				
IRGL mobility scale (scale 7–28, change from baseline)	1 implementation study (De Jong et al. 2004) (N=169)	Hip programme (pre-test vs post-test)	9 weeks, end of intervention	NS

continued

Table 5.3 Function – *continued*

Function outcome	Reference	Intervention	Assessment time	Outcome/effect size
Knee and/or hip				
WOMAC physical functioning	1 RCT (Buszewicz et al. 2006) (N=812)	Self-management programme + education booklet vs education booklet alone	4 months and 12 months post-intervention	NS
Unspecified site				
Function (pooled estimate)	1 MA (Chodosh et al. 2005) (14 RCTs)	Self-management programmes vs control groups (mostly usual care or programme control)	4 to 6 months follow-up	Effect size: –0.06, 95% CI –0.10 to –0.02, p<0.05. Effect size equivalent to approximately 2 points on the WOMAC Index
WOMAC index at 3 months post-intervention (mean improvement)	1 RCT (Heuts 2005) (N=297)	Self-management programme vs usual care	3 months post-intervention and 21 months post-intervention	3 months: 2.46 (self-management) and –0.53 (usual care), p=0.030 21 months: 2.63 (self-management) and –0.88 (usual care), p=0.022 Favours intervention
Patient-specific functional status (PSFS)	1 RCT (Heuts 2005) (N=297)	Self-management programme vs usual care	21 months post-intervention	0.49 (self-management) and –0.05 (usual care), p=0.026 Favours intervention
Functional disability (weighted average standardised gain difference)	1 MA (Superio-Cabuslay et al. 1996) (9 RCTs), N=9 RCTs	Patient education vs control	Study duration between 1 to 42 months	NS
PSFS	1 RCT (Heuts 2005) (N=297)	Self-management programme vs usual care	3 months post-intervention	NS

Table 5.4 Quality of life

QoL outcome	Reference	Intervention	Assessment time	Outcome/effect size
Knee				
SF-36 (dimensions of physical function, physical role, bodily pain, general health, social function, emotional role, vitality, mental health)	1 RCT (Nunez et al. 2006) (N=100)	Therapeutic education and functional readaptation programme (TEFR) + conventional (pharmacologic) treatment vs control (waiting list) + pharmacologic treatment	9 months, 6 months post-intervention	NS
SF-36 (vitality dimension)	1 RCT (Victor and Triggs 2005) (N=193)	Education programme (nurse-led) vs control (waiting list) group	1 year (11 months post-intervention)	Mean difference: –5.5, 95% CI –10.0 to –0.9, p<0.05 Favours intervention
SF-36 (vitality dimension)	1 RCT (Victor and Triggs 2005) (N=193)	Education programme (nurse-led) vs control (waiting list) group	1 month (end of intervention)	NS
SF-36 subscales (physical, role physical, emotional, social, pain, mental, general health); Arthritis Helplessness Index (AHI) score	1 RCT (Victor and Triggs 2005) (N=193)	Education programme (nurse-led) vs control (waiting list) group	1 month (end of intervention) and at 1 year (11 months post-intervention)	NS
Knee or hip				
Total AIMS2 health status score	1 RCT (Maisiak et al. 1996) (N=405)	Treatment counselling vs usual care	9 months (end of treatment)	Effect size 0.36, 95% CI 0.06 to 0.66, p<0.05 Favours intervention
AIMS2 pain dimension	1 RCT (Maisiak et al. 1996) (N=405)	Treatment counselling vs usual care	9 months (end of treatment)	Effect size 0.44, 95% CI 0.08 to 0.80, p<0.05 Favours intervention
AIMS2 physical dimension	1 RCT (Maisiak et al. 1996) (N=405)	Treatment counselling vs usual care	9 months (end of treatment)	NS
AIMS2 affect dimension	1 RCT (Maisiak et al. 1996) (N=405)	Treatment counselling vs usual care	9 months (end of treatment)	NS
AIMS2 physical dimension	1 RCT (Maisiak et al. 1996) (N=405)	Symptom monitoring vs usual care	9 months (end of treatment)	Effect size 0.29, 95% CI 0.01 to 0.76, p<0.05 Favours intervention
Total AIMS2 health status score; AIMS2 pain dimension; AIMS2 affect dimension	1 RCT (Maisiak et al. 1996) (N=405)	Symptom monitoring vs usual care	9 months (end of treatment)	NS
Total AIMS2 health status score	1 RCT (Maisiak et al. 1996) (N=405)	Treatment counselling vs symptom monitoring	9 months (end of treatment)	Mean score 4.1 (counselling) and 4.2 (monitoring) Both groups similar

continued

Table 5.4 Quality of life – *continued*

QoL outcome	Reference	Intervention	Assessment time	Outcome/effect size
Knee and/or hip				
Hospital anxiety and depression scale (depression component)	1 RCT (Buszewicz et al. 2006) (N=812)	Self-management programme + education booklet vs education booklet alone	4 months and 12 months post-intervention	Adjusted mean difference –0.36, 95% CI –0.76 to 0.05, p<0.05 Favours intervention
Hospital anxiety and depression scale (anxiety component)	1 RCT (Buszewicz et al. 2006) (N=812)	Self-management programme + education booklet vs education booklet alone	4 months and 12 months post-intervention	Adjusted mean difference –0.62, 95% CI –1.08 to –0.16, p<0.05 Favours intervention
SF-36 mental and physical health components; hospital anxiety and depression scale	1 RCT (Buszewicz et al. 2006) (N=812)	Self-management programme + education booklet vs education booklet alone	4 months and 12 months post-intervention	NS
Unspecified site				
Pain-related fear (TSK – 19 item questionnaire)	1 RCT (Heuts 2005) (N=297)	Self-management programme vs usual care	3 months post-intervention and 21 months post-intervention	Mean improvement 3 months: 2.05 (self-management) and –1.01 (usual care), p=0.002 21 months: 2.15 (self-management) and –1.68 (usual care), p=0.000 Favours intervention
SF–36 subscales of health change, physical functioning and general health perception	1 RCT (Heuts 2005) (N=297)	Self-management programme vs usual care	3 months post-intervention and 21 months post-intervention	NS
Beck Depression Inventory (BDI), 6 months (mean difference)	RCT (Calfas et al. 1992) (N=40)	Cognitive-behavioural modification vs education	10 weeks (end of intervention) and at 2, 6 and 12 months post-intervention	10 weeks: 8.1, p=0.00 8 months: 7.6, p=0.006 6 months: 7.2, p=0.017 12 months: 7.0, p=0.006 Favours intervention
AIMS physical functioning score (mean difference)	RCT (Calfas et al. 1992) (N=40)	Cognitive-behavioural modification vs education	2 months and 6 months post-intervention	2 months: 2.59, p=0.038 6 months: 2.35, p=0.005 Favours intervention
AIMS psychological status score (mean difference)	RCT (Calfas et al. 1992) (N=40)	Cognitive-behavioural modification vs education	6 months post-intervention	2.57, p=0.038 Favours intervention
Quality of well-being scale (QWB); AIMS pain score	RCT (Calfas et al. 1992) (N=40)	Cognitive-behavioural modification vs education	10 weeks (end of intervention) and at 2, 6 and 12 months post-intervention	NS

continued

Table 5.4 Quality of life – *continued*

QoL outcome	Reference	Intervention	Assessment time	Outcome/effect size
Unspecified site – *continued*				
AIMS psychological status	RCT (Calfas et al. 1992) (N=40)	Cognitive-behavioural modification vs education	10 weeks (end of intervention) and at 2 and 12 months post-intervention	NS
AIMS physical functioning	RCT (Calfas et al. 1992) (N=40)	Cognitive-behavioural modification vs education	10 weeks (end of intervention) and at 12 months post-intervention	NS

Table 5.5 Self-efficacy

Self-efficacy outcome	Reference	Intervention	Assessment time	Outcome/effect size
Knee				
Self-efficacy pain (scale 0–5, change from baseline)	1 implementation study (De Jong et al. 2004) (N=204)	Knee programme (pre-test vs post-test)	6 weeks, end of intervention	+0.2, p=0.006 Favours intervention
Self-efficacy functioning (scale 0–5, change from baseline) and Self-efficacy other symptoms (scale 0–5, change from baseline)	1 implementation study (De Jong et al. 2004) (N=204)	Knee programme (pre-test vs post-test)	6 weeks, end of intervention	NS
Knee and/or hip				
Arthritis self-efficacy scale (pain component) (adjusted mean difference)	1 RCT (Buszewicz et al. 2006) (N=812)	Self-management programme + education booklet vs education booklet alone	4 months and 12 months post-intervention	4 months: effect size: 1.63, 95% CI 0.83 to 2.43, p<0.05 12 months: effect size 0.98, 95% CI 0.07 to 1.89, p<0.05 Favours intervention
Arthritis self-efficacy scale ('other' component)	1 RCT (Buszewicz et al. 2006) (N=812)	Self-management programme + education booklet vs education booklet alone	4 months and 12 months post-intervention	4 months: effect size 1.83, 95% CI 0.74 to 2.92, p<0.05 12 months: 1.58, 95% CI 0.25 to 2.90, p<0.05 Favours intervention

Table 5.6 Health service use

Outcome	Reference	Intervention	Assessment time	Outcome/effect size
Knee				
Mean number of visits to the GP	1 RCT (Nunez et al. 2006) (N=100)	Therapeutic education and functional readaptation programme (TEFR) + conventional (pharmacologic) treatment vs control (waiting list) + pharmacologic treatment	9 months (6 months post-intervention)	Intervention better
Knee or hip				
Number of patient visits to physicians	1 RCT (Maisiak et al. 1996) (N=405)	Treatment counselling vs usual care	9 months (end of treatment)	Mean visits: 2.7 (counselling) and 4.3 (usual care), p<0.01 Favours intervention
Number of patient visits to physicians	1 RCT (Maisiak et al. 1996) (N=405)	Symptom monitoring vs usual care	9 months (end of treatment)	NS
Number of patient visits to physicians	1 RCT (Maisiak et al. 1996) (N=405)	Treatment counselling vs symptom monitoring	9 months (end of treatment)	Mean visits: 2.7 (counselling) and 3.9 (monitoring) Counselling better

Table 5.7 Analgesic use

Analgesic use outcome	Reference	Intervention	Assessment time	Outcome/effect size
Knee				
Number of analgesics taken per week	1 implementation study (De Jong et al. 2004) (N=204)	Knee programme (pre-test vs post-test)	6 weeks, end of intervention	8.7 (pre-test) and 4.8 (post-test), p=0.036 Favours intervention
Reduction in the number of NSAIDs taken per week	1 RCT (Nunez et al. 2006) (N=100)	Therapeutic education and functional readaptation programme (TEFR) + conventional (pharmacologic) treatment vs control (waiting list) + pharmacologic treatment	9 months, 6 months post-intervention	NS
Mean usage of analgesics/week	1 RCT (Nunez et al. 2006) (N=100)	Therapeutic education and functional readaptation programme (TEFR) + conventional (pharmacologic) treatment vs control (waiting list) + pharmacologic treatment	9 months, 6 months post-intervention	Reduced from baseline in intervention but not control group Favours intervention

Table 5.8 Osteoarthritis knowledge

Osteoarthritis knowledge outcome	Reference	Intervention	Assessment time	Outcome/effect size
Knee				
Osteoarthritis knowledge (scale 0–10, change from baseline)	1 implementation study (De Jong et al. 2004) (N=204)	Knee programme (pre-test vs post-test)	6 weeks, end of intervention	+1.3, p=0.000 Favours intervention
Arthritis knowledge score	1 RCT (Victor and Triggs 2005) (N=193)	Education programme (nurse-led) vs control (waiting list) group	1 month (end of intervention) and at 1 year (11 months post-intervention)	Only small improvement in intervention group (1 month: +0.2 and 1 year: +0.3)

Table 5.9 Use of self-management methods

Use of self-management methods outcome	Reference	Intervention	Outcome/effect size
Unspecified site			
Self-management use (mean number of methods used)	1 observational study (Hampson et al. 1993) (N=61)	Worse day vs typical day at Initial assessment and 8 months follow-up	Initial: 5.0 (worse day) and 4.4 (typical day), p<0.01 8 months: 4.5 (worse day) and 4.1 (typical day), p<0.01 Favours worse day (more used)
Most frequently used management methods (used by >50% of patients for each type)	1 observational study (Hampson et al. 1993) (N=61)	–	Gentle (low-impact) activity (92%) Medication (70%) Rest (65%) Range of motion exercises (63%)
Less popular self-management methods (used by <50% of patients)	1 observational study (Hampson et al. 1993) (N=61)		Relaxation (40%) Thermotherapy, heat or cold (37%) Joint protection (25%) Massage (25%) Splinting (23%) Other methods (5%)
Use of less popular methods	1 observational study (Hampson et al. 1993) (N=61)	Worse day vs typical day	Favours worse days (more used)
Most common 'other' self-management methods	1 observational study (Hampson et al. 1993) (N=61)	–	Dietary supplements or modifications (31%); physical activity (24%); various forms of protective behaviours (19%); application of liniments to the joints (14%)
Use of cognitive-strategies or relaxation to distract from pain and discomfort	1 observational study (Hampson et al. 1993) (N=61)	–	N=0 (cognitive) N=2 (relaxation)

continued

Table 5.9 Use of self-management methods – *continued*			
Use of self-management methods outcome	Reference	Intervention	Outcome/effect size
Unspecified site – *continued*			
Medication to control osteoarthritis	1 observational study (Hampson et al. 1993) (N=61)	–	Taken by participants regardless of symptom intensity
Use of passive methods	1 observational study (Hampson et al. 1993) (N=61)	–	Use on worse days was correlated with reported pain, believing one's pain to be serious and the number of joints involved and was associated with more pain over the last month and poorer role functioning.

5.1.4 From evidence to recommendations

There is a significant body of evidence in the field of social and psychological research on health behaviours in the context of information-giving and health-seeking behaviours and subsequent attitudes to treatments offered (Ajzen and Fishbein 1980; Carr and Donovan 1998; Donovan et al. 1989). Evidence has demonstrated that patients fail to retain all the information provided during a consultation. Lay health beliefs, perceived threat of the condition or treatments prescribed as well as time taken to adjust to the diagnosis all have an effect on an individual's ability to retain information and make changes to their health behaviours of concordance with treatments.

Although it is clear that many patients want more information than they currently receive, not all individuals will wish this. The degree to which people may wish to be involved in decisions about their treatment is likely to vary. Evidence suggests individuals may adopt one of three approaches when asked to make treatment decisions on their own (Coulter and Ellins 2006), wishing to:

- select their own treatment
- choose to collaborate with the healthcare professionals in making a decision
- delegate this responsibility to others.

Patient education is an information-giving process, designed to encourage positive changes in behaviours and beliefs conducive to health (Ramos-Remus et al. 2000). Patient education varies in content, length and type of programme (planned group sessions or tailored one-to-one sessions).

There are three components to patient education.

- General information given to provide an overview of the condition to aid understanding and enable discussions about changes in health status.
- Specific information given to encourage positive health-seeking behaviours that can improve patient self management and outcomes – for example, exercise in osteoarthritis.
- Information given about benefits and risks to aid informed consent.

There is a professional responsibility to ensure that patients are provided with sufficient and appropriate information about their condition. Patient education is an integral part of informed decision-making. In addition, within the wider context patient education has been advocated as a way of limiting the impact of a long-term condition (Department of Health 2005).

RECOMMENDATION

R7   Healthcare professionals should offer accurate verbal and written information to all people with osteoarthritis to enhance understanding of the condition and its management, and to counter misconceptions, such as that it inevitably progresses and cannot be treated. Information sharing should be an ongoing, integral part of the management plan rather than a single event at time of presentation.

5.2   Patient self-management interventions

5.2.1   Clinical introduction

Self-management can be defined as any activity that individuals do to promote health, prevent disease and enhance self-efficacy. Individuals who are able to recognise and believe in their ability to control symptoms (self-efficacy) can become more active participants in managing their condition and thus potentially improve their perceived control over their symptoms. This may improve concordance with treatment options offered and reduce reliance on healthcare interventions (Cross et al. 2006; Cox et al. 2004).

Providing a framework for patients that encourages self-management is now considered an integral aspect of care for all long-term conditions. Self-management principles empower the patient to use their own knowledge and skills to access appropriate resources and build on their own experiences of managing their condition. Not all patients will wish to self-manage or be able to achieve effective strategies and practitioners should be aware of the vulnerable groups who may require additional support.

5.2.2   Evidence base

The evidence for this self-management section was searched and appraised together with that for patient information (section 5.1)

5.2.3   From evidence to recommendations

Educational initiatives that encourage self-management strategies should be encouraged, although it has to be recognised that such support appears to have limited effectiveness from eligible UK studies to date. This may relate to a number of limitations including the range and diversity of outcomes measured and disparities in severity and site of osteoarthritis. Studies exploring key concepts such as self-efficacy and wider psychological and social factors were lacking. There are also important additional factors in the context of osteoarthritis as lay expectations – and to some extent healthcare professionals' expectations – of good outcomes are somewhat negative and access to readily accessible support and advice are generally poor. These perspectives are likely to influence outcomes.

The members of this working group have considered these limitations yet accept that with the expected changes in the population – with a doubling of chronic disease and elderly patients by 2020 – the healthcare system has to consider encouraging a greater degree of self-management principles in line with current health policy. If longer-term outcomes are to be achieved, such as reduction in the use of health resources, effective use of therapeutic options and more adequately prepared and informed patients seeking interventions such as joint replacement surgery, then self-management may be an appropriate and cost-effective tool.

There will be a range of providers including voluntary and independent sectors who will be offering self-management programmes. These programmes will require a thorough evaluation of outcomes achieved at a time when primary care will also be enhancing the infrastructures and support for those with osteoarthritis requiring healthcare support.

RECOMMENDATIONS

R8   Individualised self-management strategies should be agreed between healthcare professionals and the person with osteoarthritis. Positive behavioural changes such as exercise, weight loss, use of suitable footwear and pacing should be appropriately targeted.

R9   Self-management programmes, either individually or in groups, should emphasise the recommended core treatments (see Fig 3.2) for people with osteoarthritis, especially exercise.

5.3 Rest, relaxation and pacing

5.3.1 Clinical introduction

It would seem sensible if something hurts to rest it. This may only be true in acute situations and may not hold for chronic conditions. It is counter productive to give rheumatoid arthritis patients bed rest. Muscle loss is a feature of both rheumatoid and osteoarthritis. Pain does not mean harm in many musculoskeletal conditions. We have looked at the effect of exercise on osteoarthritis especially of the knee, but where do rest, relaxation and coping strategies fit?

5.3.2 Methodological introduction

We looked for studies that investigated the efficacy and safety of rest and relaxation compared with no treatment or other interventions with respect to symptoms, function and quality of life. Three RCTs (Gay et al. 2002; Garfinkel et al. 1994; McCaffrey and Freeman 2003) were found on relaxation, yoga and listening to music. One RCT (Garfinkel et al. 1994) was excluded due to methodological limitations. No relevant cohort or case-control studies were found.

Two RCTs did not document blinding or intention to treat (ITT) analysis. One RCT (Gay et al. 2002) compared Erikson hypnosis with Jacobson relaxation technique or no treatment in N=41 patients with knee and/or hip osteoarthritis over 2 months with follow-up at 3–6 months. The second RCT (McCaffrey and Freeman 2003) compared listening to music with sitting quietly in N=66 patients with osteoarthritis. The interventions lasted for 14 days.

5.3.3 Evidence statements

▷   Symptoms: pain, knee and/or hip

One RCT (Gay et al. 2002) (N=41) found that Jacobson relaxation was significantly better than control (no treatment) for pain (VAS) at 8 weeks, end of treatment (p<0.05), but there was no significant difference between the two groups at 4 weeks (mid-treatment) and at 3 months and 6 months post-treatment. (1+)

▷ Symptoms: pain, unspecified site

One RCT (McCaffrey 2003) (N=66) found that rest and relaxation (sitting and listening to music) was significantly better than the control (sitting quietly and/or reading) for pre-post test changes of SF-MPQ pain (VAS) and SF-MPQ pain-rating index at day 1, day 7 and at 2 weeks (end of treatment), all p=0.001. Mean differences: SF-MPQ pain 23.4 18.9 and 17.3 respectively, all p=0.001; SF-MPQ pain-rating index –5.1, +3.8 and +2.2 respectively, all p=0.001. (1+)

▷ Withdrawals: knee and/or shoulder

One RCT (Gay et al. 2002) (N=41) found that Jacobson relaxation and control (no treatment) were similar for total number of study withdrawals (N=3 21% and N=4, 31% respectively). (1+)

5.3.4 From evidence to recommendations

There was little evidence in this area. Many of the studies were about modalities not relevant to the NHS (for example therapeutic touch, playing music).

The GDG felt that it was important to emphasise the role of self-management strategies. As this is done in section 5.2, no recommendation is made here.

5.4 Thermotherapy

5.4.1 Clinical introduction

Thermotherapy has for many years been advocated as a useful adjunct to pharmacological therapies. Ice is used for acute injuries and warmth is used for sprains and strains. It seems appropriate to use hot and cold packs in osteoarthritis.

5.4.2 Methodological introduction

We looked for studies that investigated the efficacy and safety of local thermotherapy versus no treatment or other interventions with respect to symptoms, function and quality of life in adults with osteoarthritis. One systematic review and meta-analysis (Brosseau et al. 2003), one RCT (Evcik et al. 2007) and one non-comparative study (Martin et al. 1998) were found on thermotherapy. No relevant cohort or case-control studies were found. The RCT (Evcik et al. 2007) was excluded due to methodological limitations.

The meta-analysis assessed the RCTs for quality and pooled together all data for the outcomes of symptoms and function.

The meta-analysis included three single blind, parallel group RCTs (with N=179 participants) on comparisons between ice massage, cold packs and placebo, electroacupuncture (EA), short wave diathermy (SWD) or AL-TENS in patients with knee osteoarthritis.

Studies included in the analysis differed with respect to:

- types of thermotherapy and comparisons used (one RCT ice application; one RCT ice massage)
- type of comparison used (1 RCT SWD or placebo SWD; 1 RCT EA, AL-TENS or placebo AL-TENS)

- treatment regimen (3 or 5 days/week)
- trial size and length.

The non-comparative study (Martin et al. 1998) looked at pre- and post-treatment effects of liquid nitrogen cryotherapy (3 weeks of treatment) in N=26 patients with knee osteoarthritis.

5.4.3 Evidence statements

Table 5.10 Symptoms: pain

Pain outcome	Reference	Intervention	Assessment time	Outcome/effect size
Knee osteoarthritis				
Ice massage				
Pain at rest, PPI score	1 MA (Brosseau et al. 2003) 1 RCT, N=50	Ice massage vs control	Week 2, end of treatment	NS
Pain at rest, PPI score	1 MA (Brosseau et al. 2003) 1 RCT, N=50	Ice massage vs AL-TENS	Week 2, end of treatment	NS
Pain at rest, PPI score	1 MA (Brosseau et al. 2003) 1 RCT, N=50	Ice massage vs electroacupuncture	Week 2, end of treatment	NS
Ice packs				
Pain difference	1 MA (Brosseau et al. 2003) 1 RCT, N=26	Ice packs vs control	3 weeks (end of treatment) and at 3 months post-treatment	NS
Liquid nitrogen cryotherapy (pre-treatment vs post-treatment)				
Pain rating index total (McGill pain questionnaire, change from baseline)	1 non-comparative study (Martin et al. 1998), N=26	Liquid nitrogen cryotherapy (pre-treatment vs post-treatment)	3 weeks (end of treatment)	p=0.013 Favours cryotherapy
Present pain intensity (McGill pain questionnaire, change from baseline)	1 non-comparative study (Martin et al. 1998), N=26	Liquid nitrogen cryotherapy (pre-treatment vs post-treatment)	3 weeks (end of treatment)	p=0.002 Favours cryotherapy

Table 5.11 Function

Function outcome	Reference	Intervention	Assessment time	Outcome/effect size
Knee osteoarthritis				
Ice massage				
Increasing quadriceps strength	1 MA (Brosseau et al. 2003) 1 RCT, N=50	Ice massage vs control	Week 2, end of treatment	WMD 2.30, 95% CI 1.08 to 3.52, p=0.0002 Favours ice massage
Knee flexion, ROM (degrees)	1 MA (Brosseau et al. 2003) 1 RCT, N=50	Ice massage vs control	Week 2, end of treatment	WMD 8.80, 95% CI 4.57 to 13.03, p=0.00005 Favours ice massage
50-foot walk time (mins)	1 MA (Brosseau et al. 2003) 1 RCT, N=50	Ice massage vs control	Week 2, end of treatment	WMD −9.70, 95% CI −12.40 to −7.00, p<0.00001 Favours ice massage
Increasing quadriceps strength	1 MA (Brosseau et al. 2003) 1 RCT, N=50	Ice massage vs control	Week 2, end of treatment	29% relative difference Ice massage better
ROM, degrees (change from baseline)	1 MA (Brosseau et al. 2003) 1 RCT, N=50	Ice massage vs control	Week 2, end of treatment	8% relative difference – no clinical benefit for ice massage
50-foot walk time, mins (change from baseline)	1 MA (Brosseau et al. 2003) 1 RCT, N=50	Ice massage vs control	Week 2, end of treatment	11% relative difference – no clinical benefit for ice massage
Knee flexion, ROM (degrees)	1 MA (Brosseau et al. 2003) 1 RCT, N=50	Ice massage vs AL-TENS	Week 2, end of treatment	NS
50-foot walk time (mins)	1 MA (Brosseau et al. 2003) 1 RCT, N=50	Ice massage vs AL-TENS	Week 2, end of treatment	NS
Increasing quadriceps strength	1 MA (Brosseau et al. 2003) 1 RCT, N=50	Ice massage vs AL-TENS	Week 2, end of treatment	WMD −3.70, 95% CI −5.70 to −1.70, p=0.0003 Favours AL-TENS
Increasing quadriceps strength	1 MA (Brosseau et al. 2003) 1 RCT, N=50	Ice massage vs electroacupuncture	Week 2, end of treatment	WMD −2.80, 95% CI −4.14 to −1.46, p=0.00004 Favours EA
50-foot walk time (mins)	1 MA (Brosseau et al. 2003) 1 RCT, N=50	Ice massage vs electroacupuncture	Week 2, end of treatment	WMD 6.00, 95% CI 3.19 to 8.81, p=0.00003 Favours EA
Knee flexion, ROM (degrees)	1 MA (Brosseau et al. 2003) 1 RCT, N=50	Ice massage vs electroacupuncture	Week 2, end of treatment	NS

continued

Table 5.11 Function – *continued*

Function outcome	Reference	Intervention	Assessment time	Outcome/effect size
Knee osteoarthritis – *continued*				
Cold packs				
Change on knee circumference (oedema)	1 MA (Brosseau et al. 2003) 1 RCT, N=23	Cold packs vs control	After the first application	NS
Change on knee circumference (oedema)	1 MA (Brosseau et al. 2003) 1 RCT, N=23	Cold packs vs control	After 10 applications, end of treatment	WMD –1.0, 95% CI -1.98 to –0.02, p=0.04 Favours ice packs
Liquid nitrogen cryotherapy (pre-treatment vs post-treatment)				
Right and left knee extension	1 non-comparative study (Martin et al. 1998), N=26	Liquid nitrogen cryotherapy (pre-treatment vs post-treatment)	3 weeks (end of treatment)	p=0.04 and p=0.02 Favours cryotherapy
Right and left quadriceps strength (respectively)	1 non-comparative study (Martin et al. 1998), N=26	Liquid nitrogen cryotherapy (pre-treatment vs post-treatment)	3 weeks (end of treatment)	p=0.01 and 0.006 Favours cryotherapy
Right and left knee flexion	1 non-comparative study (Martin et al. 1998), N=26	Liquid nitrogen cryotherapy (pre-treatment vs post-treatment)	3 weeks (end of treatment)	NS

5.4.4 From evidence to recommendations

The evidence base on thermotherapy is limited to three small RCTs, only one of which assesses pain relief. All the thermotherapy studies in osteoarthritis are on applying cold rather than heat. The RCT looking at pain found no significant difference between cold thermotherapy and control. The results in the RCTs assessing function are mixed when compared with controls, with electroacupuncture and with AL-TENS. There is no economic evidence available on the subject.

Despite the scarcity of evidence, in the GDG's experience, local heat and cold are widely used as part of self-management. They may not always take the form of packs or massage, with some patients simply using hot baths to the same effect. As an intervention this has very low cost and is extremely safe. The GDG therefore felt that a positive recommendation was justified.

RECOMMENDATION

R10 The use of local heat or cold should be considered as an adjunct to core treatment.

6 Non-pharmacological management of osteoarthritis

6.1 Exercise and manual therapy

6.1.1 Clinical introduction

Exercise is widely used by health professionals and patients to reduce pain (Fransen et al. 2002; Minor 1999) and improve function. Exercise and physical activity can be targeted at the affected joint(s) and also at improving general mobility, function, well-being and self-efficacy. More intensive exercise can strengthen muscles around the affected joint. However, people often receive confused messages about when to exercise if they experience pain on physical activity or find that resting eases the pain. Often people believe that activity 'wears out' joints. Patients who have followed an exercise programme sometimes report they have experienced an exacerbation of their symptoms and are reluctant to continue. While some individuals may experience an exacerbation of symptoms the vast majority of people, including those severely affected, will not have any adverse reaction to controlled exercise (Hurley et al. 2007). For example, patients with significant osteoarthritis can ride a bicycle, go swimming or exercise at a gym with often no or minimal discomfort.

The goals of prescribed exercise must be agreed between the patient and the health professional. Changing health behaviour with education and advice are positive ways of enabling patients to exercise regularly. Pacing, where patients learn to incorporate specific exercise sessions with periods of rest interspersed with activities intermittently throughout the day, can be a useful strategy. Analgesia may be needed so that people can undertake the advised or prescribed exercise.

The majority of the evidence is related to osteoarthritis of the knee, few studies have considered the hip and even fewer hand osteoarthritis. This section looks at the research evidence for different types of exercise for the joints usually affected by osteoarthritis.

Manual therapies are passive or active assisted movement techniques that use manual force to improve the mobility of restricted joints, connective tissue or skeletal muscles. Manual therapies are directed at influencing joint function and pain. Techniques include mobilisation, manipulation, soft tissue massage, stretching and passive movements to the joints and soft tissue. Manipulation is defined as high velocity thrusts, and mobilisation as techniques excluding high velocity thrusts, graded as appropriate to the patient's signs and symptoms. Manual therapy may work best in combination with other treatment approaches, such as exercise.

6.1.2 Methodological introduction: exercise

We looked firstly at studies that investigated the effects of exercise therapy in relation to:
- sham exercise or no treatment control groups
- other osteoarthritis therapies.

Secondly we searched for studies that compared the risks and benefits of different exercise therapies with no treatment. Due to the high number of studies in this area, only randomised controlled trials (RCTs) were included as evidence. Knee osteoarthritis RCTs with N=30 or fewer study completers were also excluded due to the high number of studies relevant to the osteoarthritis population.

▷ Land-based exercise

For the first question, we found one meta-analysis of 13 randomised controlled trials dealing specifically with aerobic and strengthening land-based exercise therapies in the knee osteo-arthritis population (Roddy et al. 2005), and an additional 25 RCTs (Borjesson et al. 1996; Brismee et al. 2007; Chamberlain and Care 1982; Evcik and Sonel 2002; Focht et al. 2005; Fransen et al. 2007; Hay et al. 2006; Huang et al. 2003, 2005; Hughes et al. 2006; Hurley 2007; Keefe and Blomenthal 2004; Kuptniratsaikul et al. 2002; Lefler and Armstrong 2004; Messier et al. 1997, 2000, 2004; Ones et al. 2006; Peloquin et al. 1999; Penninx et al. 2001, 2002; Rejeski et al. 2002; Tak et al. 2005; Thorstensson et al. 2005; van Baar et al. 2001) of land-based exercise.

Five of these RCTs (Chamberlain and Care 1982, Evcik and Sonel 2002, Huang et al. 2005, Hughes et al. 2006; Kuptniratsaikul et al. 2002) were excluded due to multiple methodological limitations, while the remaining 16 were included as evidence.

For the second question, we found ten RCTs that compared different land-based exercise programs to a no-exercise control group (Eyigor et al. 2004; Huang et al. 2003; Lim et al. 2002; Mangione and McCully 1999; McCarthy et al. 2004a; Messier et al. 1997; 2000; Penninx et al. 2001, 2002; Tuzun 2004). Nine studies were included as evidence, with one study (Tuzun et al. 2004) excluded due to multiple methodological limitations.

▷ Hydrotherapy and manual therapy

Ten RCTs (Belza et al. 2002; Cochrane et al. 2005; Deyle et al. 2005; Dracoglu et al. 2005; Foley et al. 2003; Fransen et al. 2007; Henderson et al. 1994; Hoeksma et al. 2004; Hinman et al. 2007; Wang et al. 2007) were identified on hydrotherapy vs no treatment control or other land-based exercise programs. Four of these (Green et al. 1993; Minor et al. 1989; Wang et al. 2007; Wyatt et al. 2001) were excluded due to multiple methodological limitations. One study (Cochrane et al. 2005) did not report between-group outcome comparisons adjusted for baseline values, but was otherwise well conducted, and so was included as evidence along with the remaining two studies (Belza et al. 2002, Foley et al. 2003).

A further five RCTs were found (Deyle et al. 2000, 2005; Dracoglu et al. 2005; Hoeksma et al. 2004) comparing manual therapy with land-based exercise or a control group. All studies were methodologically sound.

▷ Study quality

Many of the included RCTs on land-based hydrotherapy and manual therapy categories had the following methodological characteristics:
- single-blinded or un-blinded
- randomisation and blinding were flawed or inadequately described
- did not include power calculations, had small sample sizes or had no ITT analysis details.

6.1.3   Methodological introduction: manual therapy

We looked for studies that investigated the efficacy and safety of manual therapies vs no treatment or other interventions with respect to symptoms, function, quality of life in patients with osteoarthritis. Five RCTs (Bennell et al. 2005; Deyle et al. 2000; Hoeksma et al. 2004; Perlman et al. 2006; Tucker et al. 2003), one cohort study (Cliborne et al. 2004) and one non-analytic study (MacDonald 2006) were found on manual therapy (joint manipulation, mobilisation, stretching, with or without exercise).

The five RCTs were all randomized, parallel group studies (apart from one study which was cross-over (Perlman et al. 2006)) and were methodologically sound. Studies differed with respect to:

* osteoarthritis site (four RCTs knee, one RCT hip)
* blinding, sample size, trial duration and follow-up.

The two non-RCTs were methodologically sound. The cohort study (Cliborne et al. 2004) compared the effects of one session of manual therapy (oscillatory mobilisations of the hip) on symptoms and function vs pre-treatment values in N=39 patients with knee osteoarthritis. The case-series compared the effects of 2–5 weeks of manual therapy (mobilisation and manipulation) on symptoms and function vs pre-treatment values in N=7 patients with hip osteoarthritis.

6.1.4   Evidence statements: land-based exercise

Table 6.1 Symptoms

Pain outcome	Reference	Intervention	Assessment time	Outcome/effect size
Exercise vs control				
Pain	1 MA (Roddy et al. 2005), 4 RCTs (N=449)	Aerobic walking vs no-exercise control interventions	Trial duration: mean 7.2 months, range 8 weeks to 2 years	Effect size 0.52, % CI 0.34 to 0.70, p<0.05 Favours exercise
Pain	1 MA (Roddy et al. 2005), 8 RCTs (N=2004)	Home-based quadriceps strengthening exercise vs no-exercise control interventions	Trial duration: mean 7.2 months, range 8 weeks to 2 years	Effect size 0.32,% CI 0.23 to 0.42, p<0.05 Favours exercise
Pain (VAS score)	1 RCT (Huang et al. 2003) (N=132)	Isokinetic, isotonic, and isometric exercise vs no exercise	One year follow-up	p<0.05 Favours exercise
Self-reported pain (VAS score)	1 RCT (Tak 2005) (N=94)	Exercise (strength training and home exercises) vs no treatment	3 months follow-up	p=0.019 Favours exercise
Observed pain (HHS pain scale)	1 RCT (Tak 2005) (N=94)	Exercise (strength training and home exercises) vs no treatment	3 months follow-up	p=0.047 Favours exercise
Transfer pain intensity and frequency (getting in and out of bed, chair, car etc)	1 RCT (Messier et al. 1997) (N=103)	Aerobic training exercise groups vs health education	18 months follow-up	P<0.001 Favours exercise

continued

Table 6.1 Symptoms – *continued*

Pain outcome	Reference	Intervention	Assessment time	Outcome/effect size
Exercise vs control – *continued*				
Transfer pain intensity and frequency (getting in and out of bed, chair, car etc)	1 RCT (Messier et al. 1997) (N=103)	Weight training exercise groups vs health education	18 months follow-up	P=0.04 Favours exercise
Mean overall knee pain (VAS)	1 RCT (Brismee et al. 2007) (N=41)	Tai chi exercise vs attention control	9 weeks (mid-treatment) and 12 weeks (end of treatment)	Both: p<0.05 Favours exercise
Mean maximum knee pain (VAS)	1 RCT (Brismee et al. 2007) (N=41)	Tai chi exercise vs attention control	6 weeks (mid-treatment) and 9 weeks (mid-treatment)	Both: p<0.05 Favours exercise
Pain for ambulation intensity and frequency	1 RCT (Messier et al. 1997) (N=103)	Aerobic training exercise groups vs health education	18 months follow-up	NS
Pain for ambulation intensity and frequency	1 RCT (Messier et al. 1997) (N=103)	Weight training exercise groups vs health education	18 months follow-up	NS
Pain (KOOS subscale)	1 RCT (Thorstensson et al. 2005) (N=61)	Weight-bearing exercise vs no treatment	6 months follow-up	NS
Pain scores (VAS)	1 RCT (van Baar et al. 2001) (N=183)	Strengthening exercise vs educational advice	9 months follow-up.	NS
Pain during walking (Borg 11-grade scale)	1 RCT (Borjesson et al. 1996) (N=68)	Strengthening exercise vs no treatment	Study end-point (3 months)	NS
Pain (six-point rating scale)	1 RCT (Lefler and Armstrong 2004) (N=19)	Strength training vs usual treatment	Study end-point (6 weeks)	NS
Mean overall knee pain (VAS)	1 RCT (Brismee et al. 2007) (N=41)	Tai chi exercise vs attention control	3 and 6 weeks (mid-treatment) and 4 weeks and 6 weeks post-treatment	NS
Mean maximum knee pain (VAS)	1 RCT (Brismee et al. 2007) (N=41)	Tai chi exercise vs attention control	3 weeks (mid-treatment), at 12 weeks (end of treatment) and at 4 weeks and 6 weeks post-treatment	NS
WOMAC pain	1 RCT (Fransen et al. 2007) (N=152)	Tai chi exercise vs attention control	0–12 weeks (end of treatment)	NS

continued

Table 6.1 Symptoms – *continued*

Pain outcome	Reference	Intervention	Assessment time	Outcome/effect size
Exercise + other therapy vs control or exercise				
WOMAC pain	1 RCT (Messier et al. 2004) (N=316)	Diet + exercise (aerobic and resistance) vs healthy lifestyle	18 months post-randomisation	$p \leq 0.05$ Favours diet + exercise
WOMAC pain; pain (VAS); walking pain; pain at rest	1 RCT (Ones et al. 2006) (N=80)	Exercise (isometric, insotonic, stepping) + hotpacks + ultrasound vs exercise only	16 weeks (end of study)	All $p<0.05$ Favours exercise + hotpacks + ultrasound
WOMAC pain (change from baseline)	1 RCT (Hay et al. 2006) (N=325)	Community physiotherapy + advice leaflet vs control (no exercise, advice leaflet + telephone call)	3 months, (2 weeks post-treatment)	Mean difference 1.15,% CI 0.2 to 2.1, $p=0.008$ Favours physiotherapy + leaflet
Change in pain severity (NRS)	1 RCT (Hay et al. 2006) (N=325)	Community physiotherapy + advice leaflet vs control (no exercise, advice leaflet + telephone call)	3 months (2 weeks post-treatment)	Mean difference −0.84,% CI −1.5 to −0.2, $p=0.01$
Change in severity of main problem (NRS)	1 RCT (Hay et al. 2006) (N=325)	Community physiotherapy + advice leaflet vs control (no exercise, advice leaflet + telephone call)	3 months (2 weeks post-treatment) and at 6 months (4 months post-treatment)	3 months: mean difference −1.06,% CI −1.8 to −0.3, $p=0.005$ 6 months: mean difference −1.22,% CI −2.0 to −0.4, $p=0.002$
WOMAC pain (change from baseline)	1 RCT (Hurley et al. 2007)	Rehabilitation programme (progressive exercise + group discussion) + usual primary care vs usual primary care	6 months (4.5 months post-treatment)	Mean difference −1.01,%CI −1.84 to −0.19, $p=0.016$ Favours intervention
WOMAC pain, (change from baseline)	1 RCT (Hay et al. 2006)	Community physiotherapy + advice leaflet vs control (no exercise, advice leaflet + telephone call)	6 months and 12 months (approximately 4 months and 10 months post-treatment	NS
Change in severity of main problem (NRS)	1 RCT (Hay et al. 2006)	Community physiotherapy + advice leaflet vs control (no exercise, advice leaflet + telephone call)	12 months (approximately 10 months post-treatment).	NS

Stiffness outcome	Reference	Intervention	Assessment time	Outcome/effect size
Exercise + other therapy vs control or exercise				
WOMAC stiffness	1 RCT (Ones et al. 2006) (N=80)	Exercise (isometric, insotonic, stepping) + hotpacks + ultrasound vs exercise only	Study endpoint (16 weeks)	$p<0.05$ Favours intervention

Table 6.2 Patient function

Function outcome	Reference	Intervention	Assessment time	Outcome/effect size
Exercise vs control				
Self-reported disability	1 MA (Roddy et al. 2005) 2 RCTs (N=385)	Aerobic walking vs no-exercise control interventions	Trial duration: mean 7.2 months, range 8 weeks to 2 years	Effect size: 0.46,% CI 0.25 to 0.67, p<0.05 Favours exercise
Self-reported disability	1 MA (Roddy et al. 2005), 8 RCTs (N=2004)	Home-based quadriceps strengthening exercise vs no-exercise control interventions	Trial duration: mean 7.2 months, range 8 weeks to 2 years	Effect size: 0.32,% CI 0.23 to 0.41, p<0.05 Favours exercise
Self-reported disability (LI 17 questionnaire)	1 RCT (Huang et al. 2003) (N=132)	Isokinetic, isotonic, and isometric exercise groups vs no exercise	1 year follow-up	p<0.05 Favours exercise
Self-reported disability (GARS)	1 RCT (Tak 2005) (N=94)	Exercise (strength training and home exercises) vs no treatment	3 months follow-up	NS
Hip function (Harris hip score)	1 RCT (Tak 2005) (N=94)	Exercise (strength training and home exercises) vs control	3 months follow-up	NS
Functional performance	1 RCT (Thorstensson et al. 2005) (N=61)	Weight-bearing exercise vs control (no treatment)	6 months follow-up	NS
Level of physical activity (Zutphen Physical Activity Questionnaire); observed disability (video of patient standard tasks)	1 RCT (van Baar et al. 2001) (N=183)	Strengthening exercise vs educational advice control group	After 9 months of follow-up	NS
Risk of activities of daily living (ADL) disability (30-item questionnaire)	1 RCT (Penninx et al. 2001) (N=250)	Aerobic exercise vs attention control	18 months follow-up	Cox proportional hazards: RR 0.53,%CI 0.33 to 0.85, p=0.009 Favours exercise
Risk of activities of daily living (ADL) disability (30-item questionnaire)	1 RCT (Penninx et al. 2001) (N=250)	Resistance exercise vs attention control	18 months follow-up	Cox proportional hazards: RR 0.60,%CI 0.38 to 0.97, p=0.04 Favours exercise
Risk of moving from a non-ADL disabled to an ADL-disabled state over this period	1 RCT (Penninx et al. 2001) (N=250)	Aerobic exercise vs attention control	18 months follow-up	RR 0.45,%CI 0.26 to 0.78, p=0.004 Favours exercise
Risk of moving from a non-ADL disabled to an ADL-disabled state over this period	1 RCT (Penninx et al. 2001) (N=250)	Resistance exercise vs attention control	18 months follow-up	RR 0.53%CI 0.31 to 0.91, p=0.02 Favours exercise

continued

Table 6.2 Patient function – *continued*

Function outcome	Reference	Intervention	Assessment time	Outcome/effect size
Exercise vs control – *continued*				
WOMAC function	1 RCT (Fransen et al. 2007) (N=152)	Tai chi exercise vs attention control	0–12 weeks (end of treatment)	Standardised response mean: 0.63,% CI 0.50 to 0.76, p<0.05. Favours exercise
WOMAC overall score	1 RCT (Brismee et al. 2007) (N=41)	Tai chi exercise vs attention control	9 weeks (mid-treatment)	p<0.05 Favours exercise
WOMAC overall score	1 RCT (Brismee et al. 2007) (N=41)	Tai chi exercise vs attention control	3 and 6 weeks (mid-treatment), at 12 weeks (end of treatment) and at 4 weeks and 6 weeks post-treatment	NS
Activities of daily living scores (KOOS subscale)	1 RCT (Thorstensson et al. 2005) (N=61)	Weight-bearing exercise vs control (no treatment)	6 months follow-up	NS
WOMAC function	1 RCT (Messier et al. 2004) (N=316)	Exercise vs healthy lifestyle	18 months post-randomisation	NS
WOMAC function	1 RCT (Messier et al. 2004) (N=316)	Diet vs healthy lifestyle	18 months post-randomisation	NS
Exercise + other therapy vs control or exercise				
WOMAC function	1 RCT (Messier et al. 2004) (N=316)	Diet + exercise (aerobic and resistance) vs healthy lifestyle	18 months post-randomisation	p<0.05 Favours exercise
WOMAC function	1 RCT (Ones et al. 2006) (N=80)	Exercise (isometric, insotonic, stepping) + hotpacks + ultrasound vs exercise only	Study endpoint (16 weeks)	p<0.05 Favours intervention
WOMAC function	1 RCT (Hay et al. 2006)	Community physiotherapy + advice leaflet vs control (no exercise, advice leaflet + telephone call)	3 months, (2 weeks post-treatment)	Mean difference 3.99,% CI 1.2 to 6.8, p=0.008 Favours intervention
WOMAC function (change from baseline)	1 RCT (Hurley et al. 2007)	Rehabilitation programme (progressive exercise + group discussion) + usual primary care vs usual primary care	6 months (4.5 months post-treatment)	Mean difference −3.33,% CI −5.88 to −0.78, p=0.01 Favours intervention
WOMAC total (change from baseline)	1 RCT (Hurley et al. 2007)	Rehabilitation programme (progressive exercise + group discussion) + usual primary care vs usual primary care	6 months (4.5 months post-treatment)	Mean difference −4.59,%CI −8.30 to −0.88, p=0.015 Favours intervention
WOMAC function, (change from baseline)	1 RCT (Hay et al. 2006)	Community physiotherapy + advice leaflet vs control (no exercise, advice leaflet + telephone call)	6 months and 12 months (approximately 4 months and 10 months post-treatment)	NS

Table 6.3 Examination findings

Examination findings outcome	Reference	Intervention	Assessment time	Outcome/effect size
Exercise vs control				
Knee flexion and extension (ascending steps)	1 RCT (Borjesson et al. 1996) (N=68)	Strengthening exercise vs control groups	3 months (end of study)	NS
Step-down ability	1 RCT (Borjesson et al. 1996) (N=68)	Strengthening exercise vs control groups	3 months (end of study)	Improved: 38% (exercise) and 12% (control) Worse: 3% (exercise) and 24% (control) Exercise better
Stair climbing	1 RCT (Tak 2005) (N=94)	Exercise (strength training and home exercises) vs control	3 months follow-up	NS
Stair climb (seconds)	1 RCT (Fransen et al. 2007) (N=152)	Tai chi vs attention control	0–12 weeks (end of treatment)	Standardised response mean: 0.36,% CI 0.23 to 0.49, p<0.05 Favours exercise
Mean peak torque values for knee extensor and flexor muscles at 60 and 180 degrees	1 RCT (Huang et al. 2003) (N=132)	Exercise (isokinetic, isotonic, and isometric exercise) vs no exercise	One-year follow-up	p<0.05 Favours exercise
Improvements in muscle strength for leg extensions; leg flexions; bicep curls	1 RCT (Keefe and Blumenthal 2004) (N=72)	Exercise (strength plus endurance training) vs no-treatment	Study endpoint (12 weeks)	Extension and flexion:p<0.001 Bicep curls p=0.004 Favours exercise
Knee mean angular velocity	1 RCT (Messier et al. 1997) (N=103)	Aerobic exercise vs health education control	18 months follow-up	p=0.04 Favours exercise
Knee mean angular velocity	1 RCT (Messier et al. 1997) (N=103)	Weight training exercise vs health education control	18 months follow-up	NS
Improvements in quadriceps strength (isometric strength 30°and 60° angle)	1 RCT (Peloquin et al. 1999) (N=137)	Exercise (aerobic plus strengthening plus stretching) vs educational advice control	3 months (end of treatment)	30°: p=0.008 60°: p=0.007 Favours exercise
Hamstring strength	1 RCT (Peloquin et al. 1999) (N=137)	Exercise (aerobic plus strengthening plus stretching) vs educational advice control	3 months (end of treatment)	30°: NS 60°p= 0.013; 30° velocity p=0.017; 90° velocity p=0.048 Favours exercise
Mean peak torque values for knee extensor and flexor muscles	1 RCT (Borjesson et al. 1996) (N=68)	Strengthening exercise vs control	Study endpoint (3 months)	NS

continued

Table 6.3 Examination findings – *continued*

Examination findings outcome	Reference	Intervention	Assessment time	Outcome/effect size
Exercise vs control – *continued*				
Muscle strength for knee or hip	1 RCT (van Baar et al. 2001) (N=183)	Strengthening exercise vs educational advice	9 months follow-up	NS
Grip strength (dynamometer), pinch measures (pinch gauge), and finger ROM	1 RCT (Lefler and Armstrong 2004) (N=19)	Strength training vs usual treatment	Study endpoint (6 weeks)	NS
Improvement in walking distance	1 RCT (Focht et al. 2005) (N=316)	Exercise (aerobic and resistance) vs healthy lifestyle control	18 months post-randomisation	p<0.0001 Favours exercise
6-minute walking distance	1 RCT (Messier et al. 2004) (N=316)	Exercise vs healthy lifestyle control	18 months post-randomisation	p≤0.05 Favours exercise
Improvement in walking speed	1 RCT (Huang et al. 2003) (N=132)	Exercise (isokinetic, isotonic, and isometric groups) vs control	One year follow-up	All p<0.05 Favours exercise
Walking velocity; absolute and relative stride length	1 RCT (Messier et al. 1997) (N=103)	Aerobic exercise vs education control	18 months of follow-up	Walking: p=0.001 Stride: p≤0.03 Favours exercise
Walking velocity; absolute and relative stride length	1 RCT (Messier et al. 1997) (N=103)	Weight-training vs education	18 months of follow-up	Walking: p=0.03 Stride: NS Favours exercise
Improvements in 5-minute walking test	1 RCT (Peloquin et al. 1999) (N=137)	Exercise (aerobic + strengthening + stretching) vs educational advice	3 months (end of intervention)	p=0.0001 Favours exercise
Free walking speed, step frequency, stride length/lower extremity length, gait cycle, range of stance knee flexion, and range of swing knee flexion	1 RCT (Borjesson et al. 1996) (N=68)	Strengthening exercise vs control	Study endpoint (3 months)	NS
Walking 20 meters	1 RCT (Tak 2005) (N=94)	Exercise (strength training and home exercises) vs control	3 months follow-up	NS
50-foot walk time	1 RCT (Fransen et al. 2007) (N=152)	Tai chi vs attention control	0–12 weeks (end of treatment)	NS

continued

Table 6.3 Examination findings – *continued*

Examination findings outcome	Reference	Intervention	Assessment time	Outcome/effect size
Exercise vs control – *continued*				
Area, root mean square of centre of pressure and average velocity in the double leg stance with eyes closed position	1 RCT (Messier et al. 2000) (N=103)	Weight training exercise vs healthy lifestyle control	18 months of follow-up	Area and pressure: p<0.001 Velocity: p=0.001 Favours exercise
Area, root mean square of centre of pressure and average velocity in the double leg stance with eyes closed position	1 RCT (Messier et al. 2000) (N=103)	Aerobic exercise vs healthy lifestyle control	18 months of follow-up	Area and pressure: p=0.02 Velocity: NS Favours exercise
Measures taken in the double-leg stance with eyes open position	1 RCT (Messier et al. 2000) (N=103)	Weight training exercise vs healthy lifestyle control	18 months of follow-up	NS
Measures taken in the double-leg stance with eyes open position	1 RCT (Messier et al. 2000) (N=103)	Aerobic exercise vs healthy lifestyle control	18 months of follow-up	NS
Hamstring and lower back flexibility (sit-and-reach test)	1 RCT (Peloquin et al. 1999) (N=137)	Exercise (aerobic plus strengthening plus stretching) vs educational advice control	3 months (end of treatment)	p=0.003 Favours exercise
Timed up-and-go performance	1 RCT (Tak 2005) (N=94)	Exercise (strength training and home exercises) vs no intervention control	3 months follow-up	p=0.043 Favours exercise
Up-and-go time (seconds)	1 RCT (Fransen et al. 2007) (N=152)	Tai chi vs attention control	0–12 weeks (end of treatment)	Standardised response mean: 0.32,% CI 0.19 to 0.45, p<0.05 Favours exercise
Exercise + other therapy vs control or exercise				
Stair-climb time	1 RCT (Focht et al. 2005) (N=316)	Diet plus exercise (aerobic plus resistance vs healthy lifestyle control	18 months	p=0.0249 Favours intervention
Improvement in walking distance	1 RCT (Focht et al. 2005) (N=316)	Diet plus exercise (aerobic and resistance) vs healthy lifestyle control	18 months post-randomisation	p<0.0001 Favours exercise
6-minute walking distance	1 RCT (Messier et al. 2004) (N=316)	Diet + exercise vs healthy lifestyle control	18 months post-randomisation	p≤0.05 Favours exercise

Table 6.4 Quality of life

QoL outcome	Reference	Intervention	Assessment time	Outcome/effect size
Exercise vs control				
Improvements in health status (AIMS2 scale) subsets of walking and bending and arthritis pain	1 RCT (Peloquin et al. 1999) (N=137)	Exercise (aerobic plus strengthening plus stretching) vs educational advice control	At 3 months (end of treatment)	Walking/bending: p=0.03 pain: p=0.02 Favours exercise
SF-36 physical health status; SF-36 mental health status	1 RCT (Thorstensson et al. 2005) (N=61)	Weight-bearing exercise vs no treatment	Follow-up (6 months)	NS
Improvement in quality of life scores (KOOS subscale)	1 RCT (Thorstensson et al. 2005) (N=61)	Weight-bearing exercise vs no treatment	Follow-up (6 months)	p=0.02 Favours exercise
6-minute walk time	1 RCT (Focht et al. 2005) (N=316)	Exercise (aerobic and resistance) vs healthy lifestyle control	18 months post-randomisation	p<0.05 Favours exercise
Lower depression scores (CES-D scale) over time	1 RCT (Penninx et al. 2002) (N=439)	Aerobic exercise vs education	18 months follow-up	p<0.001 Favours exercise
Lower depression scores (CES-D scale) over time	1 RCT (Penninx et al. 2002) (N=439)	Resistance exercise vs education	18 months follow-up	NS
SF-36 composite mental health score and subsets of vitality and emotional role	1 RCT (Rejeski et al. 2002) (N=316)	Exercise only vs diet only or vs healthy lifestyle control	18 months post-randomisation.	NS
Improvement in health status (Sickness Impact Profile)	1 RCT (Tak 2005) (N=94)	Exercise (strength training and home exercises) vs control	3 months follow-up	p=0.041
Quality of life scores (VAS and health-related QOL scores)	1 RCT (Tak 2005) (N=94)	Exercise (strength training and home exercises) vs no intervention control	3 months follow-up	NS
SF-12 version 2, physical component	1 RCT (Fransen et al. 2007) (N=152)	Tai chi vs attention control	0–12 weeks (end of treatment)	Standardised response mean: 0.25,% CI 0.12 to 0.38, p≤0.05 Favours exercise
SF-12 version 2, mental component; Depression, Anxiety and Stress Scale (DASS21) components of anxiety, stress and depression	1 RCT (Fransen et al. 2007) (N=152)	Tai chi vs attention control	0–12 weeks (end of treatment)	NS

continued

Table 6.4 Quality of life – *continued*

QoL outcome	Reference	Intervention	Assessment time	Outcome/effect size
Exercise + other therapy vs control or exercise				
Improvement in mobility-related self-efficacy; stair-climb; 6-minute walk time	1 RCT (Focht et al. 2005) (N=316)	Diet + exercise (aerobic and resistance) vs healthy lifestyle control	18 months post-randomisation	Self-efficacy: p=0.0035 Stair: p=0.005 Walk: p=0.0006 Favours intervention
SF-36 composite physical health score and subscales of physical role, general health and social functioning	1 RCT (Rejeski et al. 2002) (N=316)	Diet plus exercise (aerobic and resistance) vs healthy lifestyle control	18 months post-randomisation	All p<0.01 Favours intervention
SF-36 subscale body pain	1 RCT (Rejeski et al. 2002)	Diet + exercise (aerobic and resistance) vs exercise vs control	18 months post-randomisation	Both: p<0.04 Favours diet + exercise
SF-36 composite physical health score and subscales of physical role, general health and social functioning	1 RCT (Rejeski et al. 2002) (N=316)	Exercise (aerobic and resistance) vs healthy lifestyle control	18 months post-randomisation	NS
Patient satisfaction with physical function (SF-36)	1 RCT (Rejeski et al. 2002) (N=316)	Diet + exercise (aerobic and resistance) vs healthy lifestyle control	18 months post-randomisation	P<0.01 Favours intervention
Patient satisfaction with physical function (SF-36)	1 RCT (Rejeski et al. 2002) (N=316)	Diet + exercise (aerobic and resistance) vs diet	18 months post-randomisation	P<0.01 Favours intervention
Patient satisfaction with physical function (SF-36)	1 RCT (Rejeski et al. 2002) (N=316)	Exercise (aerobic and resistance) vs healthy lifestyle control	18 months post-randomisation	P<0.01 Favours intervention
SF-36 composite mental health score and subsets of vitality and emotional role	1 RCT (Rejeski et al. 2002) (N=316)	Diet + exercise (aerobic and resistance) vs diet only or vs exercise only or vs healthy lifestyle control	18 months post-randomisation.	NS
HAD anxiety (change from baseline)	1 RCT (Hurley et al. 2007)	Rehabilitation programme (progressive exercise + group discussion) + usual primary care vs usual primary care	6 months (4.5 months post-treatment)	Mean difference −0.65,%CI −1.28 to −0.02, p=0.043 Favours intervention
HAD depression (change from baseline)	1 RCT (Hurley et al. 2007)	Rehabilitation programme (progressive exercise + group discussion) + usual primary care vs usual primary care	6 months (4.5 months post-treatment)	NS
MACTAR score – QoL (change from baseline)	1 RCT (Hurley et al. 2007)	Rehabilitation programme (progressive exercise + group discussion) + usual primary care vs usual primary care	6 months (4.5 months post-treatment)	Mean difference 2.20,%CI 0.36 to 4.04, p=0.019 Favours intervention

Table 6.5 Use of concomitant medication

Use of concomitant medication outcome	Reference	Intervention	Assessment time	Outcome/effect size
Exercise vs control				
Use of paracetamol	1 RCT (van Baar et al. 2001) (N=183)	Strengthening exercise vs educational advice	9 months follow-up	0.32, mean difference –17%;%CI –30% to –3%, p<0.05 Favours exercise
Use of NSAIDs	1 RCT (van Baar et al. 2001) (N=183)	Strengthening exercise vs educational advice	9 months follow-up	NS
Exercise + other therapy vs control or exercise				
Self-reported use of NSAIDs	1 RCT (Hay et al. 2006)	Community physiotherapy + advice leaflet vs control (no exercise, advice leaflet + telephone call)	Over 6 months (up to 4-months post-treatment)	Mean difference 15%, % CI 2 to 28, p=0.02 Favours intervention
Self-reported use of analgesia	1 RCT (Hay et al. 2006)	Community physiotherapy + advice leaflet vs control (no exercise, advice leaflet + telephone call)	Over 6 months (up to 4-months post-treatment)	Mean difference 16%, % CI 3 to 29, p=0.02 Favours intervention

6.1.5 Evidence statements: comparing different land-based exercise regimens

Table 6.6 Symptoms

Pain outcome	Reference	Intervention	Assessment time	Outcome/effect size
Exercise vs control/other exercise				
Reductions in pain scores (VAS and WOMAC)	1 RCT (McCarthy et al. 2004) (N=214)	Home + class-based exercise vs home-based exercise	One year of follow-up	VAS: p<0.001 WOMAC: p=0.036 Favours Home + class exercise
Reductions in pain (AIMS2)	1 RCT (Eyigor et al. 2004) (N=44)	Progressive resistance exercise vs isokinetic exercise	Study endpoint (6 weeks)	p<0.05 Favours resistance exercise
Pain severity (VAS, WOMAC); night pain and pain on standing (Lequesne Index)	1 RCT (Eyigor et al. 2004) (N=44)	Progressive resistance exercise vs isokinetic exercise	Study endpoint (6 weeks)	NS
Reduction in pain (VAS score)	1 RCT (Huang et al. 2003) (N=132)	Isotonic exercise vs isokinetic and isometric exercise	One-year follow-up	p<0.05 Favours isotonic exercise

continued

Table 6.6 Symptoms – *continued*

Pain outcome	Reference	Intervention	Assessment time	Outcome/effect size
Exercise vs control/other exercise – *continued*				
Reductions in intensity and frequency of transfer pain (getting in and out of bed, chair, car etc)	1 RCT (Messier et al. 1997) (N=103)	Aerobic exercise vs health education control	18 months follow-up	Both: p<0.001 Favours exercise
Reductions in intensity and frequency of transfer pain (getting in and out of bed, chair, car etc)	1 RCT (Messier et al. 1997) (N=103)	Weight training exercise vs health education control	18 months follow-up	Both: p=0.04 Favours exercise
Intensity and frequency of ambulation pain	1 RCT (Messier et al. 1997) (N=103)	Aerobic exercise vs health education control	18 months follow-up	NS
Intensity and frequency of ambulation pain	1 RCT (Messier et al. 1997) (N=103)	Weight training exercise vs health education control	18 months follow-up	NS
Intensity and frequency of ambulation pain	1 RCT (Messier et al. 1997) (N=103)	Weight training exercise vs aerobic exercise	18 months follow-up	NS
WOMAC pain	1 RCT (Lim 2002) (N=32)	Open kinetic chain exercise vs closed kinetic chain exercise	Study endpoint (6 weeks)	NS
Pain scores (AIMS2, VAS, WOMAC)	1 RCT (Mangione and McCully 1999) (N=39)	High intensity vs low intensity aerobic exercise	Study endpoint (10 weeks)	NS

Table 6.7 Stiffness

Stiffness outcome	Reference	Intervention	Assessment time	Outcome/effect size
Exercise vs control/other exercise				
WOMAC stiffness	1 RCT (McCarthy et al. 2004) (N=214)	Home + class-based exercise vs home-based exercise	One year of follow-up	NS
WOMAC stiffness; joint stiffness (Lequesne's scale)	1 RCT (Eyigor et al. 2004) (N=44)	Progressive resistance exercise vs isokinetic exercise	Study endpoint (6 weeks)	NS
WOMAC stiffness	1 RCT (Lim 2002) (N=32)	Open kinetic chain exercise vs closed kinetic chain exercise	Study endpoint (6 weeks)	NS

Table 6.8 Patient function

Patient function outcome	Reference	Intervention	Assessment time	Outcome/effect size
Exercise vs control/other exercise				
Aggregate locomotor function score; WOMAC function	1 RCT (McCarthy et al. 2004) (N=214)	Home + class-based exercise vs home-based exercise	One year of follow-up	Function: p<0.001 WOMAC: p=0.014 Favours home + class exercise
Functionality (Lequesne Index); physical function	1 RCT (Eyigor et al. 2004) (N=44)	Progressive resistance exercise vs isokinetic exercise	Study endpoint (6 weeks)	NS
Social activity (AIMS2)	1 RCT (Eyigor et al. 2004) (N=44)	Progressive resistance exercise vs isokinetic exercise	Study endpoint (6 weeks)	p<0.05 Favours resistance exercise
AIMS2 items (self-care, mobility, walking, family support, level of tension, mood and household tasks) items; daily activities scores (Lequesne Index)	1 RCT (Eyigor et al. 2004) (N=44)	Progressive resistance exercise vs isokinetic exercise	Study endpoint (6 weeks)	NS
WOMAC physical function	1 RCT (Lim 2002) (N=32)	Open kinetic chain exercise vs closed kinetic chain exercise	Study endpoint (6 weeks)	NS
Risk of activities of daily living (ADL) disability (30-item questionnaire)	1 RCT (Penninx et al. 2001) (N=250)	Aerobic exercise vs attention control	18 months follow-up	Cox proportional hazards: RR 0.53, %CI 0.33 to 0.85, p=0.009 Favours exercise
Risk of activities of daily living (ADL) disability (30-item questionnaire)	1 RCT (Penninx et al. 2001) (N=250)	Resistance exercise vs attention control	18 months follow-up	Cox proportional hazards: RR 0.60, %CI 0.38 to 0.97, p=0.04 Favours exercise
Cumulative incidence of ADL disability	1 RCT (Penninx et al. 2001) (N=250)	Aerobic exercise vs resistance exercise	18 months follow-up	Aerobic: 36.4% Resistance: 37.8% Both groups similar

Table 6.9 Examination findings

Examination findings outcome	Reference	Intervention	Assessment time	Outcome/effect size
Exercise vs control/other exercise				
Strength and range of knee flexion measures	1 RCT (McCarthy et al. 2004) (N=214)	Home + class-based exercise vs home-based exercise	One year of follow-up	NS
Balance scores	1 RCT (McCarthy et al. 2004) (N=214)	Home + class-based exercise vs home-based exercise	One year of follow-up	NS
Gains in 90° peak torque and 90° torque body weight	1 RCT (Eyigor et al. 2004) (N=44)	Progressive resistance exercise vs isokinetic exercise	Study endpoint (6 weeks)	Both p<0.05 Favours isokinetic exercise
All other flexor/ extensor muscle strength ratios (60–180° peak torque, 60–180° peak torque body weight, 60–180° total work, and 60–180° total work body weight)	1 RCT (Eyigor et al. 2004) (N=44)	Progressive resistance exercise vs isokinetic exercise	Study endpoint (6 weeks)	NS
Walking time (chronometer), walking distance and transfer (both Lequesne scale)	1 RCT (Eyigor et al. 2004) (N=44)	Progressive resistance exercise vs isokinetic exercise	Study endpoint (6 weeks)	NS
Mean peak torque for knee extensor muscles in concentric and eccentric contraction at 60° and flexor muscles in eccentric contraction at 60°	1 RCT (Huang et al. 2003) (N=132)	Isometric exercise vs isotonic and isokinetic exercise	One-year follow-up	All p<0.05 Favours isometric exercise
All other mean peak torque values (knee flexors in concentric contraction at 60°, knee flexor and extensor muscles in concentric and eccentric contraction at 180°)	1 RCT (Huang et al. 2003) (N=132)	Isokinetic exercise vs isotonic and isometric exercise	One-year follow-up	p<0.05 Favours isokinetic exercise
Walking speed	1 RCT (Huang et al. 2003) (N=132)	Isokinetic exercise vs isotonic and isometric exercise	One-year follow-up	p<0.05 Favours isokinetic

continued

Table 6.9 Examination findings – *continued*

Examination findings outcome	Reference	Intervention	Assessment time	Outcome/effect size
Exercise vs control/other exercise – *continued*				
Knee mean angular velocity	1 RCT (Messier et al. 1997) (N=103)	Aerobic exercise vs health education control	18 months follow-up	P=0.04 Favours exercise
Knee mean angular velocity	1 RCT (Messier et al. 1997) (N=103)	Weight training exercise vs health education control	18 months follow-up	NS
Walking velocity; absolute and relative stride	1 RCT (Messier et al. 1997) (N=103)	Aerobic exercise vs health education control	18 months follow-up	Velocity: p=0.001 Stride: p≤ 0.03 Favours exercise
Walking velocity	1 RCT (Messier et al. 1997) (N=103)	Weight training exercise vs health education control	18 months follow-up	p=0.03 Favours exercise
Absolute and relative stride	1 RCT (Messier et al. 1997) (N=103)	Weight training exercise vs aerobic exercise	18 months follow-up	NS
Area, root mean square of centre of pressure and average velocity in the double leg stance with eyes closed position	1 RCT (Messier et al. 1997) (N=103)	Weight training exercise vs aerobic exercise	18 months follow-up	Area and pressure: both p<0.001 Velocity: p=0.001 Favours exercise
Area, root mean square of centre of pressure in the double leg stance with eyes closed position	1 RCT (Messier et al. 1997) (N=103)	Aerobic exercise vs health education control	18 months follow-up	Area and pressure: both p=0.02 Favours exercise
Average velocity in the double leg stance with eyes closed position	1 RCT (Messier et al. 1997) (N=103)	Aerobic exercise vs health education control	18 months follow-up	NS
Area, root mean square of centre of pressure measures taken in the double-leg stance with eyes open position.	1 RCT (Messier et al. 1997) (N=103)	Weight training exercise vs aerobic exercise	18 months follow-up	NS
Area, root mean square of centre of pressure measures taken in the double-leg stance with eyes open position.	1 RCT (Messier et al. 1997) (N=103)	Aerobic exercise vs health education control	18 months follow-up	NS

continued

Table 6.9 Examination findings – *continued*

Examination findings outcome	Reference	Intervention	Assessment time	Outcome/effect size
Exercise vs control/other exercise – *continued*				
More balance time spent in single-leg stance with eyes open position	1 RCT (Messier et al. 1997) (N=103)	Aerobic exercise vs health education control	18 months follow-up	p=0.016 Favours exercise
More balance time spent in single-leg stance with eyes open position	1 RCT (Messier et al. 1997) (N=103)	Weight training exercise vs aerobic exercise	18 months follow-up	NS
All other measures taken in single-leg stance eyes open and shut positions	1 RCT (Messier et al. 1997) (N=103)	Aerobic exercise vs health education control	18 months follow-up	NS
All other measures taken in single-leg stance eyes open and shut positions	1 RCT (Messier et al. 1997) (N=103)	Weight training exercise vs aerobic exercise	18 months follow-up	NS
Area, root mean square of centre of pressure measures taken in the double-leg stance with eyes open position.	1 RCT (Messier et al. 1997) (N=103)	Weight training exercise vs aerobic exercise	18 months follow-up	NS
All other measures taken in single-leg stance eyes open and shut positions	1 RCT (Messier et al. 1997) (N=103)	Weight training exercise vs aerobic exercise	18 months follow-up	NS
Mean peak torque and mean torque	1 RCT (Lim 2002) (N=32)	Open kinetic chain exercise vs closed kinetic chain exercise	Study endpoint (6 weeks)	NS
Timed chair rise, 6-metre walking distance, and gait performance (AIMS2)	1 RCT (Mangione and McCully 1999) (N=39)	High intensity vs low intensity aerobic exercise	Study endpoint (10 weeks)	NS
Aerobic capacity	1 RCT (Mangione and McCully 1999) (N=39)	High intensity vs low intensity aerobic exercise	Study endpoint (10 weeks)	NS

Table 6.10 Quality of life

QoL outcome	Reference	Intervention	Assessment time	Outcome/effect size
Exercise vs control/other exercise				
SF-36 physical health status, emotional and mental health status and physical function scales	1 RCT (McCarthy et al. 2004) (N=214)	Home + class-based exercise vs home-based exercise	One year of follow-up	NS
SF-36 pain	1 RCT (McCarthy et al. 2004) (N=214)	Home + class-based exercise vs home-based exercise	One year of follow-up	p=0.003 Favours home + class exercise
Improvement in SF-36 post treatment pain scores and SF-36 pain score	1 RCT (Eyigor et al. 2004) (N=44)	Progressive resistance exercise vs isokinetic exercise	Study endpoint (6 weeks)	p<0.05 Favours resistance exercise
All other physical health quality of life outcomes (SF-36: physical function, physical role, health, and vitality scales); SF-36 mental health status (social, emotional, role physical and mental scales)	1 RCT (Eyigor et al. 2004) (N=44)	Progressive resistance exercise vs isokinetic exercise	Study endpoint (6 weeks)	NS
Lower depression scores (CES-D scale)	1 RCT (Penninx et al. 2002) (N=439)	Aerobic exercise vs education control	18 months of follow-up	p<0.001 Favours exercise
Lower depression scores (CES-D scale)	1 RCT (Penninx et al. 2002) (N=439)	Resistance exercise vs education control	18 months of follow-up	NS

6.1.6 Evidence statements: hydrotherapy

Table 6.11 Symptoms

Pain outcome	Reference	Intervention	Assessment time	Outcome/effect size
Exercise vs control/other exercise				
Pain on movement (VAS)	1 RCT (Hinman et al. 2007) (N=71)	Aquatic exercise vs no exercise (usual care)	6 weeks (end of treatment)	Effect size 0.28, p<0.001 Favours exercise
WOMAC pain	1 RCT (Hinman et al. 2007) (N=71)	Aquatic exercise vs no exercise (usual care)	6 weeks (end of treatment)	Effect size 0.24, p=0.003 Favours exercise
WOMAC pain	1 RCT (Fransen et al. 2007) (N=152)	Tai chi vs attention control	0–12 weeks (end of treatment)	Standardised response mean: 0.43,% CI 0.30 to 0.56, p<0.05 Favours exercise
WOMAC pain	1 RCT (Cochrane et al. 2005) (N=312)	Hydrotherapy vs usual care	1 year	p<0.05 Favours exercise
WOMAC pain	1 RCT (Cochrane et al. 2005) (N=312)	Hydrotherapy vs usual care	18 months	NS
WOMAC pain	1 RCT (Foley et al. 2003) (N=105)	Hydrotherapy vs land-based gym exercises or attention control	Study endpoint (6 weeks)	NS

Table 6.12 Stiffness

Stiffness outcome	Reference	Intervention	Assessment time	Outcome/effect size
Exercise vs control/other exercise				
WOMAC stiffness	1 RCT (Hinman et al. 2007) (N=71)	Aquatic exercise vs no exercise (usual care)	6 weeks (end of treatment)	Effect size 0.24, p=0.007 Favours exercise
WOMAC stiffness	1 RCT (Cochrane et al. 2005) (N=312)	Hydrotherapy vs usual care	1 year (end of treatment) and 18 months (6 months post-treatment)	NS
WOMAC stiffness	1 RCT (Foley et al. 2003) (N=105)	Hydrotherapy vs land-based gym exercises or attention control	Study endpoint (6 weeks)	NS

Table 6.13 Patient function

Function outcome	Reference	Intervention	Assessment time	Outcome/effect size
Exercise vs control/other exercise				
Function, disability and pain scores (HAQ)	1 RCT (Belza et al. 2002) (N=249)	Aquatic exercise vs usual care no-exercise control	20 weeks of treatment	p=0.02 Favours exercise
WOMAC function	1 RCT (Hinman et al. 2007) (N=71)	Aquatic exercise vs no exercise (usual care)	6 weeks (end of treatment)	Effect size 0.08, p<0.001 Favours exercise
Six-minute walk test	1 RCT (Hinman et al. 2007) (N=71)	Aquatic exercise vs no exercise (usual care)	6 weeks (end of treatment)	Effect size 0.01, p=0.001 Favours exercise
WOMAC function	1 RCT (Fransen et al. 2007) (N=152)	Tai chi vs attention control	0–12 weeks (end of treatment)	Standardised response mean: 0.62,% CI 0.49 to 0.75, p<0.05. Favours exercise
Physical Activity Scale for the Elderly (PASE); Timed up-and-go test; step test.	1 RCT (Hinman et al. 2007) (N=71)	Aquatic exercise vs no exercise (usual care)	6 weeks (end of treatment)	NS
WOMAC physical function	1 RCT (Cochrane et al. 2005) (N=312)	Hydrotherapy vs usual care	1 year (end of treatment)	p<0.05 Favours exercise
WOMAC physical function	1 RCT (Cochrane et al. 2005) (N=312)	Hydrotherapy vs usual care	18 months (6 months post-treatment)	NS
WOMAC function	1 RCT (Foley et al. 2003) (N=105)	Hydrotherapy vs land-based gym exercises or attention control	Study endpoint (6 weeks)	NS

Table 6.14 Examination findings

Examination findings outcome	Reference	Intervention	Assessment time	Outcome/effect size
Exercise vs control/other exercise				
Hip abductor strength	1 RCT (Hinman et al. 2007) (N=71)	Aquatic exercise vs no exercise (usual care)	6 weeks (end of treatment)	Left: effect size 0.07, p=0.011; right: effect size 0.16, p=0.012 Favours exercise
Quadriceps muscle strength	1 RCT (Hinman et al. 2007) (N=71)	Aquatic exercise vs no exercise (usual care)	6 weeks (end of treatment)	NS
Improvement in stair ascent and descent	1 RCT (Cochrane et al. 2005) (N=312)	Hydrotherapy vs usual care	1 year (end of treatment)	p<0.05 Favours exercise
Stair climb (seconds)	1 RCT (Fransen et al. 2007) (N=152)	Tai chi vs attention control	0–12 weeks (end of treatment)	Standardised response mean: 0.55,% CI 0.42 to 0.68, p<0.05. Favours exercise

continued

Table 6.14 Examination findings – *continued*

Examination findings outcome	Reference	Intervention	Assessment time	Outcome/effect size
Exercise vs control/other exercise – *continued*				
Improvement in stair ascent and stair descent	1 RCT (Cochrane et al. 2005) (N=312)	Hydrotherapy vs usual care	18 months (6 months post-treatment)	NS
Hamstring and quadriceps muscle strength	1 RCT (Cochrane et al. 2005) (N=312)	Hydrotherapy vs usual care	1 year (end of treatment) and 18 months (6 months post-treatment)	NS
8-foot walk	1 RCT (Cochrane et al. 2005) (N=312)	Hydrotherapy vs usual care	1 year (end of treatment)	NS
8-foot walk	1 RCT (Cochrane et al. 2005) (N=312)	Hydrotherapy vs usual care	18 months (6 months post-treatment)	ES 0.23,%CI 0.00 to 0.45 Favours exercse
50-foot walk time	1 RCT (Fransen et al. 2007) (N=152)	Tai chi vs attention control	0–12 weeks (end of treatment)	Standardised response mean: 0.49,% CI 0.36 to 0.62, p<0.05 Favours exercise
Improvements in right quadriceps muscle strength	1 RCT (Foley et al. 2003) (N=105)	Gym exercises vs hydrotherapy	Study endpoint (6 weeks)	p=0.030
Improvements in right quadriceps muscle strength	1 RCT (Foley et al. 2003) (N=105)	Gym exercises vs attention control	Study endpoint (6 weeks)	p<0.001
Improvements in left quadriceps muscle strength	1 RCT (Foley et al. 2003) (N=105)	Gym exercises or vs attention control	Study endpoint (6 weeks)	p=0.018
Improvements in left quadriceps muscle strength	1 RCT (Foley et al. 2003) (N=105)	Hydrotherapy vs attention control	Study endpoint (6 weeks)	p<0.001
Improvements in walking distance	1 RCT (Foley et al. 2003) (N=105)	Hydrotherapy vs attention control	Study endpoint (6 weeks)	P=0.048 Favours hydrotherapy
Improvements in walking distance	1 RCT (Foley et al. 2003) (N=105)	Gym exercise vs attention control	Study endpoint (6 weeks)	NS
Walking speed	1 RCT (Foley et al. 2003) (N=105)	Gym exercise vs attention control	Study endpoint (6 weeks)	p=0.009 Favours exercise
Walking speed	1 RCT (Foley et al. 2003) (N=105)	Hydrotherapy vs attention control	Study endpoint (6 weeks)	NS
Up-and-go time (seconds) at 0–12 weeks, end of treatment	1 RCT (Fransen et al. 2007) (N=152)	Tai chi vs attention control	0–12 weeks (end of treatment)	Standardised response mean: 0.76,% CI 0.63 to 0.89, p<0.05. Favours exercise

Table 6.15 Quality of life

QoL outcome	Reference	Intervention	Assessment time	Outcome/effect size
Exercise vs control/other exercise				
Self-efficacy pain and self-efficacy function scores (Arthritis Self-Efficacy Scale), SF-12 mental component scores	1 RCT (Foley et al. 2003) (N=105)	Hydrotherapy, land-based gym exercises vs attention control	Study endpoint (6 weeks)	NS
Improvement in self-efficacy satisfaction score (Arthritis Self-Efficacy Scale)	1 RCT (Foley et al. 2003) (N=105)	Hydrotherapy vs control	Study endpoint (6 weeks)	p=0.006 Favours exercise
Arthritis Self-Efficacy Scale dimensions of: self-efficacy pain; self-efficacy function; improvement in self-efficacy satisfaction score	1 RCT (Foley et al. 2003) (N=105)	Hydrotherapy vs control	Study endpoint (6 weeks)	NS
SF-12 physical component score	1 RCT (Foley et al. 2003) (N=105)	Hydrotherapy vs control	Study endpoint (6 weeks),	Exercise significantly better (p value not given)
SF-12 physical and mental component scores	1 RCT (Foley et al. 2003) (N=105)	Hydrotherapy vs control	Study endpoint (6 weeks)	NS
Improved health status (Quality of Well-Being Scale	1 RCT (Belza et al. 2002) (N=249)	Aquatic exercise vs usual care (no-exercise)	20 weeks (end of treatment)	p=0.02 Favours exercise
Improved quality of life scores (Arthritis QOL)	1 RCT (Belza et al. 2002) (N=249)	Aquatic exercise vs usual care (no-exercise)	20 weeks (end of treatment)	p=0.01 Favours exercise
AQoL	1 RCT (Hinman et al. 2007) (N=71)	Aquatic exercise vs no exercise (usual care)	6 weeks (end of treatment)	Effect size 0.17, p=0.018 Favours exercsie
SF-36 dimensions of: vitality, general health, physical function and physical role	1 RCT (Cochrane et al. 2005) (N=312)	Hydrotherapy vs usual care	1 year (end of treatment) and at 18 months (6 months post-treatment)	NS
SF-12 version 2, physical component	1 RCT (Fransen et al. 2007) (N=152)	Tai chi vs attention control	0–12 weeks (end of treatment)	Standardised response mean: 0.34,% CI 0.21 to 0.47, p<0.05. Favours exercise

continued

Table 6.15 Quality of life – *continued*

QoL outcome	Reference	Intervention	Assessment time	Outcome/effect size
Exercise vs control/other exercise – *continued*				
SF-36 pain	1 RCT (Cochrane et al. 2005) (N=312)	Hydrotherapy vs usual care	1 year (end of treatment)	p<0.05 Favours exercise
SF-36 pain	1 RCT (Cochrane et al. 2005) (N=312)	Hydrotherapy vs usual care	18 months (6 months post-treatment)	NS
SF-12 version 2, mental component summary and depression, Anxiety and Stress scale (DASS21) components of anxiety, stress and depression	1 RCT (Fransen et al. 2007) (N=152)	Tai chi vs attention control	0–12 weeks (end of treatment)	NS

6.1.7   Evidence statements: exercise vs manual therapy

Table 6.16 Symptoms

Symptoms outcome	Reference	Intervention	Assessment time	Outcome/effect size
Manual therapy vs other exercise				
Improvement in participants' main symptoms (either pain, stiffness, walking disability measured by VAS)	1 RCT (Hoeksma et al. 2004) (N=109)	Manual therapy vs strengthening exercise	Study endpoint (5 weeks)	Or 1.92,%CI 1.30 to 2.60
Pain at rest (VAS)	1 RCT (Hoeksma et al. 2004) (N=109)	Manual therapy vs strengthening exercise	Study endpoint (5 weeks) and 6 months follow-up	5 weeks: p<0.05 6 months: NS
Walking pain (VAS)	1 RCT (Hoeksma et al. 2004) (N=109)	Manual therapy vs strengthening exercise	Study endpoint (5 weeks) and 6 months follow-up	Both: p<0.05
Starting stiffness (VAS)	1 RCT (Hoeksma et al. 2004) (N=109)	Manual therapy vs strengthening exercise	Study endpoint (5 weeks)	p<0.05
Starting stiffness (VAS)	1 RCT (Hoeksma et al. 2004) (N=109)	Manual therapy vs strengthening exercise	6 months follow-up	NS

Table 6.17 Patient function

Function outcome	Reference	Intervention	Assessment time	Outcome/effect size
Manual therapy vs other exercise				
Harris Hip scores	1 RCT (Hoeksma et al. 2004) (N=109)	Manual therapy vs strengthening exercise	Study endpoint (5 weeks) and 6 months follow-up	Both: p<0.05 Favours manual
Improvements in WOMAC physical function scores	1 RCT (Dracoglu et al. 2005) (N=66)	Kinaesthesia + balancing + strengthening exercises vs strengthening exercises	Study endpoint (8 weeks)	p=0.042 Favours manual
Improvement in mean total WOMAC scores	1 RCT (Deyle et al. 2000) (N=83)	Manual therapy + strengthening exercise vs control group (sub-therapeutic US)	Study endpoint (8 weeks)	Mean improvement mm, % CI 197 to 1002 mm
Improvement in total WOMAC scores (change from baseline)	1 RCT (Deyle et al. 2005) (N=134)	Clinic-based manual therapy + strengthening exercises vs home-based strengthening exercise	1 year follow-up	32% (manual) vs 28% (home)

Table 6.18 Examination findings

Examination findings outcome	Reference	Intervention	Assessment time	Outcome/effect size
Manual therapy vs other exercise				
Walking speed	1 RCT (Hoeksma et al. 2004) (n=109)	Manual therapy vs strengthening exercise	Study endpoint (5 weeks)	p<0.05 Favours manual
Walking speed	1 RCT (Hoeksma et al. 2004) (n=109)	Manual therapy vs strengthening exercise	6 months follow-up	NS
10 stairs climbing time	1 RCT (Dracoglu et al. 2005 2) (N=66)	Kinaesthesia + balancing + strengthening exercises vs strengthening exercises	Study endpoint (8 weeks)	p<0.05 Favours manual
Improvement in 10 metre walking time	1 RCT (Dracoglu et al. 2005 2) (N=66)	Kinaesthesia + balancing + strengthening exercises vs strengthening exercises	Study endpoint (8 weeks)	p=0.039 Favours manual
Improvement in mean 6-minute walk distance	1 RCT (Deyle et al. 2000) (N=83)	Manual therapy + strengthening exercise vs control group (sub-therapeutic US)	Study endpoint (8 weeks)	Mean improvement 170 metres, % CI 71 to 270 metres
Improvement in mean 6-minute walking test distance	1 RCT (Deyle et al. 2005 10) (N=134)	Clinic-based manual therapy + strengthening exercises vs home-based strengthening exercise	Study endpoint (4 weeks)	Both groups the same (9% improvement)

Table 6.19 Quality of life

QoL outcome	Reference	Intervention	Assessment time	Outcome/effect size
Manual therapy vs other exercise				
SF-36 role physical	1 RCT (Hoeksma et al. 2004) (N=109)	Manual therapy vs strengthening exercise	Study endpoint (5 weeks)	p<0.05 Favours manual
SF-36 role physical	1 RCT (Hoeksma et al. 2004) (N=109)	Manual therapy vs strengthening exercise	6 months follow-up	NS
SF-36 bodily pain and physical function	1 RCT (Hoeksma et al. 2004) (N=109)	Manual therapy vs strengthening exercise	Study endpoint (5 weeks) and 6 months follow-up	NS
SF-36 vitality and energy/fatigue scores	1 RCT (Dracoglu et al. 2005) (N=66)	Kinaesthesia + balancing + strengthening exercises vs strengthening exercises	Study endpoint (8 weeks)	p=0.046 Favours manual
SF-36 physical function	1 RCT (Dracoglu et al. 2005) (N=66)	Kinaesthesia + balancing + strengthening exercises vs strengthening exercises	Study endpoint (8 weeks)	p=0.006 Favours manual
SF-36 physical role limitations	1 RCT (Dracoglu et al. 2005) (N=66)	Kinaesthesia + balancing + strengthening exercises vs strengthening exercises	Study endpoint (8 weeks)	p=0.048 Favours manual
Number of patients satisfied with the treatment	1 RCT (Deyle et al. 2005) (N=134)	Clinic-based manual therapy + strengthening exercises vs home-based strengthening exercise	1 year follow-up	52% (clinic) and 25% (home) p=0.018 Favours clinic

Table 6.20 Use of concomitant medication

Medication use outcome	Reference	Intervention	Assessment time	Outcome/effect size
Manual therapy vs other exercise				
Use of rescue paracetamol	1 RCT (Dracoglu et al. 2005) (N=66)	Kinaesthesia + balancing + strengthening exercises vs strengthening exercises	Study endpoint (8 weeks)	NS
Use of concomitant medication	1 RCT (Deyle et al. 2005) (N=134)	Clinic-based manual therapy + strengthening exercises vs home-based strengthening exercise	1 year follow-up	48% (clinic) and 68% (home) p=0.03 Favours clinic

6.1.8 Evidence statements: manual therapy

Table 6.21 Symptoms

Pain outcome	Reference	Intervention	Assessment time	Outcome/effect size
Knee osteoarthritis				
Manual therapy vs sham ultrasound				
Pain on movement, VAS (change from baseline)	1 RCT (Bennell et al. 2005), N=140	Manual therapy (knee taping, mobilisation, massage + exercise) vs control (sham ultrasound)	12 weeks post-treatment	Manual better than control: −2.1 (manual) and −1.6 (control)
WOMAC pain (change from baseline)	1 RCT (Bennell et al. 2005), N=140	Manual therapy (knee taping, mobilisation, massage + exercise) vs control (sham ultrasound)	12 weeks post-treatment	Manual better than control: −2.4 (manual) and −2.0 (control)
Pain severity, KPS (change from baseline)	1 RCT (Bennell et al. 2005), N=140	Manual therapy (knee taping, mobilisation, massage + exercise) vs control (sham ultrasound)	12 weeks (end of treatment and 12 weeks post-treatment	Manual better than control 12 weeks: −3.3 (manual) and −2.6 (control) 12 weeks post-treatment: −3.1 (manual) and −2.1 (control)
Pain frequency, KPS (change from baseline)	1 RCT (Bennell et al. 2005), N=140	Manual therapy (knee taping, mobilisation, massage + exercise) vs control (sham ultrasound)	12 weeks (end of treatment and 12 weeks post-treatment	Manual better than control 12 weeks: −4.3 (manual) and −3.0 (control) 12 weeks post-treatment: −4.1 (manual) and −2.5 (control)
Clinically relevant reduction in pain (≥1.75 cm), VAS	1 RCT (Bennell et al. 2005), N=140	Manual therapy (knee taping, mobilisation, massage + exercise) vs control (sham ultrasound	12 weeks post-treatment	NS
Pain on movement, VAS (change from baseline)	1 RCT (Bennell et al. 2005), N=140	Manual therapy (knee taping, mobilisation, massage + exercise) vs control (sham ultrasound	12 weeks (end of treatment)	Both groups similar −2.2 (manual) and −2.0 (control)
WOMAC pain (change from baseline)	1 RCT (Bennell et al. 2005), N=140	Manual therapy (knee taping, mobilisation, massage + exercise) vs control (sham ultrasound	12 weeks (end of treatment)	Both groups similar −2.1 (manual) and −2.0 (control)
Manual therapy vs meloxicam				
Pain (VAS); pain Intensity (NRS-101); pressure pain tolerance, PPT (kg/sec)	1 RCT (Tucker et al. 2003), N=60	Manual therapy (motion palpation, thrust movement, manipulation) vs meloxicam	Mid-treatment and at 3 weeks (end of treatment)	NS

continued

Table 6.21 Symptoms – *continued*

Pain outcome	Reference	Intervention	Assessment time	Outcome/effect size
Knee osteoarthritis – *continued*				
Manual therapy (pre-treatment vs post-treatment)				
Functional squat pain (NPRS)	1 cohort study (Cliborne et al. 2004), (N=39)	Manual therapy (hip oscillatory mobilizations) – pre-treatment vs post-treatment	Immediate	p<0.01 Favours manual
FABER pain (NPRS)	1 cohort study (Cliborne et al. 2004), (N=39)	Manual therapy (hip oscillatory mobilizations) – pre-treatment vs post-treatment	Immediate Favours manual	p<0.05
Hip flexion pain (NPRS)	1 cohort study (Cliborne et al. 2004), (N=39)	Manual therapy (hip oscillatory mobilizations) – pre-treatment vs post-treatment	Immediate Favours manual	p<0.05
Hip scour pain (NPRS)	1 cohort study (Cliborne et al. 2004), (N=39)	Manual therapy (hip oscillatory mobilizations) – pre-treatment vs post-treatment	Immediate	p<0.01 Favours manual
Manual therapy vs usual care				
WOMAC pain, VAS (change from baseline)	1 RCT (Perlman et al. 2006) (N=68)	Swedish massage vs usual care	8 weeks (end of treatment)	–23.2mm (manual) and –3.1mm (usual care), p<0.001 Favours manual
Pain, VAS (change from baseline)	1 RCT (Perlman et al. 2006) (N=68)	Swedish massage vs usual care	8 weeks (end of treatment)	–22.6mm (manual) and –2.0mm (usual care) Manual better
Manual therapy vs manual contact				
Knee PPT	1 RCT (Moss et al. 2007) (N=38)	Manual therapy (large-amplitutde AP glide) vs control (manual contact)	Immediate	27.3% (manual) and 6.4% (control), p=0.008 Favours manual
Heel PPT	1 RCT (Moss et al. 2007) (N=38)	Manual therapy (large-amplitutde AP glide) vs control (manual contact)	Immediate	15.3% (manual) and 6.9% (control), p<0.001 Favours manual
WOMAC pain; pain during timed up-and-go test (VAS)	1 RCT (Moss et al. 2007) (N=38)	Manual therapy (large-amplitutde AP glide) vs control (manual contact)	Immediate	NS
Manual therapy vs no contact				
Knee PPT	1 RCT (Moss et al. 2007) (N=38)	Manual therapy (large-amplitutde AP glide) vs control (no contact)	Immediate	27.3% (manual) and 9.5% (control), p=0.01 Favours manual

continued

Table 6.21 Symptoms – *continued*

Pain outcome	Reference	Intervention	Assessment time	Outcome/effect size
Knee osteoarthritis – *continued*				
Manual therapy vs no contact – *continued*				
Heel PPT	1 RCT (Moss et al. 2007) (N=38)	Manual therapy (large-amplitutde AP glide) vs control (no contact)	Immediate	15.3% (manual) and 0.4% (control), p<0.019 Favours manual
WOMAC pain; pain during timed up-and-go test (VAS)	1 RCT (Moss et al. 2007) (N=38)	Manual therapy (large-amplitutde AP glide) vs control (no contact)	Immediate	NS
Hip				
Manual therapy vs exercise				
Pain at rest (VAS)	1 RCT (Hoeksma et al. 2004), (N=109)	Manual therapy (manipulation + stretching) vs exercise	5 weeks, end of study	Effect size 0.5,% CI –16.4 to –1.6, p<0.05 Favours manual
Pain walking (VAS)	1 RCT (Hoeksma et al. 2004), (N=109)	Manual therapy (manipulation + stretching) vs exercise	5 weeks, end of study	Effect size 0.5,% CI –17.3 to –1.8, p<0.05 Favours manual
Manual therapy (pre-treatment vs post-treatment)				
Pain (NPRS), change from baseline	1 case-series (MacDonald et al. 2006), (N=7)	Manual therapy (thrust movement, manipulation) pre-treatment vs post-treatment	Between 2–5 weeks	Mean change –4.7 Favours manual

Table 6.22 Stiffness

Stiffness outcome	Reference	Intervention	Assessment time	Outcome/effect size
Knee osteoarthritis				
Manual therapy vs usual care				
WOMAC stiffness, VAS (change from baseline)	1 RCT (Perlman et al. 2006) (N=68)	Swedish massage vs usual care	8 weeks (end of treatment)	–21.6 mm (manual) and –4.3 mm (usual care), p<0.007 Favours manual
Hip				
Manual therapy vs exercise				
Starting stiffness (VAS)	1 RCT (Hoeksma et al. 2004), N=109	Manual therapy (manipulation + stretching) vs exercise	5 weeks, end of study	Effect size 0.5,% CI –23.5 to –2.8, p<0.05 Favours manual

Table 6.23 Function

Function outcome	Reference	Intervention	Assessment time	Outcome/effect size
Knee osteoarthritis				
Manual therapy vs sham ultrasound				
6-minute walk distance	1 RCT (Deyle et al. 2000), N=83	Manual therapy (movements, mobilisation and stretching) + exercise vs control (sham ultrasound)	8 weeks (4 weeks post-treatment)	170m difference, % CI 71 to 270 m, p<0.05
WOMAC score	1 RCT (Deyle et al. 2000), N=83	Manual therapy (movements, mobilisation and stretching) + exercise vs control (sham ultrasound)	8 weeks (4 weeks post-treatment)	599m difference, % CI 197 to 1002m, p<0.05
Restriction of activity, VAS (change from baseline)	1 RCT (Bennell et al. 2005), N=140	Manual therapy (knee taping, mobilisation, massage) + exercise vs control (sham ultrasound)	12 weeks post-treatment	−1.9 (manual) and −1.7 (control) Manual better
WOMAC physical function (change from baseline)	1 RCT (Bennell et al. 2005), N=140	Manual therapy (knee taping, mobilisation, massage) + exercise vs control (sham ultrasound	12 weeks post-treatment	−7.5 (manual) and −6.7 (control) Manual better
Step test, number of steps (change from baseline)	1 RCT (Bennell et al. 2005), N=140	Manual therapy (knee taping, mobilisation, massage) + exercise vs control (sham ultrasound)	12 weeks post-treatment	2.1 (manual) and 1.8 (control) Manual better
Quadriceps strength, N/kg (change from baseline) at 12 weeks (end of treatment), 0.3 and 0.0 respectively and at, 0.3 and 0.1 respectively	1 RCT (Bennell et al. 2005), N=140	Manual therapy (knee taping, mobilisation, massage) + exercise vs control (sham ultrasound)	12 weeks (end of treatment) and 12 weeks post-treatment	12 weeks: 0.3 (manual) and 0.0 (control) 12 weeks post-treatment: 0.3 (manual) and 0.1 (control) Manual better
Step test, number of steps (change from baseline)	1 RCT (Bennell et al. 2005), N=140	Manual therapy (knee taping, mobilisation, massage) + exercise vs control (sham ultrasound)	12 weeks (end of treatment)	1.5 (manual) and 1.4 (control) Both groups similar
Restriction of activity, VAS (change from baseline	1 RCT (Bennell et al. 2005), N=140	Manual therapy (knee taping, mobilisation, massage) + exercise vs control (sham ultrasound)	12 weeks (end of treatment)	−1.6 (manual) and −1.9 (control) Control better
WOMAC physical function (change from baseline)	1 RCT (Bennell et al. 2005), N=140	Manual therapy (knee taping, mobilisation, massage) + exercise vs control (sham ultrasound)	12 weeks (end of treatment)	−7.8 (manual) and −8.2 (control) Control better

continued

Table 6.23 Function – *continued*

Function outcome	Reference	Intervention	Assessment time	Outcome/effect size
Knee osteoarthritis – *continued*				
Manual therapy vs meloxicam				
Flexion (degrees); Extension (degrees) and Patient-Specific Functional Scale, PSFS (1–11 scale).	1 RCT (Tucker et al. 2003), (N=60)	Manual therapy (motion palpation, thrust movement, manipulation) vs meloxicam	Mid-treatment and at 3 weeks (end of treatment)	NS
Manual therapy vs manual contact				
Sit-to-stand time	1 RCT (Moss et al. 2007) (N=38)	Manual therapy (large-amplitutde AP glide) vs control (manual contact)	Immediate	–5.06 (manual) and –0.35 (control), p<0.001 Favours manual
Total up-and-go time	1 RCT (Moss et al. 2007) (N=38)	Manual therapy (large-amplitutde AP glide) vs control (manual contact)	Immediate	NS
Manual therapy vs no contact				
Sit-to-stand time	1 RCT (Moss et al. 2007) (N=38)	Manual therapy (large-amplitutde AP glide) vs control (no contact)	Immediate	–5.06 (manual) and –7.92 (control), p<0.001 Favours manual
Total up-and-go time	1 RCT (Moss et al. 2007) (N=38)	Manual therapy (large-amplitutde AP glide) vs control (no contact)	Immediate	NS
Manual therapy (pre-treatment vs post-treatment)				
Functional squat ROM (degrees)	1 cohort study (Cliborne et al. 2004), N=39	Manual therapy (hip oscillatory mobilizations) – pre-treatment vs post-treatment	Immediate	p<0.05 Favours manual
Hip flexion ROM (degrees)	1 cohort study (Cliborne et al. 2004), N=39	Manual therapy (hip oscillatory mobilizations) – pre-treatment vs post-treatment	Immediate	p<0.01 Favours manual
FABER ROM (degrees), change from baseline	1 cohort study (Cliborne et al. 2004), N=39	Manual therapy (hip oscillatory mobilizations) – pre-treatment vs post-treatment	Immediate	+3.6 Favours manual
Manual therapy vs usual care				
WOMAC total, VAS (change from baseline)	1 RCT (Perlman et al. 2006) (N=68)	Swedish massage vs usual care	8 weeks (end of treatment)	–21.2mm (manual) and –4.6mm (control), p<0.001 Favours manual

continued

Table 6.23 Function – *continued*

Function outcome	Reference	Intervention	Assessment time	Outcome/effect size
Knee osteoarthritis – *continued*				
Manual therapy vs usual care – *continued*				
WOMAC physical functional disability, VAS (change from baseline	1 RCT (Perlman et al. 2006) (N=68)	Swedish massage vs usual care	8 weeks (end of treatment)	–20.5 mm (manual) and –0.02 mm (control), p=0.002 Favours manual
ROM, degrees (change from baseline	1 RCT (Perlman et al. 2006) (N=68)	Swedish massage vs usual care	8 weeks (end of treatment)	7.2 (manual) and –1.1 mm (control) Manual better
50-foot walk time, seconds (change from baseline	1 RCT (Perlman et al. 2006) (N=68)	Swedish massage vs usual care	8 weeks (end of treatment)	–1.8 (manual) and 0.2 (control) Manual better
Hip				
Manual therapy vs exercise				
Walking speed (seconds)	1 RCT (Hoeksma et al. 2004), N=109	Manual therapy (manipulation + stretching) vs exercise	5 weeks, end of study	Effect size 0.3, % CI –16.7 to –0.5, p<0.05 Favours manual
ROM flexion-extension (degrees)	1 RCT (Hoeksma et al. 2004), N=109	Manual therapy (manipulation + stretching) vs exercise	5 weeks, end of study	Effect size 1.0,% CI 8.1 to 22.6, p<0.05 Favours manual
ROM external-internal rotation (degrees)	1 RCT (Hoeksma et al. 2004), N=109	Manual therapy (manipulation + stretching) vs exercise	5 weeks, end of study	Effect size 0.9,% CI 6.1 to 17.3, p<0.05 Favours manual
ROM flexion-extension (degrees)	1 RCT (Hoeksma et al. 2004), N=109	Manual therapy (manipulation + stretching) vs exercise	5 weeks, end of study	Effect size 1.0,% CI 8.1 to 22.6, p<0.05 Favours manual
Manual therapy (pre- treatment vs post-treatment)				
Passive ROM (degrees)	1 case-series (MacDonald et al. 2006), N=7	Manual therapy (thrust movement, manipulation) pre-treatment vs post-treatment	2 to 5 weeks	Mean change +23.3 Favours manual
Passive ROM internal rotation (degrees)	1 case-series (MacDonald et al. 2006), N=7	Manual therapy (thrust movement, manipulation) pre-treatment vs post-treatment	2 to 5 weeks	Mean change +16.3 Favours manual
Total hip passive ROM (degrees)	1 case-series (MacDonald et al. 2006), N=7	Manual therapy (thrust movement, manipulation) pre-treatment vs post-treatment	2 to 5 weeks	Mean change +84.3 Favours manual
Disability (Harris Hip Score)	1 case-series (MacDonald et al. 2006), N=7	Manual therapy (thrust movement, manipulation) pre-treatment vs post-treatment	2 to 5 weeks	Mean change +20.0 Favours manual

Table 6.24 Global assessment

Global assessment outcome	Reference	Intervention	Assessment time	Outcome/effect size
Knee osteoarthritis				
Manual therapy vs sham ultrasound				
Patient global assessment of improvement	1 RCT (Bennell et al. 2005), N=140	Manual therapy (knee taping, mobilisation, massage) + exercise vs control (sham ultrasound)	12 weeks post-treatment	NS
Hip				
Manual therapy vs exercise				
Main complaint	1 RCT (Hoeksma et al. 2004), N=109	Manual therapy (manipulation + stretching) vs exercise	5 weeks, end of study	Effect size 0.5,% CI –20.4 to –2.7 Favours manual
Improvement of the main complaint at 5 weeks, end of study	1 RCT (Hoeksma et al. 2004), N=109	Manual therapy (manipulation + stretching) vs exercise	5 weeks, end of study	81% and 50% respectively; OR 1.92,% CI 1.30 to 2.60 Favours manual
Worsening of the main complaint at 5 weeks, end of study	1 RCT (Hoeksma et al. 2004), N=109	Manual therapy (manipulation + stretching) vs exercise	5 weeks, end of study	19% and 50% Favours manual

Table 6.25 Quality of life

QoL outcome	Reference	Intervention	Assessment time	Outcome/effect size
Knee osteoarthritis				
Manual therapy vs sham ultrasound				
SF-36 bodily pain (change from baseline)	1 RCT (Bennell et al. 2005), N=140	Manual therapy (knee taping, mobilisation, massage) + exercise vs control (sham ultrasound)	12 weeks (end of treatment) and 12 weeks post-treatment	12 weeks: –11.4 (manual) and –9.4 (control) 12 weeks post-treatment: –6.7 (manual) and –4.9 (control) Manual better
SF-36 physical function (change from baseline)	1 RCT (Bennell et al. 2005), N=140	Manual therapy (knee taping, mobilisation, massage) + exercise vs control (sham ultrasound)	12 weeks (end of treatment) and 12 weeks post-treatment	12 weeks: –12.2 (manual) and –7.9 (control) 12 weeks post-treatment: –9.7 (manual) and –5.4 (control) Manual better

continued

Table 6.25 Quality of life – *continued*

QoL outcome	Reference	Intervention	Assessment time	Outcome/effect size
Knee osteoarthritis				
Manual therapy vs sham ultrasound – *continued*				
SF-36 physical role (change from baseline)	1 RCT (Bennell et al. 2005), N=140	Manual therapy (knee taping, mobilisation, massage) + exercise vs control (sham ultrasound)	12 weeks post-treatment	−13.3 (manual) and −11.8 (control) Manual better
AQoL (change from baseline)	1 RCT (Bennell et al. 2005), N=140	Manual therapy (knee taping, mobilisation, massage) + exercise vs control (sham ultrasound)	12 weeks post-treatment	0.07 (manual) and 0.001 (control) Manual better
AQoL (change from baseline)	1 RCT (Bennell et al. 2005), N=140	Manual therapy (knee taping, mobilisation, massage) + exercise vs control (sham ultrasound)	12 weeks (end of treatment)	0.05 (manual) and 0.04 (control) Both groups similar
SF-36 physical role (change from baseline)	1 RCT (Bennell et al. 2005), N=140	Manual therapy (knee taping, mobilisation, massage) + exercise vs control (sham ultrasound)	12 weeks (end of treatment)	14.8 (manual) and 16.0 (control) Control better
Hip				
Manual therapy vs exercise				
SF-36 role physical function	1 RCT (Hoeksma et al. 2004), N=109	Manual therapy (manipulation + stretching) vs exercise	5 weeks, end of study	Effect size 0.4,% CI −21.5 to −1.1, p<0.05 Favours manual
SF-36 bodily pain and physical function	1 RCT (Hoeksma et al. 2004), N=109	Manual therapy (manipulation + stretching) vs exercise	5 weeks, end of study	NS

Table 6.26 Adverse events

AEs outcome	Reference	Intervention	Assessment time	Outcome/effect size
Knee osteoarthritis				
Manual therapy vs sham ultrasound				
Number of patients with AEs	1 RCT (Bennell et al. 2005), N=140	Manual therapy (knee taping, mobilisation, massage) + exercise vs control (sham ultrasound)	12 weeks (end of treatment)	Control better
Manual therapy vs meloxicam				
Number of AEs (N=0, 0% and N=3 10% respectively).	1 RCT (Tucker et al. 2003), N=60	Manual therapy (motion palpation, thrust movement, manipulation) vs meloxicam	3 weeks (end of treatment)	0% (manual) and 10% (meloxicam) Manual better

Table 6.27 Study withdrawals

Withdrawals outcome	Reference	Intervention	Assessment time	Outcome/effect size
Knee osteoarthritis				
Manual therapy vs sham ultrasound				
Number of withdrawals	1 RCT (Bennell et al. 2005), N=140	Manual therapy (knee taping, mobilisation, massage) + exercise vs control (sham ultrasound)	12 weeks (end of treatment) and 12 weeks post-treatment	12 weeks: 18% (manual) and 3% (control) 12 weeks post-treatment: 23% (manual) and 6% (control) Control better
Number of withdrawals	1 RCT (Deyle et al. 2000), N=83	Manual therapy (movements, mobilisation and stretching) + exercise vs control (sham ultrasound)	4 weeks (end of treatment)	12% (manual) and 21% (control) Manual better
Hip				
Manual therapy vs exercise				
Number of withdrawals + number lost to follow-up	1 RCT (Hoeksma et al. 2004), N=109	Manual therapy (manipulation + stretching) vs exercise	End of study (week 5) and 6 months (5 months post-intervention)	N=15 (manual) and N=13 (exercise) Both groups similar
Withdrawals due to AEs, increase of complaints	1 RCT (Hoeksma et al. 2004), N=109	Manual therapy (manipulation + stretching) vs exercise	End of study (week 5)	N=3 (manual) and N=2 (exercise) Both groups similar

6.1.9 Health economic evidence overview

We looked at studies that focused on economically evaluating exercise programmes compared with other exercise interventions, or with no treatment/placebo for the treatment of adults with osteoarthritis. Thirteen studies were identified through the literature search as possible cost-effectiveness analyses in this area. On closer inspection nine of these studies (Callaghan et al. 1995; Cochrane et al. 2005; Fioravanti et al. 2003; Hughes et al. 2004; Hurley and Scott 1998; Kettunen and Kujala 2004; Maurer et al. 1999; McCarthy et al. 2004; Patrick et al. 2001; Ververeli et al. 1995) were excluded for:

- not directly answering the question
- not including sufficient cost data to be considered a true economic analyses
- involving a study population of less than 30 people.

Four papers were found to be methodologically sound and were included as health economics evidence. After the re-run search, two more papers were included as health economic evidence.

One recent UK study involved a full pragmatic, single-blind randomised clinical trial accompanied by a full economic evaluation (McCarthy et al. 2004a). The study duration was 1 year, and the study population included 214 patients meeting the American College of Rheumatology's classification of knee OA, selected from referrals from the primary and secondary care settings. The interventions considered were:

- group 1: a home exercise programme aimed at increasing lower-limb strength, endurance, and improving balance
- group 2: a group supplemented with 8 weeks of twice-weekly knee classes run by a physiotherapist. Classes represented typical knee class provision in the UK.

Effectiveness data were taken from the accompanying RCT. An NHS perspective was taken meaning that costs included resource use gathered from patient records and questionnaires, the cost of the intervention estimated from resource-use data and national pay-scale figures, capital and overhead costs and one-off expenses incurred by the patient. Travel costs were considered in sensitivity analysis. QALYs were calculated through converting EuroQol 5-dimensional outcomes questionnaire (EQ-5D) scores obtained at baseline 1, 6, and 12 months into utilities.

One recent UK study (Thomas et al. 2005) conducted a cost-effectiveness analysis of exercise, telephone support, and no intervention. The study duration was 2 years and the study population involved adults aged over 45 years old reporting current knee pain (exclusion criteria included having had a total knee replacement, lower limb amputation, cardiac pacemaker, unable to give informed consent, or no current knee pain). Four intervention groups were used.

- *Exercise therapy.* This included quadriceps strengthening, aerobic exercise taught in a graded programme, and resistance exercises using a rubber exercise band. A research nurse taught the programme in the participants' homes. The initial training phase consisted of 4 visits lasting ~30 minutes in the first 2 months, with follow-up visits scheduled every 6 months thereafter. Participants were encouraged to perform the programme daily, taking 20–30 minutes.

- *Monthly telephone support.* This was used to monitor symptoms and to offer simple advice on the management of knee pain. This aimed to control the psychological impact of the exercise programme.

- *Combination of exercise and telephone support.* As above, in combination.

- *No intervention.* Patients in this group received no contact between the biannual assessment visits.

Effectiveness data were obtained from an accompanying RCT (786 participants). Health provider and patient perspectives were considered regarding costs. However, patient specific costs were only considered in terms of time, and a monetary cost was not placed on this. This means that costs reported are those relevant for the health provider perspective (direct treatment costs, medical costs).

A limitation of the study is that it does not distinguish between medical costs incurred due to knee pain and medical costs incurred due to any other type of illness. This may bias results because changes in costs may not reflect changes in costs associated with knee pain.

One US study (Sevick et al. 2000) conducted an economic analysis comparing exercise interventions and an education intervention. The study was 18 months long and focused on people aged 60 or over who have pain on most days of the month in one or both knees; and who have difficulty with one of a variety of everyday activities; radiographic evidence of knee OA in the tibial-femoral compartments on the painful knee(s) as judged by a radiologist. The interventions included were:

- *Aerobic exercise programme.* This included a 3-month facility-based programme and a 15-month home-based programme. At each session exercise lasted 60 minutes including warm-up, stimulus, and cool-down phases. Exercise was prescribed three times per week. During the 3-month period, training was under the supervision of a trained exercise leader. Between 4 and 6 months participants were instructed to continue the exercise at home and were contacted biweekly by the programme leader who made four home visits and six follow-up telephone calls to participants. For months 7–9 telephone contact was made every 3 weeks, and during months 10–18 monthly follow-up telephone calls were made.

- *Resistance exercise programme.* This included a 3-month facility based and a 15-month home-based programme. Duration of session, the number, timing, and type of follow-up were consistent with the aerobic exercise. Weights were used.

- *Health education.* This was used as a control to minimise attention and social interaction bias. During months 1–3 participants received a monthly 1.5 hour educational session, and during months 4–18 participants were regularly contacted by a nurse to discuss the status of their arthritis and any problems with medications. Telephone contacts were bi-weekly during months 4–6 and monthly for months 7–18.

Efficacy estimates were from the single-blind Fitness and Arthritis in Seniors Trial (FAST) RCT. A healthcare-payer perspective was adopted. Limitations of the study include that it only reported results comparing each exercise programme individually with the education control, rather than also comparing the exercise programmes with one another. Also, incremental cost-effectiveness ratios (ICERs) were calculated incorrectly.

An Australian study (Segal et al. 2004) economically evaluated a number of different interventions for the treatment of OA. The population considered varied for the different comparisons. The interventions considered were:

- comprehensive mass media programme for weight loss
- intensive primary care weight-loss programme delivered by GP or dietician for overweight or obese
- intensive primary care weight-loss programme delivered by GP or dietician for overweight or obese with previous knee injury
- surgery for obese people
- lay-led group education
- primary care: GP or clinical nurse educator plus phone support
- exercise/strength training
    - home-based basic
    - home-based intensive
    - clinic-based primary care
    - clinic based outpatients
- specially fitted knee brace
- non-specific NSAIDs (naproxen, diclofenac)
- COX2s (celecoxib)

- glucosamine sulfate
- avocado
- topical capsaicin/soy unsaponifiable
- total knee replacement
- total hip replacement
- knee arthroscopy with lavage.

The paper required published outcomes and costs of the considered interventions to be found. At a minimum the papers used had to include a precise programme description and quantitative evidence of effectiveness derived from an acceptable research design and preferably health endpoints, a usual care or placebo control, and a suitable follow-up period. Costs included resources applied to the intervention and to the management of treatment side effects, and for primary prevention estimated savings in 'downstream' healthcare service use. Intervention costs were calculated as the product of programme inputs multiplied by current published unit costs.

The paper is limited with regards to its technique applied to compare health outcomes. A 'transfer-to-utility' (TTU) technique was used, which has been criticised in the literature (Viney et al. 2004). This involves transforming health outcome scores found in the original trials into QALY scores.

One study from the Netherlands investigated behavioural graded activity and usual physiotherapy treatment for 200 patients with osteoarthritis of the hip or knee (Coupe et al. 2007).

The behavioural graded activity group received a treatment integrating the concepts of operant conditioning with exercise treatment comprising booster sessions. Graded activity was directed at increasing the level of activity in a time-contingent manner, with the goal of integrating these activities in the daily lives of patients. Treatment consisted of a 12-week period with a maximum of 18 sessions, followed by five preset booster moments with a maximum of seven sessions (in weeks 18, 25, 34, 42 and 55).

The usual care group received treatment according to Dutch physiotherapy guidelines for patients with OA of the hip and/or knee. This recommends provision of information and advice, exercise treatment and encouragement of coping positively with the complaints. Treatment consisted of a 12-week period with a maximum of 18 sessions and could be discontinued within this 12-week period if, according to the physiotherapist, all treatment goals had been achieved.

6.1.10 Health economic evidence statements

▷ Home-based exercise vs home-based exercise supplemented with class-based exercise

One UK study (McCarthy et al. 2004a) conducted an economic analysis into the effects on supplementing a home-based exercise programme with a class-based programme.

Table 6.28 McCarthy's cost–benefit estimates		
Intervention	QALYs gained	Cost (1999/2000 £)
Home-based	0.022	£445.52
Class-based	0.045	£440.04

These results show that the class-based supplement dominates the home-based intervention alone. However, neither the cost or the effect data were statistically significantly different, so cost-effectiveness acceptability curves (CEACs) were presented. These showed that for all plausible threshold willingness to pay (WTP) values, the class-based regime was more likely to be cost effective than the home-based regime. The CEAC showed that the probability of the class-based programme being cost-saving was just over 50%. At a WTP of £30,000 the probability of the class-based programme being cost effective was over 70%.

Additional sensitivity analysis was undertaken. When considering only patients for whom complete cost data were available (N=74, 30 in home-based groups and 44 in class-based groups) the class-based group had a higher probability of being cost effective (approximately 95% at WTP £20,000 to £30,000). Sensitivity analysis also included adding travel costs to the class-based regime. In this case the class-based programme was still likely (65% probability) to be cost effective compared with the home-based programme with a WTP threshold per additional QALY of £20,000–£30,000. However, there is considerable uncertainty with a probability of 30–35% that the class-based programme will not be cost effective.

It should be noted that as a one-year time horizon is used, the results are biased against the more effective intervention, or the intervention for which benefits are likely to be prolonged the most. This is because these patients will benefit from an increased QALY score for some time going into the future, assuming that the QALY improvement does not disappear immediately after the intervention is stopped.

In conclusion, it is likely that supplementing a home-based exercise programme with a class-based programme will be cost saving or cost effective and will improve outcomes. If travel costs are included this becomes less likely but it is probable that the class-based supplement will remain cost effective.

▷ Exercise vs no exercise vs telephone

One 2005 UK study (Thomas et al. 2005) compared exercise interventions, no treatment and telephone interventions, essentially from the healthcare provider perspective. All costs were reported in pound sterling at 1996 prices.

Table 6.29 Thomas's cost–benefit estimates

Intervention	% of patients showing a ≥50% improvement in knee pain	Bootstrapped total costs (95% CI)
Exercise intervention (exercise, exercise + telephone, exercise + telephone + placebo)	27%	1,354 (1,350 to 1,358)
No-exercise control (telephone, placebo, no intervention)	20% (p=0.1)	1,129 (1,125 to 1,132)

It should be noted that this paper has a bias against the exercise intervention if it is assumed that the benefits of the exercise programme continue for some time after the intervention has been stopped. This is because the intervention would no longer be paid for but some of the benefits may remain.

There is no evidence of telephone interventions being more effective than no-telephone interventions, so it is unclear whether adding telephone contact would be cost effective.

▷ Home-based exercise vs clinic-based exercise vs control

An Australian study (Segal et al. 2004) undertakes an economic analysis of a number of different interventions for the treatment of OA, using a transfer-to-utility technique which allows each intervention to be analysed regarding their cost per QALY gain.

Table 6.30 Segal's cost-effectiveness estimates

Intervention	Mean QALY gain per person	Mean programme cost per person (2003 Australian $, converted to 2003 £*)	Cost/QALY best estimate versus control (no intervention)	ICER
Home-based exercise – basic	0.022	$400 (£164)	$18,000 (£7,377) to equivocal	Extendedly dominated
Clinic-based exercise – primary care	0.091	$480 (£197)	$5,000 (£2,049)	$5,000 (£2,049)
Clinic-based exercise – outpatients	0.078	$590 (£242)	$8,000 (£3,279)	Dominated
Home-based exercise – intensive	0.100	$1,420 (£582)	$15,000 (£6,148)	$104,444 (£42,805)

* Currencies were converted using current exchange rates (0.41 for Australian $).

Note that the effectiveness data these estimates are based on were generally from studies of around 12 weeks, but these estimates calculate costs and QALYs for a 1-year time period – that is, as if the intervention was continued for one full year.

Compared with one another clinic-based exercise in a primary care setting (between one and three 30 minute exercise sessions per week for 12 weeks given on an individual basis by a physiotherapist, which included strengthening and lengthening exercises for muscle functions, mobility, coordination and elementary movement plus locomotion abilities) is cost effective if there is a WTP per additional QALY gained of between approximately £2049 and £42,805. For a WTP higher than £42,805 the evidence suggests that intensive home-based exercise may be cost effective. Home-based basic exercise is extendedly dominated by clinic-based exercise in primary care. Clinic-based exercise in an outpatient setting is dominated by clinic-based exercise in primary care.

▷ Aerobic exercise versus resistance exercise vs education control

One US study (Sevick et al. 2000) considers the cost effectiveness of aerobic exercise and resistance exercise compared with an education control from the healthcare payer perspective.

Table 6.31 Sevick's cost-effectiveness estimates

	Education	Aerobic exercise	Resistance exercise	Cost effectiveness
Cost per participant (1994 US$)	$343.98	$323.55	$325.20	Aerobic cheaper
Self-reported disability score (points)	1.90	1.72	1.74	Aerobic dominant
6-minute walking distance (feet)	1,349	1,507	1,406	Aerobic dominant
Stair climb (seconds)	13.9	12.7	13.2	Aerobic dominant
Lifting and carrying task (seconds)	10.0	9.1	9.3	Aerobic dominant
Car task (seconds)	10.6	8.7	9.0	Aerobic dominant
Transfer pain frequency (points)	3.18	2.89	2.99	Aerobic dominant
Ambulatory pain frequency (points)	3.46	3.12	3.06	Resistance CE if WTP $27.5 per additional point
Transfer pain intensity (points)	2.28	2.10	2.11	Aerobic dominant
Ambulatory pain intensity (points)	2.45	2.27	2.34	Aerobic dominant

Note that the resistance and aerobic exercise programmes were undertaken in the same setting, that is, 3 months facility-based and 15 months home-based, and cost differences were only from medical referrals and adverse events, despite the fact that weights were used in the resistance exercise group. The authors state that the educational control arm of the study would be equivalent to a 'no special instruction' group in the real world. They state that the cost for this would be zero, but that it is possible outcomes would be slightly worse for these patients.

Also, similarly to other studies with relatively short time horizons, and which stop recording outputs as soon as the intervention is stopped, this paper may bias against the intervention as the benefits of the intervention may not disappear as soon as the intervention is discontinued.

In conclusion, aerobic exercise has been shown to result in lower costs than a resistance exercise group and an educational control group in the USA, while incurring lower medical costs. Exercise programmes are likely to be cost effective compared with an educational programme involving regular telephone follow-up with patients.

The Dutch study (Coupe et al. 2007) found that the behavioural graded activity group was less costly than the usual care group, but not statistically significantly so. It is notable that more joint replacement operations took place in the usual care group, and it is unclear whether this is related to the interventions under consideration. The difference in effect of the two treatments was minimal for all outcomes. The study was excluded from the clinical review for this guideline, and given the uncertainty in the results no evidence statements can be made based on it.

A recent UK study which is soon to be published investigates the Enabling Self-management and Coping with Arthritic knee Pain through Exercise (ESCAPE-knee pain) Programme in 418 patients with chronic knee pain (Hurley et al. 2007). The interventions studied were:
- usual primary care
- usual primary care plus individual rehabilitation (individual ESCAPE)
- usual primary care plus rehabilitation in groups of about eight participants (group ESCAPE).

The content and format of ESCAPE was the same for the individual and group patients. They consisted of 12 sessions (twice weekly for 6 weeks) involving self-management advice and exercises to improve lower limb function.

The results of the study suggest that the group patients achieved very similar results as the individual patients, but the group costs were less. The probability that ESCAPE (individual and group combined) is cost effective compared with usual care based on QALYs, with £20,000 WTP threshold for an additional QALY = 60%.

The probability that ESCAPE (individual and group combined) is cost effective compared with usual care based on a 15% improvement in WOMAC function, with £1900 WTP threshold for an additional person with a 15% improvement is 90%. With a WTP threshold of £800 the probability is 50%. Based on the WOMAC outcome, the probability of Individual ESCAPE being more cost effective than Group ESCAPE reached 50% at a WTP threshold of £6000.

6.1.11 From evidence to recommendations

Exercise

The GDG recognised the need to distinguish between exercise therapy aimed at individual joints and general activity-related fitness. Evidence from a large, well-conducted systematic review (Roddy et al. 2005) and one large RCT (Miller et al. 2005) for knee osteoarthritis demonstrated the beneficial effects of exercise compared with no exercise. Exercise in this context included aerobic walking, home quadriceps exercise, strengthening and home exercise, aerobic exercise with weight training, and diet with aerobic and resisted exercise. Exercise reduced pain, disability, medication intake and improved physical functioning, stair climbing, walking distance, muscle strength, balance, self-efficacy and mental health and physical functioning (SF-36). The majority of these beneficial outcomes were seen at 18 months.

The strengths of these effects were not evident for hip and hand osteoarthritis. However, there is limited evidence for hip and hand osteoarthritis and the mechanisms of exercise on the hip and hand may be different to those for knee osteoarthritis (Garfinkel et al. 1994).

There is limited evidence for the benefits of one type of exercise over another but delivery of exercise in a class setting supplemented by home exercise may be superior to home exercise alone in terms of pain reduction, improved disability and increased walking speed (McCarthy et al. 2004b). Classes were also shown to be cost effective. A class-based exercise programme was superior to a home exercise programme at 12 months for pain, disability and walking speed in knee osteoarthritis (McCarthy 2004). This study was conducted in a secondary care setting and patients were referred from primary and secondary care.

There is limited evidence to suggest exercise in water may be beneficial in the short term. There is difficulty in interpreting the study findings (one in pool-based sessions in the community in the UK, a second of hydrotherapy in the USA) for current practice in the NHS.

Exercise therapies given by health professionals to individuals and to groups of patients (for example, exercise classes) may both be effective and locally available. Individual patient preferences can inform the design of exercise programmes.

Adverse events were not consistently studied, but the risk of adverse events is considered low if the suitability of the exercise for the individual is appropriately assessed by a trained health professional.

The GDG considered that the choice between individual and group exercise interventions has to be informed by patient preference, and tailoring it to the individual will achieve longer-term positive behavioural change.

The GDG also considered adding reference to the Expert Patient Programme but NICE guidelines do not specify the service model used to deliver effective interventions, and therefore an open recommendation is made focussing on the intervention shown to be of benefit.

Manual therapy

The majority of studies evaluated manual therapy for osteoarthritis in combination with other treatment approaches, for example exercise. This reflected current practice in physiotherapy, where manual therapy would not be used as a sole treatment for osteoarthritis but as part of a package of care.

There was strong evidence for the benefit of manual therapy alone compared with exercise (Hoeksma et al. 2004). Again the design of this study reflects usual physiotherapy practice, where there is limited evidence for the benefit of exercise for hip osteoarthritis. The exercise programme was based on that reported by van Barr (van Baar et al. 1998). Manual therapy included stretching techniques of the identified shortened muscles around the hip joint and manual traction which was repeated at each visit until the therapist concluded optimal results. Patients were treated twice weekly for 5 weeks with a total of nine treatments. The duration of this programme is somewhat longer than that usually available in the NHS. However, the benefit of the manual therapy would indicate that such a programme should be considered in individuals who are not benefiting from home stretching exercises.

There have been few reported adverse events of manual therapy, pain on massage being one.

RECOMMENDATIONS

R11   Exercise should be a core treatment (see Fig 3.2) for people with osteoarthritis, irrespective of age, comorbidity, pain severity or disability. Exercise should include:
- local muscle strengthening
- general aerobic fitness.

It has not been specified whether exercise should be provided by the NHS or the healthcare professional should provide advice and encouragement to the patient to obtain and carry out the intervention themselves. Exercise has been found to be beneficial but the clinician needs to make a judgement in each case on how to effectively ensure patient participation. This will depend on the patient's individual needs, circumstances, self-motivation and the availability of local facilities.

R12   Manipulation and stretching should be considered as an adjunct to core treatment, particularly for osteoarthritis of the hip.

6.2   Weight loss

6.2.1   Clinical introduction

Excess or abnormal mechanical loading of the joint appears to be one of the main factors leading to the development and progression of osteoarthritis. This is apparent in secondary forms of osteoarthritis, such as that related to developmental dysplasia of the hip. It also occurs in primary osteoarthritis, where abnormal or excess loading may be related to obesity or even relatively minor degrees of mal-alignment (varus or valgus deformity) at the knee.

The association of obesity with the development and progression of osteoarthritis, especially at the knee, provides the justification for weight reduction. Weight loss is usually achieved with either dietary manipulation and/or exercise, where the independent effect of the latter must also be considered.

6.2.2 Methodological introduction

We looked for studies that investigated the efficacy and safety of weight loss vs no weight loss with respect to symptoms, function and quality of life in adults with osteoarthritis. One systematic review and meta-analysis (Christensen et al. 2007) and four additional RCTs (Huang et al. 2000; Miller et al. 2006; Rejeski et al. 2002; Toda 2001) were found. One of these RCTs (Rejeski et al. 2002) was a subgroup analysis of another trial (Messier et al. 2004). Three RCTs (Huang et al. 2000; Miller et al. 2006; Toda 2001) were excluded due to methodological limitations. No relevant cohort or case-control studies were found.

The systematic review and meta-analysis (Christensen et al. 2007) on weight loss vs no weight loss in patients with knee osteoarthritis. The MA included five RCTs (with N=454 participants). All RCTs were methodologically sound. Studies included in the analysis differed with respect to:

- intervention – weight loss method (four RCTs exercise and cognitive-behavioural therapy; one RCT low-energy diet; one RCT Mazindol weight loss drug and low-energy diet)
- study size and length.

The one RCT (Rejeski et al. 2002) not included in the systematic review was methodologically sound and compared weight loss (exercise vs diet vs exercise + diet) with no weight loss (healthy lifestyle education) in N=316 patients with knee osteoarthritis in an 18-month treatment phase.

6.2.3 Evidence statements

Table 6.32 Symptoms				
Pain outcome	**Reference**	**Intervention**	**Assessment time**	**Outcome/effect size**
Knee osteoarthritis				
Weight loss vs no weight loss				
Pain	1MA (Christensen et al. 2007) 4 RCTs, N=417	Weight loss vs no weight loss	Between 8 weeks to 18 months	NS
Predictors of significant change in pain score – body weight change (%) or rate of weight change per week	1MA (Christensen et al. 2007) 4 RCTs, N=417	Weight loss vs no weight loss	Between 8 weeks to 18 months	Not predictors

Table 6.33 Function

Function outcome	Reference	Intervention	Assessment time	Outcome/effect size
Knee osteoarthritis				
Weight loss vs no weight loss				
Self-reported disability	1 MA (Christensen et al. 2007) 4 RCTs, N=417	Weight loss vs no weight loss	Between 8 weeks to 18 months	Weight loss 6.1 kg; effect size 0.23,% CI 0.04 to 0.42, p=0.02 Favours weight loss
Lequesne's Index	1 MA (Christensen et al. 2007) 2 RCTs, N=117	Weight loss vs no weight loss	6 to 8 weeks	NS
Predictors of significant reduction in self-reported disability – body weight change (weight reduction of at least 5.1%)	1 MA (Christensen et al. 2007) 4 RCTs, N=417	Weight loss vs no weight loss	Between 8 weeks to 18 months	Predictor
Predictors of significant reduction in self-reported disability – weight change per week (at least 0.24%)	1 MA (Christensen et al. 2007) 4 RCTs, N=417	Weight loss vs no weight loss	Between 8 weeks to 18 months	Not predictor

Table 6.34 Quality of life

Function outcome	Reference	Intervention	Assessment time	Outcome/effect size
Knee osteoarthritis				
Weight loss vs minimal weight loss				
SF-36 dimensions of composite mental health, composite physical health score, patient satisfaction with function, body pain, physical role, general health, social functioning, vitality, emotional role	1 RCT (Rejeski et al. 2002), N=316	Weight loss (diet) vs minimal weight loss (healthy lifestyle)	18-months (end of treatment)	NS
SF-36 patient satisfaction with function	1 RCT (Rejeski et al. 2002), N=316	Weight loss (exercise) vs minimal weight loss (healthy lifestyle)	18-months (end of treatment)	p<0.01 Favours weight loss

continued

Table 6.34 Quality of life – *continued*

Function outcome	Reference	Intervention	Assessment time	Outcome/effect size
Knee osteoarthritis				
Weight loss vs minimal weight loss – *continued*				
SF-36 dimensions composite mental health, composite physical health score, body pain, physical role, general health, social functioning, vitality, emotional role	1 RCT (Rejeski et al. 2002), N=316	Weight loss (exercise) vs minimal weight loss (healthy lifestyle)	18-months (end of treatment)	NS
SF-36 dimensions of composite physical health score, patient satisfaction with function, physical role, general health, social functioning	1 RCT (Rejeski et al. 2002), N=316	Weight loss (diet + exercise) vs minimal weight loss (healthy lifestyle)	18-months (end of treatment)	All: p< 0.01 Favours weight loss
SF-36 dimensions of composite mental health, vitality and emotional role	1 RCT (Rejeski et al. 2002), N=316	Weight loss (diet + exercise) vs minimal weight loss (healthy lifestyle)	18-months (end of treatment)	NS
Weight loss vs weight loss				
SF-36 patient satisfaction with function	1 RCT (Rejeski et al. 2002), N=316	Weight loss (diet + exercise) vs weight loss (diet)	18-months (end of treatment)	p<0.01 Favours diet + exercise
SF-36 body pain	1 RCT (Rejeski et al. 2002), N=316	Weight loss (diet + exercise) vs weight loss (exercise)	18-months (end of treatment)	p<0.01 Favours diet + exercise

Table 6.35 Weight loss

Weight loss outcome	Reference	Intervention	Assessment time	Outcome/effect size
Knee osteoarthritis				
Weight loss (%)	1 RCT (Rejeski et al. 2002), N=316	Weight loss (diet vs exercise vs diet + exercise) vs control, minimal weight loss (healthy lifestyle)	18 months (end of treatment)	Diet (5.7%), diet + exercise (4.4%), exercise (2.6%), control – healthy lifestyle (1.3%)

6.2.4 From evidence to recommendations

Published data suggest that interventions reducing excess load, including weight loss, lead to improvement in function, providing the magnitude of weight loss is sufficient. In contrast, the effect of weight loss on pain is inconsistent. The only study to show an unequivocal effect on WOMAC pain as a primary outcome measure included exercise as one part of a complex intervention (Messier et al. 2004). Other studies suggest exercise might achieve this outcome in the absence of weight loss (see 7.1), although the exercise only arm in this study did not show a statistically significant reduction in pain.

Furthermore, there is no clear evidence so far that weight loss, either alone or in combination with exercise, can slow disease progression. Although only one of the studies reviewed specifically addressed this question, (Messier et al. 2004), it was small (N=84), of relatively short duration and therefore underpowered for this outcome. Nor is there a definite threshold of weight below which the beneficial effect of weight loss on function is reduced or diminished, although all of the studies were restricted to those who were overweight (BMI>26.4 kg.m^{-2}). Also, all of the studies have been conducted in knee osteoarthritis, with consequent difficulties in generalising the results to other joints, where mechanical influence may be less. The other health benefits of sustained weight loss are generally assumed to justify its widespread recommendation, but there is a paucity of trials showing that the kind of sustainable weight loss which would achieve metabolic and cardiovascular health benefits is achievable in clinical practice. The NICE guideline for obesity provides information on this evidence and the most effective weight loss strategies (National Institute for Health and Clinical Excellence 2006b).

Despite the limitations of the available evidence, the benefits of weight loss in people with osteoarthritis who are overweight are generally perceived to be greater than the risks. The GDG therefore advocate weight loss in all obese and overweight adults with osteoarthritis of the knee and hip who have associated functional limitations.

RECOMMENDATION

R13   Interventions to achieve weight loss should be a core treatment for people who are obese or overweight.[*]

6.3   Electrotherapy

6.3.1   Clinical introduction

Electrotherapy and electrophysical agents include pulsed short wave diathermy (pulsed electromagnetic field, PEMF), interferential therapy, laser, transcutaneous electrical nerve stimulation (TENS) and ultrasound. All are commonly used to treat the signs and symptoms of OA such as pain, trigger point tenderness and swelling. These modalities involve the introduction of energy into affected tissue resulting in physical changes in the tissue as a result of thermal and non-thermal effects.

---

[*] See 'Obesity: guidance on the prevention, identification, assessment and management of overweight and obesity in adults and children.' NICE clinical guideline 43.

▷ Ultrasound

The therapeutic effects of ultrasound have been classifed as relating to thermal and non-thermal effects (Dyson 2007). Thermal effects cause a rise in temperature in the tissue and non-thermal effects (cavitation, acoustic streaming) can alter the permeability of the cell membrane (Baker et al. 2001; ter Haar 1999), which is thought to produce therapeutic benefits (Zhang et al. 2007). The potential therapeutic benefits seen in clinical practice may be more likely in tissue which has a high collagen content, for example a joint capsule rather than cartilage and bone which has a lower collagen content.

▷ Pulsed electromagnetic field (also termed pulsed short wave diathermy)

Pulsed electromagnetic field (PEMF) has been purported to work by increasing blood flow, facilitating the resolution of inflammation and increasing deep collagen extensibility (Scott 1996). The application of this type of therapy can also produce thermal and non-thermal effects. The specific effect may be determined by the specific dose.

▷ Transcutaneous electrical nerve stimulation or TENS (also termed TNS)

TENS produces selected pulsed currents which are delivered cutaneously via electrode placement on the skin. These currents can activate specific nerve fibres potentially producing analgesic responses (Cheing et al. 2003a; Cheing 2003b). TENS is recognised as a treatment modality with minimal contraindications (Walsh 1997). The term AL-TENS is not commonly used in the UK. It involves switching between high and low frequency electrical stimulation and many TENS machines now do this. The term is more specific to stimulating acupuncture points.

▷ Interferential therapy

Interferential therapy can be described as the transcutaneous application of alternating medium-frequency electrical currents, and may be considered a form of TENS. Interferential therapy may be useful in pain relief, promoting healing and producing muscular contraction (Martin 1996).

▷ LASER

LASER is an acronym for light amplification by the stimulated emission of radiation. Therapeutic applications of low intensity or low level laser therapy at doses considered too low to effect any detectable heating of the tissue have been applied to treat musculoskeletal injury (Baxter 1996).

6.3.2 Methodological introduction

We looked for studies that investigated the efficacy and safety of electrotherapy (ultrasound, laser, transcutaneous electrical nerve stimulation [TENS, TNS, AL-TENS], pulsed shortwave diathermy, interferential therapy) vs no treatment, placebo or other interventions with respect to symptoms, function and quality of life in adults with osteoarthritis. Five systematic reviews and meta-analyses (Brosseau et al. 2006; Hulme et al. 2002; McCarthy et al. 2006; Osiri et al.

2000; Robinson et al. 2001) were found on electrotherapy (laser, electromagnetic fields, ultrasound and TENS) and six additional RCTs (Battisti et al. 2004; Cheing et al. 2002; Cheing and Hui-Chan 2004; Paker et al. 2006; Tascioglu et al. 2004; Yurtkuran et al. 2007) on electrotherapy (laser, electromagnetic fields and TENS). Due to the large volume of evidence, trials with a sample size of less than 40 were excluded.

The meta-analyses assessed the RCTs for quality and pooled data for the outcomes of symptoms and function. However, the outcomes of quality of life and adverse events (AEs) were not always reported. Results for quality of life have been taken from the individual RCTs included in this section.

▷ Ultrasound

One systematic review (SR)/meta-analysis (MA) (Robinson et al. 2001) was found on ultrasound in patients with knee or hip osteoarthritis. The MA included three RCTs (with N=294 participants) on comparisons between therapeutic ultrasound (continuous or pulsed) vs placebo or galvanic current or short wave diathermy (SWD). All RCTs were randomised and of parallel group design. Studies included in the analysis differed with respect to:

- comparison used (one RCT placebo – sham ultrasound; one RCT short wave diathermy; one RCT galvanic current)
- treatment regimen (stimulation frequency and intensity; placement of electrodes; lengths of stimulation time and how often TENS was applied)
- trial size, blinding, length, follow-up and quality.

▷ LASER

One SR/MA (Brosseau et al. 2006) and two RCTs (Tascioglu et al. 2004, Yurtkuran et al. 2007) were found that focused on laser therapy.

The MA (Brosseau 2006) included seven RCTs (with N=345 participants) on comparisons between laser therapy vs placebo in patients with osteoarthritis. All RCTs were randomised, double-blind and parallel group studies. Studies included in the analysis differed with respect to:

- site of osteoarthritis (four RCTs knee, one RCT thumb, one RCT hand, one RCT not specified)
- type of laser used (two RCTs He-Ne laser of 632.8 nm; one RCT space laser 904 nm; four RCTs Galenium-Arsenide laser – either 830 or 860 nm)
- treatment regimen (two RCTs two to three sessions/week; one RCT every day; one RCT twice a day; one RCT three times a week)
- trial size, length and quality.

The first RCT (Tascioglu et al. 2004) not in the systematic review focused on the outcomes of symptoms, function and AEs in N=60 patients with knee osteoarthritis. The RCT was a single blind, parallel group study and compared low-power laser treatment with placebo laser treatment (given once a day, five times a week) in a 10-day treatment phase with 6 months follow-up. The second RCT (Yurtkuran et al. 2007) not in the systematic review focused on the outcomes of symptoms, function and AEs in N=55 patients with knee osteoarthritis. The RCT was a triple blind, parallel group study and compared laser acupuncture (laser at acupuncture sites) and exercise with placebo laser acupuncture + exercise (given once a day, five times a week) in a 2-week treatment phase with 12 weeks follow-up.

▷ TENS

One SR/MA (Osiri et al. 2000) and three RCTs (Cheing et al. 2002; Cheing and Hui-Chan 2004; Paker et al. 2006) were found that focused on TENS.

The MA (Osiri 2000) included seven RCTs (with N=294 participants) that focused on comparisons between TENS and AL-TENS vs placebo in patients with knee osteoarthritis. Studies included in the analysis differed with respect to:

- type of TENS used (four RCTs high frequency TENS; one RCT strong burst TENS; one RCT high frequency and strong burst TENS; one RCT AL-TENS)
- treatment regimen (modes of stimulation, optimal stimulation levels, pulse frequencies, electrode placements, lengths of stimulation time and how often TENS was applied)
- trial size, blinding, length, follow-up and quality
- trial design (four RCTs were parallel-group studies; three RCTs were cross-over studies).

The three RCTs (Cheing et al. 2002; Cheing and Hui-Chan 2004; Paker et al. 2006) not in the systematic review were parallel studies that focused on the outcomes of symptoms, function and quality of life in patients with knee osteoarthritis. The two studies by Cheing et al (Cheing 2002, Cheing 2004) refer to the same RCT with different outcomes published in each paper. This RCT did not mention blinding or ITT analysis but was otherwise methodologically sound. AL-TENS was compared with placebo AL-TENS or exercise (all given 5 days a week) in N=66 patients in a 4-week treatment phase with 4 weeks follow-up. The second RCT (Paker et al. 2006) was methodologically sound (randomised and double-blind) and compared TENS (given 5 times a week) with intra-articular Hylan GF-20 injection (given once a week) in N=60 patients with knee osteoarthritis in a 3-week treatment phase with 6 months follow-up.

▷ PEMF

Two SRs/MAs (Hulme et al. 2002; McCarthy et al. 2006) were found on PEMF.

The first MA (Hulme et al. 2002) included three RCTs (with N=259 participants) that focused on comparisons between PEMF and placebo PEMF in patients with knee osteoarthritis. All RCTs were high quality, double-blind parallel group studies. Studies included in the analysis differed with respect to:

- type of electromagnetic field used and treatment regimen (two RCTs pulsed electromagnetic fields, PEMF, using a non-contact device delivering three signals ranging from 5–12 Hz frequency at 10 G to 25 G of magnetic energy. These used 9 hours of stimulation over a 1-month period; one RCT used a pulsed electric device delivering 100 Hz low-amplitude signal via skin surface electrodes for 6–10 hrs/day for 4 weeks)
- trial size and length.

The second MA (McCarthy et al. 2006) included five RCTs (with N=276 participants) that focused on comparisons between PEMF and placebo PEMF in patients with knee osteoarthritis. All RCTs were high quality, randomised, double-blind parallel group studies. Studies included in the analysis differed with respect to:

- type of electromagnetic field used and treatment regimen (two RCTs low frequency PEMF ranging from 3–50 Hz requiring long durations of treatment range 3–10 hrs/week; three RCTs used 'pulsed short wave' high frequency devices with shorter treatment durations)
- trial size and length.

6.3.3   Evidence statements: ultrasound

Table 6.36 Symptoms

Pain outcome	Reference	Intervention	Assessment time	Outcome/effect size
Knee or hip osteoarthritis				
Pain (VAS), change from baseline	1 SR/MA (Robinson et al. 2001) 1 RCT, N=74	Ultrasound vs placebo	4–6 weeks (end of therapy) and at 3 months (2 months post-treatment).	NS
Decrease in pain (VAS) change from baseline	1 SR/MA (Robinson et al. 2001) 1 RCT, N=120	Ultrasound vs galvanic current	3 weeks	WMD –5.10,% CI –9.52 to –0.68, p=0.02 Favours galvanic current
Pain (number of knees with subjective improvement), change from baseline; pain (number of knees with objective improvement), change from baseline	1 SR/MA (Robinson et al. 2001) 1 RCT, N=100	Ultrasound vs diathermy	Single assessment – immediate	NS
Decrease in pain (VAS) change from baseline	1 SR/MA (Robinson et al. 2001) 1 RCT, N=120	Ultrasound vs diathermy	Single assessment – immediate	NS

Table 6.37 Patient function

Function outcome	Reference	Intervention	Assessment time	Outcome/effect size
Knee or hip osteoarthritis				
Knee ROM (flexion and extension, degrees), change from baseline	1 SR/MA (Robinson et al. 2001) 1 RCT, N=74	Ultrasound vs placebo	4–6 weeks (end of therapy) and at 3 months (2 months post-treatment)	NS

Table 6.38 Global assessment

Global assessment outcome	Reference	Intervention	Assessment time	Outcome/effect size
Knee or hip osteoarthritis				
Patient and clinician global assessment (number of patients 'good' or 'excellent'), change from baseline	1 SR/MA (Robinson et al. 2001) 1 RCT, N=108	Ultrasound vs galvanic current	3 weeks	NS
Patient and clinician global assessment (number of patients 'good' or 'excellent'), change from baseline	1 SR/MA (Robinson et al. 2001) 1 RCT, N=120	Ultrasound vs diathermy	Single assessment – immediate	NS

6.3.4   Evidence statements: LASER

Table 6.39 Symptoms

Pain outcome	Reference	Intervention	Assessment time	Outcome/effect size
Knee				
Pain intensity at rest (VAS); pain intensity on activation (VAS); WOMAC pain	1 RCT (Tascioglu et al. 2004) (N=60)	Laser vs placebo laser	3 weeks and 6 months follow-up	NS
Pain (VAS); medical tenderness score	RCT (Yurtkuran et al. 2007) (N=55)	Laser acupuncture + exercise vs placebo laser acupuncture + exercise	2 Weeks (end of treatment) and 12 weeks (10 weeks post-treatment	NS
Mixed (Knee or hand or thumb or unspecified sites)				
Number of patients with no pain relief	1 MA (Brosseau et al. 2006)1 RCT, N=8	Laser vs placebo laser	Not mentioned	Peto OR 0.06,% CI0.00 to 0.88, p=0.04 Favours laser
Patient pain – different scales	1 MA (Brosseau et al. 2006)3 RCTs, N=145	Laser vs placebo laser	Not mentioned	Significant heterogeneity

Table 6.40 Stiffness

Stiffness outcome	Reference	Intervention	Assessment time	Outcome/effect size
Knee				
WOMAC stiffness	1 RCT (Tascioglu et al. 2004) (N=60)	Laser vs placebo laser	3 weeks and 6 months follow-up	NS

Table 6.41 Patient function

Function outcome	Reference	Intervention	Assessment time	Outcome/effect size
Knee				
WOMAC function	1 RCT (Tascioglu et al. 2004) (N=60)	Laser vs placebo laser	3 weeks and 6 months follow-up	NS
WOMAC total; 50-foot walk time	RCT (Yurtkuran et al. 2007) (N=55)	Laser acupuncture + exercise vs placebo laser acupuncture + exercise	2 weeks (end of treatment) and 12 weeks (10 weeks post-treatment	NS

Table 6.42 Global assessment

Global assessment outcome	Reference	Intervention	Assessment time	Outcome/effect size
Mixed (knee or hand or thumb or unspecified sites)				
Patient global assessment – improved	1 MA (Brosseau et al. 2006) 2 RCTs, N=110	Laser vs placebo laser	Not mentioned	NS
Number of patients improved on pain or global assessment	1 MA (Brosseau et al. 2006) 4 RCTs, N=147	Laser vs placebo laser	Not mentioned	NS

Table 6.43 Quality of life

QoL outcome	Reference	Intervention	Assessment time	Outcome/effect size
Knee				
Quality of life (NHP score)	RCT (Yurtkuran et al. 2007) (N=55)	Laser acupuncture + exercise vs placebo laser acupuncture + exercise	2 weeks (end of treatment) and 12 weeks (10 weeks post-treatment	NS

Table 6.44 Adverse events

AEs outcome	Reference	Intervention	Assessment time	Outcome/effect size
Knee				
Number of AEs	1 RCT (Tascioglu et al. 2004) (N=60)	Laser vs placebo laser	3 weeks and 6 months follow-up	Both groups same (N=0)

6.3.5   Evidence statements: TENS

Table 6.45 Symptoms

Pain outcome	Reference	Intervention	Assessment time	Outcome/effect size
TENS/AL-TENS				
Knee				
Pain relief (VAS)	1 MA (Osiri et al. 2000) 6 RCTs, N=264	TENS/AL-TENS vs Placebo	Study length: range single treatment to 9 weeks treatment; Follow-up: range immediate to 1 year	WMD −0.79, % CI −1.27 to −0.30, p=0.002 Favours TENS/AL-TENS

continued

Table 6.45 Symptoms – *continued*

Pain outcome	Reference	Intervention	Assessment time	Outcome/effect size
TENS				
Number of patients with pain improvement	1 MA (Osiri et al. 2000) 5 RCTs, N=214	TENS vs placebo	Study length: range single treatment to 9 weeks treatment; follow-up: range immediate to 1 year	Peto OR 3.91,% CI 2.13 to 7.17, p=0.00001 Favours TENS
Pain relief (VAS)	1 MA (Osiri et al. 2000) 5 RCTs, N=214	TENS vs placebo	Study length: range single treatment to 9 weeks treatment; Follow-up: range immediate to 1 year	Significant heterogeneity
WOMAC pain	1 RCT (Paker et al. 2006) (N=60)	TENS vs intra-articular Hylan GF-20	3 weeks (end of treatment) and 1 month and 6 months post-treatment.	NS
AL-TENS				
Pain at rest (pain intensity score, PPI)	1 MA (Osiri et al. 2000); 1 RCT (Yurt-kuran et al. 1999) (N=100)	AL-TENS vs ice massage	End of treatment (2 weeks)	NS
Pain relief (VAS)	1 MA (Osiri et al. 2000) 1 RCT, N=50	AL-TENS vs placebo	2 weeks (end of treatment)	WMD –0.80,% CI –1.39 to –0.21, p=0.007
Pain, VAS (difference between pre-and post-treatment scores)	1 RCT (Cheing et al. 2002) (N=66)	AL-TENS vs placebo (sham AL-TENS)	Day 1, 2 weeks (mid-treatment) and 4 weeks (end of treatment)	Day 1: –35.9 (AL-TENS) and –15.5 (sham) 2 weeks: –7.9 (AL-TENS) and +2.7 (sham) 4 weeks: –11.9 (AL-TENS) and –6.2 (sham) AL-TENS better
Pain, VAS (difference between pre-and post-treatment scores	1 RCT (Cheing et al. 2002) (N=66)	AL-TENS vs placebo (sham AL-TENS)	4 weeks post-treatment	–7.8 (AL-TENS) and –19.3 (sham) Placebo better
Pain, VAS (difference between pre-and post-treatment scores)	1 RCT (Cheing et al. 2002) (N=66)	AL-TENS vs exercise	Day 1, 4 weeks (end of treatment) and 4 weeks post-treatment	Day 1: -35.9 (AL-TENS) and +21.6 (exercise) 4 weeks: –11.9 (AL-TENS) and –7.6 (exercise) 4 weeks post-treatment: –7.8 (AL-TENS) and +42.0 (exercise) AL-TENS better
Pain, VAS (difference between pre-and post-treatment scores)	1 RCT (Cheing et al. 2002) (N=66)	AL-TENS vs exercise	2 weeks (mid-treatment)	2 weeks: –7.9 (AL-TENS) and –9.1 (exercise) Exercise better

Table 6.46 Stiffness

Pain outcome	Reference	Intervention	Assessment time	Outcome/effect size
Knee				
TENS/AL-TENS				
Knee stiffness	1 MA (Osiri et al. 2000) 2 RCTs, N=90	TENS/AL-TENS vs placebo	Immediate and 2 weeks (end of treatment)	WMD −6.02,% CI −9.07 to −2.96, p=0.0001 Favours TENS/AL-TENS
TENS				
WOMAC stiffness	1 RCT (Paker et al. 2006) (N=60)	TENS vs intra-articular Hylan GF-20	3 weeks (end of treatment	NS
WOMAC stiffness	1 RCT (Paker et al. 2006) (N=60)	TENS vs intra-articular Hylan GF-20	1 month post-treatment (p<0.007) and 6 months post-treatment (p<0.05)	1 month post-treatment (p<0.007) and 6 months post-treatment (p<0.05). Favours intra-articular Hylan
AL-TENS				
Knee stiffness	1 MA (Osiri et al. 2000) 1 RCT, N=50	AL-TENS vs placebo	2 weeks (end of treatment)	WMD −7.90,% CI −11.18 to −4.62, p<0.00001 Favours AL-TENS

Table 6.47 Patient function

Pain outcome	Reference	Intervention	Assessment time	Outcome/effect size
TENS/AL-TENS				
Knee				
Pain relief (VAS)	1 MA (Osiri et al. 2000) 6 RCTs, N=264	TENS/AL-TENS vs placebo	Study length: range single treatment to 9 weeks treatment; Followup: range immediate to 1 year	WMD −0.79,% CI −1.27 to −0.30, p=0.002 Favours TENS/AL-TENS
TENS				
Number of patients with pain improvement	1 MA (Osiri et al. 2000) 5 RCTs, N=214	TENS vs placebo	Study length: range single treatment to 9 weeks treatment; Followup: range immediate to 1 year	Peto OR 3.91,% CI 2.13 to 7.17, p=0.00001 Favours TENS
Pain relief (VAS)	1 MA (Osiri et al. 2000) 5 RCTs, N=214	TENS vs placebo	Study length: range single treatment to 9 weeks treatment; Followup: range immediate to 1 year	Significant heterogeneity

continued

Table 6.47 Patient function – *continued*

Pain outcome	Reference	Intervention	Assessment time	Outcome/effect size
TENS – *continued*				
Lequesne function	1 RCT (Paker et al. 2006) (N=60)	TENS vs intra-articular Hylan GF-20	3 weeks (end of treatment)	p<0.05 Favours TENS
WOMAC function	1 RCT (Paker et al. 2006) (N=60)	TENS vs intra-articular Hylan GF-20	3 weeks (end of treatment) and 1 month post-treatment	NS
Lequesne function	1 RCT (Paker et al. 2006) (N=60)	TENS vs intra-articular Hylan GF-20	1 and 6 months post-treatment	NS
Lequesne total	1 RCT (Pakeret al. 2006) (N=60)	TENS vs intra-articular Hylan GF-20	3 weeks (end of treatment) and 1 month and 6 months post-treatment	NS
WOMAC function	1 RCT (Paker et al. 2006) (N=60)	TENS vs intra-articular Hylan GF-20	6 months post-treatment	p<0.05 Intra-articular Hylan G-F20 better
AL-TENS				
50-foot walk time; quadriceps muscle strength (kg); Flexion (degrees)	1 MA (Osiri et al. 2000); 1 RCT Yurtkuran et al. 1999) (N=100)	AL-TENS vs ice massage	End of treatment (2 weeks)	NS
50-foot walking time (minutes)	1 MA (Osiri et al. 2000) 1 RCT, N=50	AL-TENS vs placebo	2 weeks (end of treatment)	WMD –22.60,% CI –43.01 to –2.19, p=0.03 Favours AL-TENS
Quadriceps muscle strength (kg)	1 MA (Osiri et al. 2000) 1 RCT, N=50	AL-TENS vs placebo	2 weeks (end of treatment)	WMD –5.20,% CI –7.85 to –2.55, p=0.0001 Favours AL-TENS
Knee flexion (degrees)	1 MA (Osiri et al. 2000) 1 RCT, N=50	AL-TENS vs placebo	2 weeks (end of treatment)	WMD –11.30,% CI –17.59 to –5.01, p=0.0004 Favours AL-TENS
Stride length (m) at 4 weeks	1 RCT (Cheing et al. 2002) (N=66)	AL-TENS vs placebo (sham AL-TENS)	4 weeks (end of treatment) and 4 weeks post-treatment	4 weeks: 1.06 (AL-TENS) and 1.02 (sham) 4 weeks post-treatment: 1.07 (AL-TENS) and 1.04 (sham) AL-TENS better
Cadence (steps/min)	1 RCT (Cheing et al. 2002) (N=66)	AL-TENS vs placebo (sham AL-TENS)	4 weeks (end of treatment) and 4 weeks post-treatment	4 weeks: 109 (AL-TENS) and 108 (sham) 4 weeks post-treatment: 110 (AL-TENS) and 107 (sham) AL-TENS better

continued

Table 6.47 Patient function – *continued*

Pain outcome	Reference	Intervention	Assessment time	Outcome/effect size
AL-TENS – *continued*				
Velocity (m/s) at 4 weeks	1 RCT (Cheing et al. 2002) (N=66)	AL-TENS vs placebo (sham AL-TENS)	4 weeks (end of treatment) and 4 weeks post-treatment	4 weeks: 0.97 (AL-TENS) and 0.92 (sham) 4 weeks post-treatment: 0.98 (AL-TENS) and 0.93 (sham)
				AL-TENS better
ROM during walking (degrees)	1 RCT (Cheing et al. 2002) (N=66)	AL-TENS vs placebo (sham AL-TENS)	4 weeks (end of treatment) and 4 weeks post-treatment	4 weeks: 51.8 (AL-TENS) and 51.5 (sham) 4 weeks post-treatment: 53.1 (AL-TENS) and 51.2 (sham) AL-TENS better
ROM at rest (degrees) at 4 weeks post-treatment (106 and 103 respectively).	1 RCT (Cheing et al. 2002) (N=66)	AL-TENS vs placebo (sham AL-TENS)	4 weeks post-treatment	106 (AL-TENS) and 103 (sham) AL-TENS better
ROM at rest (degrees)	1 RCT (Cheing et al. 2002) (N=66)	AL-TENS vs placebo (sham AL-TENS)	4 weeks, end of treatment	Both groups the same
Isometric peak torque of knee extensors and flexors at specified knee positions	1 RCT (Cheing et al. 2002) (N=66)	AL-TENS vs placebo (sham AL-TENS)	Day 1 2 weeks (mid-treatment), 4 weeks (end of treatment) and at 4 weeks post-treatment	NS
Stride length (m)	1 RCT (Cheing et al. 2002) (N=66)	AL-TENS vs placebo (sham AL-TENS)	Day 1 and 2 weeks, mid-treatment	Day 1: 0.95 (AL-TENS) and 0.99 (sham) 2 weeks: 1.01 (AL-TENS) and 1.02 (sham) Sham better
Cadence (steps/min) at velocity (m/s)	1 RCT (Cheing et al. 2002) (N=66)	AL-TENS vs placebo (sham AL-TENS)	Day 1 and 2 weeks, mid-treatment	Day 1: 100 (AL-TENS) and 103 (sham) 2 weeks: 105 (AL-TENS) and 108 (sham) Sham better
ROM during walking (degrees)	1 RCT (Cheing et al. 2002) (N=66)	AL-TENS vs placebo (sham AL-TENS)	Day 1 and 2 weeks, mid-treatment	Day 1: 50.3 (AL-TENS) and 51.3 (sham) 2 weeks: 51.7 (AL-TENS) and 52.3 (sham) Sham better

continued

Table 6.47 Patient function – *continued*				
Pain outcome	**Reference**	**Intervention**	**Assessment time**	**Outcome/effect size**
AL-TENS – *continued*				
ROM at rest (degrees)	1 RCT (Cheing et al. 2002) (N=66)	AL-TENS vs placebo (sham AL-TENS)	Day 1 and 2 weeks, mid-treatment	Day 1: 104 (AL-TENS) and 107 (sham) 2 weeks: 102 (AL-TENS) and 104 (sham) Sham better
Stride length (m)	1 RCT (Cheing et al. 2002) (N=66)	AL-TENS vs exercise	4 weeks, end of treatment and 4 weeks post-treatment	4 weeks: 1.06 (AL-TENS) and 1.03 (exercise) 4 weeks post-treatment: 1.07 (AL-TENS) and 1.03 (exercise) AL-TENS better
Cadence (steps/min)	1 RCT (Cheing et al. 2002) (N=66)	AL-TENS vs exercise	4 weeks, end of treatment and 4 weeks post-treatment	4 weeks: 109 (AL-TENS) and 104 (exercise) 4 weeks post-treatment: 110 (AL-TENS) and 107 (exercise) AL-TENS better
Velocity (m/s)	1 RCT (Cheing et al. 2002) (N=66)	AL-TENS vs exercise	4 weeks, end of treatment and 4 weeks post-treatment	4 weeks: 0.97 (AL-TENS) and 0.89 (exercise) 4 weeks post-treatment: 0.98 (AL-TENS) and 0.92 (exercise) AL-TENS better
ROM during walking (degrees)	1 RCT (Cheing et al. 2002) (N=66)	AL-TENS vs exercise	Day 1, 2 weeks (mid-treatment), 4 weeks (end of treatment) and 4 weeks post-treatment	Day 1: 50.3 (AL-TENS) and 48.7 (exercise) 2 weeks: 51.7 (AL-TENS) and 48.6 (exercise) 4 weeks: 51.8 (AL-TENS) and 48.7 (exercise) 4 weeks post-treatment: 53.1 (AL-TENS) and 48.3 (exercise) AL-TENS better
ROM at rest (degrees)	1 RCT (Cheing et al. 2002) (N=66)	AL-TENS vs exercise	4 weeks, end of treatment and 4 weeks post-treatment	4 weeks: 107 (AL-TENS) and 106 (exercise) 4 weeks post-treatment: 106 (AL-TENS) and 104 (exercise) AL-TENS better

continued

Table 6.47 Patient function – *continued*

Pain outcome	Reference	Intervention	Assessment time	Outcome/effect size
AL-TENS – *continued*				
Peak torque of knee extensors and flexors at specified knee positions	1 RCT (Cheing et al. 2002) (N=66)	AL-TENS vs exercise	Day 1, 2 weeks (mid-treatment), 4 weeks (end of treatment) and at 4 weeks post-treatment.	NS
Stride length (m)	1 RCT (Cheing et al. 2002) (N=66)	AL-TENS vs exercise	Day 1 and 2 weeks (mid-treatment)	Day 1: 0.95 (AL-TENS) and 1.00 (exercise) 2 weeks: 1.01 (AL-TENS) and 1.02 (exercise) Exercise better
Cadence (steps/min)	1 RCT (Cheing et al. 2002) (N=66)	AL-TENS vs exercise	Day 1 and 2 weeks (mid-treatment)	Day 1: 100 (AL-TENS) and 104 (exercise) 2 weeks: 105 (AL-TENS) and 106 (exercise) Exercise better
Velocity (m/s)	1 RCT (Cheing et al. 2002) (N=66)	AL-TENS vs exercise	Day 1 and 2 weeks (mid-treatment)	Day 1: 0.81 (AL-TENS) and 0.87 (exercise) 2 weeks: 0.89 (AL-TENS) and 0.90 (exercise) Exercise better
ROM at rest (degrees) at day 1 (104 and 105 respectively) and 2 weeks, mid-treatment (102 and 105 respectively)	1 RCT (Cheing et al. 2002) (N=66)	AL-TENS vs exercise	Day 1 and 2 weeks (mid-treatment)	Day 1: 104 (AL-TENS) and 105 (exercise) 2 weeks: 102 (AL-TENS) and 105 (exercise) Exercise better

Table 6.48 Quality of life

QoL outcome	Reference	Intervention	Assessment time	Outcome/effect size
Knee				
TENS				
SF-36 all dimensions	1 RCT (Paker et al. 2006) (N=60)	TENS vs intra-articular hylan GF-20	3 weeks (end of treatment 1 month and 6 months post-treatment	NS

Table 6.49 Study withdrawals

Withdrawals outcome	Reference	Intervention	Assessment time	Outcome/effect size
Knee				
TENS				
Number of withdrawals	1 RCT (Paker et al. 2006) (N=60)	TENS vs intra-articular hylan G-F20	6 months post-treatment	10% (TENS) and 17% (intra-articular hylan G-F20) TENS better
Number of withdrawals	1 RCT (Paker et al. 2006) (N=60)	TENS vs intra-articular hylan G-F20	6 months post-treatment	N=0 (TENS) and N=2 (intra-articular hylan G-F20) AL-TENS better

6.3.6 Evidence statements: PEMF

Table 6.50 Symptoms

Pain outcome	Reference	Intervention	Assessment time	Outcome/effect size
Knee				
PEMF				
Joint pain on motion	1 MA (Hulme et al. 2002)	PEMF vs placebo PEMF	4 weeks and 1 month	SMD: -0.59,% CI –0.98 to –2.0 Favours PEMF
Improvements in knee tenderness	MA (Hulme et al. 2002)	PEMF vs placebo PEMF	4 weeks and 1 month	SMD –0.91,% CI –1.20 to –0.62) Favours PEMF
Pain (ADL)	1 MA (Hulme et al. 2002)	PEMF vs placebo PEMF	4 weeks and 1 month	SMD –0.41,% CI –0.79 to –0.02 Favours PEMF
Pain (WOMAC and VAS)	1 MA (McCarthy et al. 2006) 5 RCTs, N=276	PEMF vs placebo PEMF	2–6 weeks	NS

Table 6.51 Stiffness

Stiffness outcome	Reference	Intervention	Assessment time	Outcome/effect size
Knee				
PEMF				
>15 minutes improvement in morning stiffness and 0–14 minutes improvement in morning stiffness.	1 MA (Hulme et al. 2002) 1 RCT, N=71	PEMF vs placebo PEMF	4 weeks and 1 month	NS

Table 6.52 Function

Function outcome	Reference	Intervention	Assessment time	Outcome/effect size
Knee				
PEMF				
Number of patients with 5 degrees improvement in flexion	1 MA (Hulme et al. 2002) 1 RCT, N=71	PEMF vs placebo PEMF	4 weeks and 1 month	OR 0.27,% CI 0.09 to 0.82, p=0.02 Favours PEMF
Difficulty (ADL)	MA (Hulme et al. 2002)	PEMF vs placebo PEMF	4 weeks and 1 month	SMD −0.71,% CI −1.11 to −0.31 Favours PEMF
Number of patients with 0–4 degrees improvement in flexion	1 MA (Hulme et al. 2002) 1 RCT, N=71	PEMF vs placebo PEMF	4 weeks and 1 month	Favours PEMF
Function (WOMAC and AIMS)	1 MA (McCarthy et al. 2006) 5 RCTs, N=228	PEMF vs placebo PEMF	2–6 weeks	NS

Table 6.53 Global assessment

Global assessment outcome	Reference	Intervention	Assessment time	Outcome/effect size
Knee				
PEMF				
Physician's global assessment	1 MA (Hulme et al. 2002) 1 RCT, N=71	PEMF vs placebo PEMF	4 weeks and 1 month	SMD −0.71,% CI −1.11 to −0.31 Favours PEMF
Patient's global assessment	1 MA (McCarthy et al. 2006) 2 RCTs, N=108	PEMF vs placebo PEMF	2–6 weeks	NS

Table 6.54 Quality of life

QoL assessment outcome	Reference	Intervention	Assessment time	Outcome/effect size
Knee				
PEMF				
Improvement in EuroQoL perception of health status	1 MA (Hulme et al. 2002) 1 RCT (Pipitone and Scott 2001), N=75	PEMF vs placebo PEMF	6 weeks (end of treatment)	SMD –0.71,% CI –1.11 to –0.31 Favours PEMF
AIMS score	1 MA (McCarthy et al. 2006) 1 RCT (Callaghan et al. 2005), N=27	PEMF vs placebo PEMF	2 weeks (end of treatment)	+0.3 (low and high dose PEMF) and –0.2 (placebo PEMF) PEMF better
Pattern of change in GHQ score over time	1 MA (McCarthy et al. 2006) 1 RCT (Klaber Moffett et al. 1996), N=90	PEMF vs placebo PEMF	Over 12 weeks (8 weeks post-treatment)	NS

Table 6.55 Adverse events

AEs assessment outcome	Reference	Intervention	Assessment time	Outcome/effect size
Knee				
PEMF				
Number of patients with AEs	1 MA (McCarthy et al. 2006) 1 RCT (Pipitone and Scott 2001), N=75	PEMF vs placebo PEMF	6 weeks (end of treatment)	2.7% (PEMF) and 5.3% placebo PEMF Favours PEMF
Adverse skin reactions	1 MA (Hulme et al. 2002) 1 RCT, N=71	PEMF vs placebo PEMF	4 weeks and 1 month	NS
Number of patients with mild AEs	1 MA (McCarthy et al. 2006) 1 RCT (Thamsborg et al. 2005), N=90	PEMF vs placebo PEMF	2 weeks (mid-teatment)	13.3% (PEMF) and 6.7% (placebo PEMF) Placebo better

Table 6.56 Study withdrawals

Withdrawals outcome	Reference	Intervention	Assessment time	Outcome/effect size
Knee				
PEMF				
Total withdrawals	1 MA (Hulme et al. 2002) 3 RCTs, N=184	PEMF vs placebo PEMF	4 weeks and 1 month	NS

6.3.7 From evidence to recommendations

Studies had varying methodological quality and detail on treatment dosages. There was evidence that ultrasound provided no benefits beyond placebo ultrasound or other electrotherapy agents in the treatment of knee and hip osteoarthritis (Robinson et al. 2001). There was no evidence for the benefit of LASER for pain relief at mixed sites of osteoarthritis from a systematic review (Brosseau et al. 2000), but a recent study (Yurtkuran et al. 2007) suggests a benefit of LASER at acupuncture points in reducing knee swelling. Evidence for the benefits of pulsed electromagnetic field for osteoarthritis was limited in knee osteoarthritis (McCarthy et al. 2006). In the hip and hand no studies were identified. Ultrasound, LASER and pulsed electromagnetic field are well suited for small joints such as hand and foot, but there is insufficient evidence to support their efficacy or clinical effectiveness in osteoarthritis. Further research would be helpful in these areas because it is not clear if efficacy or safety can be extrapolated from knee studies, and a research recommendation is included on this area. Given that there is no evidence on harm caused by laser, ultrasound or pulsed electromagnetic fields, the GDG have not made a negative recommendation on these.

There is evidence that TENS is clinically beneficial for pain relief and reduction of stiffness in knee osteoarthritis, especially in the short term. However, this was not shown in a community setting. There is no evidence that efficacy tails off over time, or that periodic use for exacerbations is helpful. Proper training for people with osteoarthritis in the placing of pads and selection of stimulation intensity could make a difference to the benefit they obtain. Good practice guidance recommends an assessment visit with the health professional with proper training in the selection of stimulation intensity (for example, low intensity, once a day, 40 minutes duration, 80Hz 140 microseconds pulse) with reinforcement with an instruction booklet. People with osteoarthritis should be encouraged to experiment with intensities and duration of application if the desired relief of symptoms is not initially achieved. This enables patients control of their symptoms as part of a self-management approach. A further follow-up visit is essential in allowing the health professional to check patients' usage of TENS and problem solve. No adverse events or toxicity have been reported with TENS. Contraindications include active implants (pacemakers, devices with batteries giving active medication); the contraindication of the first 3 months of pregnancy is currently under review (CSP guidelines). Although adverse events from TENS such as local skin reactions and allergies to the adhesive pads are known, they are rare.

As with all therapies adjunctive to the core treatments (see Fig 3.2), it is important that the individual with osteoarthritis is able to assess the benefit they obtain from electrotherapy and take part in treatment decisions.

RECOMMENDATION

R14   Healthcare professionals should consider the use of transcutaneous electrical nerve stimulation (TENS) as an adjunct to core treatment for pain relief.[*]

---

[*] TENS machines are generally loaned to the patient by the NHS for a short period, and if effective the patient is advised where they can purchase their own. There is therefore very little cost to the NHS associated with the use of TENS.

6.4 Acupuncture

6.4.1 Clinical introduction

The Chinese discovered acupuncture about 2000 years ago, and their explanation of how it works has changed over time, as world views evolved. In the 1950s, all these explanations were combined into the system currently known as 'traditional Chinese acupuncture'. This approach uses concepts that cannot be explained by conventional physiology, but remains the most common form of acupuncture practised throughout the world. In the UK, doctors and physiotherapists are increasingly using acupuncture on the basis of neurophysiological mechanisms, known as 'Western medical acupuncture', whereas acupuncturists outside the NHS tend to use traditional Chinese acupuncture, and sometimes add Chinese herbs.

Acupuncture involves treatment with needles, and is most commonly used for pain relief. Typically, about six needles are placed near the painful area and possibly elsewhere. They will be either manipulated to produce a particular 'needle sensation', or stimulated electrically (electroacupuncture) for up to 20 minutes. Some practitioners also use moxa, a dried herb which is burned near the point to provide heat. A course of treatment usually consists of six or more sessions during which time, if a response occurs, pain relief gradually accumulates. The response of individuals is variable, for reasons that are not well understood but may be related to differences in activity of opioid receptors.

The potential mechanisms of action of acupuncture are complex in terms of neurophysiology, and involve various effects including the release of endogenous opioids.

Research into acupuncture has also proved complex. As with surgery and physiotherapy, it is impossible to blind the practitioner, and difficult to blind the participant. Sham acupuncture is usually done by putting needles in the wrong site and not stimulating them, but there is some doubt whether this is a completely inactive 'placebo'. Blunt, retractable sham needles have been devised, but even these stimulate the limbic system and might have some activity in reducing pain.

6.4.2 Methodological introduction

We looked at studies that investigated the efficacy and safety of acupuncture compared with placebo (sham acupuncture) and other interventions with respect to symptoms, function, and quality of life in adults with osteoarthritis. One systematic review and meta-analysis (White et al. 2007) and 12 additional RCTs (Dickens and Lewith 1989, Fink et al. 2001, Gaw et al. 1975, Haslam 2001, Junnila 1982, McIndoe and Young 1995, Salim 1996, Stener et al. 2004, Tillu et al. 2001, Tillu et al. 2002, Witt et al. 2006, Yurtkuran and Kocagil 1999) were found that addressed the question. Six RCTs (McIndoe and Young 1995, Junnila 1982, Stener et al. 2004, Salim 1996, Tillu et al. 2002, Haslam 2001) were excluded due to methodological limitations.

The systematic review and meta-analysis (White et al. 2007) focused on acupuncture and electroacupuncture vs true sham acupuncture in people with knee osteoarthritis. The MA included eight RCTs (with N=2362 participants). All RCTs were high quality. Studies included in the analysis differed with respect to:
- interventions and comparisons
- study size and trial length.

The six included RCTs were similar in terms of trial design: all were randomised parallel group studies and all were methodologically sound. They differed with respect to:

- sample size, blinding, length of treatment and follow-up periods
- osteoarthritis site (two RCTs knee, one RCT hip, one RCT thumb, one RCT hip and knee and one RCT mixed sites)
- interventions and comparisons.

6.4.3 Evidence statements

Table 6.57 Symptoms: pain

Pain outcome	Reference	Intervention	Assessment time	Outcome/effect size
Knee osteoarthritis				
Acupuncture vs sham/no treatment				
WOMAC pain (outlier study removed to remove heterogeneity)	1MA (White et al. 2007) 4 RCTs, N=1246	Acupuncture vs sham acupuncture	Short term (up to 25 weeks)	WMD 0.87,% CI 0.40 to 1.34, p=0.0003
WOMAC pain	1MA (White et al. 2007) 3 RCTs, N=1178	Acupuncture vs sham acupuncture	Long term (up to 52 weeks)	WMD 0.54,% CI 0.05 to 1.04, p<0.05
WOMAC pain	1MA (White et al. 2007) 2 RCTs, N=403	Acupuncture vs true sham acupuncture	Short term (up to 25 weeks)	Significant heterogeneity
WOMAC pain	1MA (White et al. 2007) 4 RCTs, N=927	Acupuncture vs no additional treatment	Short term (up to 25 weeks)	WMD 3.42,% CI 2.58 to 4.25, p<0.05
WOMAC pain	1MA (White et al. 2007)	Acupuncture vs other sham treatment (sham TENS)	Short term (up to 25 weeks)	Insufficient data
WOMAC pain	1MA (White et al. 2007)	Acupuncture vs other sham treatment (sham AL-TENS or education)	Short term (up to 25 weeks)	Insufficient data
Unilateral acupuncture vs bilateral acupuncture				
Pain (VAS)	1 RCT (Tillu et al. 2001 2207)	Unilateral acupuncture vs bilateral acupuncture	2 weeks and at 4.5 months post-intervention.	NS
Electroacupuncture vs ice massage				
Pain at rest, PPI scale of 1–5	1 RCT (Yurtkuran and Kocagil 1999)	Electroacupuncture vs ice massage	2 weeks (end of treatment)	NS
Electroacupuncture vs AL-TENS				
Pain at rest PPI scale of 1–5	1 RCT (Yurtkuran and Kocagil 1999)	Electroacupuncture vs AL-TENS	2 weeks (end of treatment)	NS

continued

Table 6.57 Symptoms: pain – *continued*

Pain outcome	Reference	Intervention	Assessment time	Outcome/effect size
Hip				
Acupuncture vs sham acupuncture				
Pain intensity (VAS)	1 RCT (Fink et al. 2001) (N=67)	Acupuncture vs placebo (sham acupuncture)	1 week, 6 weeks and 6 months post-intervention.	NS
Thumb				
Acupuncture vs mock TNS				
Pain reduction, VAS (change from baseline and change from end-of treatment scores)	1 RCT (Dickens and Lewis 1989) (N=13)	Acupuncture was better than placebo (mock TNS)	2 weeks post-intervention	Acupuncture better
Pain reduction, VAS (change from baseline)	1 RCT (Dickens and Lewis 1989) (N=13)	Acupuncture was better than placebo (mock TNS)	2 weeks post-intervention	NS
Pain reduction, VAS (change from baseline)	1 RCT (Dickens and Lewis 1989) (N=13)	Acupuncture was better than placebo (mock TNS)	End of treatment	Acupuncture worse
Knee or hip				
Acupuncture vs no acupuncture				
WOMAC pain (change from baseline)	1 RCT (Witt et al. 2006) (N=712)	Acupuncture vs no acupuncture	3 months, end of treatment	Mean change 43.7% (acupuncture) and 6.2% (no acupuncture), p<0.001
Mixed (knee, hip, finger, lumbar, thoracic or cervical)				
Acupuncture vs sham acupuncture				
Pain (patient's assessment, scale 1–4, change from baseline) and tenderness (physician's evaluation, scale 1–4, change from baseline)	1 RCT (Gaw et al. 1975) (N=40)	Acupuncture vs placebo (sham acupuncture)	End of treatment (8 weeks) and at 2 weeks and 6 weeks post-intervention	NS

Table 6.58 Symptoms: stiffness

Stiffness outcome	Reference	Intervention	Assessment time	Outcome/effect size
Knee osteoarthritis				
Electroacupuncture vs Ice massage				
Stiffness (verbal rating)	1 RCT (Yurtkuran and Kocagil 1999)	Electroacupuncture vs ice massage	2 weeks (end of treatment)	NS
Electroacupuncture vs AL-TENS				
Stiffness (verbal rating)	1 RCT (Yurtkuran and Kocagil 1999)	Electroacupuncture vs AL-TENS	2 weeks (end of treatment)	NS
Knee or hip				
Acupuncture vs no acupuncture				
WOMAC stiffness (change from baseline)	1 RCT (Witt et al. 2006) (N=712)	Acupuncture vs no acupuncture	3 months, end of treatment	Mean change 31.7% (acupuncture) and 1.5% (no acupuncture), p<0.001
Mixed (knee, hip, finger, lumbar, thoracic or cervical)				
Acupuncture vs sham acupuncture				
Pain (patient's assessment, scale 1–4, change from baseline) and tenderness (physician's evaluation, scale 1–4, change from baseline)	1 RCT (Gaw et al. 1975) (N=40)	Acupuncture vs placebo (sham acupuncture)	End of treatment (8 weeks) and at 2 weeks and 6 weeks post-intervention	NS

Table 6.59 Symptoms: function and stiffness

Function outcome	Reference	Intervention	Assessment time	Outcome/effect size
Knee osteoarthritis				
Acupuncture vs sham/no treatment				
WOMAC function – outlier study removed to remove heterogeneity	1MA (White et al. 2007) 4 RCTs, N=1245	Acupuncture vs sham acupuncture	Short term (up to 25 weeks)	WMD 2.41,% CI 0.60 to 4.21, p=0.009 Favours acupuncture
WOMAC function	1MA (White et al. 2007) 3 RCTs, N=1178	Acupuncture vs sham acupuncture	Long term (up to 52 weeks)	WMD 2.01,% CI 0.36 to 3.66, p<0.05 Favours acupuncture
WOMAC function	1MA (White et al. 2007) 2 RCTs, N=403	Acupuncture vs true sham acupuncture	Short term (up to 25 weeks)	Significant heterogeneity

continued

Table 6.59 Symptoms: function and stiffness – *continued*

Function outcome	Reference	Intervention	Assessment time	Outcome/effect size
Knee osteoarthritis				
Acupuncture vs sham/no treatment – *continued*				
WOMAC function	1MA (White et al. 2007) 3 RCTs, N=907	Acupuncture vs no additional treatment	Short term (up to 25 weeks)	Significant heterogeneity
WOMAC function	1MA (White et al. 2007)	Acupuncture vs other sham treatment (sham TENS)	Short term (up to 25 weeks)	Insufficient data
WOMAC function	1MA (White et al 2007)	Acupuncture vs other sham treatment (sham AL-TENS or education)	Short term (up to 25 weeks)	Insufficient data
Unilateral acupuncture vs bilateral acupuncture				
Hospital for special surgery knee score, HSS (composite outcomes, max. score 100); 50 m walk time (seconds); 20 stair climb time (seconds)	1 RCT (Tillu et al. 2001 2207)	Unilateral acupuncture vs bilateral acupuncture	2 weeks and at 4.5 months post-intervention.	NS
Electroacupuncture vs Ice massage				
50-foot walk time (seconds); quadriceps muscle strength; active knee flexion (degrees)	1 RCT (Yurtkuran and Kocagil 1999)	Electroacupuncture vs Ice massage	2 weeks (end of treatment)	NS
Electroacupuncture vs AL-TENS				
50-foot walk time (seconds); quadriceps muscle strength; active knee flexion (degrees)	1 RCT (Yurtkuran and Kocagil 1999)	Electroacupuncture vs AL-TENS	2 weeks (end of treatment)	NS
Hip				
Acupuncture vs sham acupuncture				
Lequesne function	1 RCT (Fink et al. 2001) (N=67)	Acupuncture vs placebo (sham acupuncture)	1 week, 6 weeks and 6 months post-intervention.	NS

continued

Table 6.59 Symptoms: function and stiffness – *continued*

Function outcome	Reference	Intervention	Assessment time	Outcome/effect size
Thumb				
Acupuncture vs mock TNS				
Function score at end of treatment (change from baseline and change from end of treatment scores); pinch grip and joint tenderness	1 RCT (Dickens and Lewis 1989) (N=13)	Acupuncture vs placebo (mock TNS)	End of treatment and 2 weeks post-intervention	NS
Knee or hip				
Acupuncture vs no acupuncture				
WOMAC total (change from baseline)	1 RCT (Witt et al. 2006) (N=712)	Acupuncture vs no acupuncture	3 months, end of treatment	Mean change 37.3% (acupuncture) and 2.8% (no acupuncture), p<0.001 Favours acupuncture
WOMAC function (change from baseline)	1 RCT (Witt et al. 2006) (N=712)	Acupuncture vs no acupuncture	3 months, end of treatment	Mean change 35.8% (acupuncture) and 2.5% (no acupuncture), p<0.001 Favours acupuncture
Mixed (knee, hip, finger, lumbar, thoracic or cervical)				
Acupuncture vs sham acupuncture				
Activity (patient's evaluation, scale 1–4, change from baseline)	1 RCT (Gaw et al. 1975) (N=40)	Acupuncture vs placebo (sham acupuncture)	End of treatment (8 weeks) and at 2 weeks and 6 weeks post-intervention	NS

Table 6.60 Global assessment

Global assessment outcome	Reference	Intervention	Assessment time	Outcome/effect size
Hip				
Acupuncture vs sham acupuncture				
Patient's overall assessment of satisfaction (Carlsson comparative scale)	1 RCT (Fink et al. 2001) (N=67)	Acupuncture vs placebo (sham acupuncture)	6 weeks post-intervention	NS
Patient's overall assessment of satisfaction (Carlsson comparative scale)	1 RCT (Fink et al. 2001) (N=67)	Acupuncture vs placebo (sham acupuncture)	6 months post-intervention	Score: 105 (acupuncture) and 98 (sham) Acupuncture better

Table 6.61 Quality of life

QoL outcome	Reference	Intervention	Assessment time	Outcome/effect size
Hip				
Acupuncture vs sham acupuncture				
QoL (Bullinger's Everyday Life questionnaire)	1 RCT (Fink et al. 2001) (N=67)	Acupuncture vs placebo (sham acupuncture)	1 week, 6 weeks and 6 months post-intervention	NS
Knee or hip				
Acupuncture vs no acupuncture				
SF-36 physical (change from baseline)	1 RCT (Witt et al. 2006) (N=712)	Acupuncture vs no acupuncture	3 months, end of treatment	Mean change 6.1 (acupuncture) and 0.6 (no acupuncture) p<0.001 Favours acupuncture
SF-36 mental (change from baseline)	1 RCT (Witt et al. 2006) N=712	Acupuncture vs no acupuncture	3 months, end of treatment	Mean change 1.3 (acupuncture) and −0.3 (no acupuncture) p<0.045 Favours acupuncture

Table 6.62 Adverse events: mixed (knee, hip, finger, thoracic or cervical)

AEs outcome	Reference	Intervention	Assessment time	Outcome/effect size
Mixed (knee, hip, finger, lumbar, thoracic or cervical)				
Acupuncture vs sham acupuncture				
Number of AEs	1 RCT (Gaw et al. 1975) (N=40)	Acupuncture vs placebo (sham acupuncture)	8 weeks	N=2 (acupuncture) and N=1 (sham) Similar in both groups

Table 6.63 Withdrawals

Withdrawals outcome	Reference	Intervention	Assessment time	Outcome/effect size
Knee osteoarthritis				
Unilateral acupuncture vs bilateral acupuncture				
Number of withdrawals	1 RCT (Tillu et al. 2001 2207)	Unilateral acupuncture vs bilateral acupuncture	6 months (4.5 months post-treatment)	N=4 18% (unilateral) and N=2, 9% (bilateral) Unilateral worse

continued

Table 6.63 Withdrawals – *continued*

Withdrawals outcome	Reference	Intervention	Assessment time	Outcome/effect size
Hip				
Acupuncture vs sham acupuncture				
Number of withdrawals	1 RCT (Fink et al. 2001) (N=67)	Acupuncture vs placebo (sham acupuncture)	6 months post-treatment	48% (acupuncture) and 29% (sham), Acupuncture worse
Thumb				
Acupuncture vs mock TNS				
Number of withdrawals	1 RCT (Dickens and Lewis 1989) (N=13)	Acupuncture vs placebo (mock TNS)	2 weeks (end of treatment)	N=0 (acupuncture) and N=1 (mock TNS) Both groups similar

Table 6.64 Other outcomes

Other outcome	Reference	Intervention	Assessment time	Outcome/effect size
Knee or hip				
Acupuncture vs no acupuncture				
Proportion of responders (≥50% reduction in WOMAC total)	1 RCT (Witt et al. 2006) (N=712)	Acupuncture vs no acupuncture	3 months, end of treatment	34.5% (acupuncture) and 6.5% (no acupuncture) p<0.001 Favours acupuncture
Thumb				
Acupuncture vs mock TNS				
Number of patients reporting verbal rating of improvement	1 RCT (Dickens and Lewis 1989) (N=13)	Acupuncture vs placebo (mock TNS)	2 weeks (end of treatment)	85.7% (acupuncture) and 40% (mock TNS) Both groups similar

6.4.4   Health economic evidence statements

We looked at studies that conducted economic evaluations involving electrotherapy and acupuncture. One paper suitable for evidence statements was found.

One German paper (Witt et al. 2006a) was found which addressed the cost effectiveness of acupuncture in patients with headache, low back pain and osteoarthritis of the hip and knee. The study does not give precise data on the costs and utility of the acupuncture programme, but instead concentrates on the incremental cost-effectiveness ratio, which for osteoarthritis patients was €17,845 per additional QALY compared with the control group. Acupuncture was concluded to be less cost effective for osteoarthritis patients compared with patients with headache and low back pain. This suggests that acupuncture along with usual care is cost effective compared with usual care alone for a 3-month time period, from the societal perspective. The cost year was not reported in the study

The overall study was large (304,674 patients) but the number of OA patients included in the economic analysis was much smaller (421 patients). The study adopted a societal perspective, but no further details are given on this. Because of this the results can only be interpreted from a societal perspective, which presumably includes costs which are not relevant for the healthcare payer perspective which is used by NICE.

It is of note that a study analysing the cost effectiveness of long-term outcomes following acupuncture treatment for osteoarthritis of the knee is being funded as one of the National Institutes of Health (NIH) Center of Research in Alternative Medicine core projects.

6.4.5 From evidence to recommendations

There is a fairly extensive evidence base, and for pragmatic reasons, the GDG considered only those studies with sample size greater than 40. The studies are evenly divided between acupuncture and electro-acupuncture, mostly using a comparison of sham acupuncture where a needle does not pierce the skin. This is a widely accepted placebo in studies of acupuncture. Trial participants cannot feel a difference between acupuncture and electro-acupuncture so this comparison should be well controlled.

The results from acupuncture studies are mixed. Certainly the studies which have shown superiority of acupuncture over placebo have shown this only in the short term (6–12 weeks). At 26 weeks there are few studies, and overall they do not support a benefit over placebo. It therefore seems likely that acupuncture can provide short- to medium-term relief for some people. Acupuncture of peripheral joints appears safe. The question that remains unclear is whether a specific group of people with osteoarthritis, who will particularly benefit from acupuncture, can be identified. A research recommendation is made in section 9 to this effect.

The health economic literature is limited and not based in the UK NHS or similar healthcare systems. Acupuncture was therefore included in the cost-consequence table (see Appendix C available online at www.rcplondon.ac.uk/pubs/brochure.aspx?e=242). The incremental cost-effectiveness ratio for acupuncture is often higher than the threshold of £20–£30K per QALY that is typically quoted as what the NHS can afford. However, there is considerable uncertainty about this estimate because of the limitations in the data. However, electro-acupuncture was consistently above the threshold of cost effectiveness.

RECOMMENDATION

R15   Electro-acupuncture should not be used to treat people with osteoarthritis.*

---

* There is not enough consistent evidence of clinical or cost-effectiveness to allow a firm recommendation on the use of acupuncture for the treatment of osteoarthritis.

6.5 Aids and devices

6.5.1 Clinical introduction

Walking aids are commonly prescribed for hip and knee OA and their mechanism of efficacy is assumed to be via a biomechanical effect. Chan et al. conducted a small trial of cane use (on either side) and examined walking speed and cadence as mediators of effect (Chan and Smith 2005). Van der Esch et al. identified that 44% of an OA cohort possessed a walking aid (commonly canes), and that being older and greater pain and disability were determinants of use (Van der Esch et al. 2003). Non-use is associated with negative views of walking aids, suggesting that careful attention is needed to clients' attitudes to cane use.

People with more severe hip and knee OA are commonly provided with or obtain long-handled reachers, personal care aids (for example, sock aids to reduce bending), bath aids, chair and bed raisers, raised toilet seats, perch stools, half steps and grab rails, additional stair rails and may also have home adaptations to improve access internally and externally. Wielandt et al. highlighted the importance of carefully matching assistive devices to the patients' needs (Wielandt et al. 2006). Factors significantly associated with assistive technology (AT) non-use are: poor perceptions of AT and their benefits; anxiety; poor ability to recall AT training; poor perception of disability/illness; and lack of choice during the selection process. Many people do obtain AT without professional advice and may waste money if their choice is inappropriate due to lack of information.

Splints are commonly used for hand problems, especially OA of the thumb base. Practical advice is given to balance activity and rest during hand use; to avoid *repetitive* grasp, pinch and twisting motions; and to use appropriate assistive devices to reduce effort in hand function (for example, using enlarged grips for writing, using small non-slip mats for opening objects, electric can openers).

6.5.2 Methodological introduction

▷ Footwear, bracing and walking aids

We looked for studies that investigated the efficacy and safety of aids and devices compared with other aids and devices or no intervention/usual care with respect to symptoms, function and quality of life. One Cochrane systematic review and meta-analysis (Brouwer et al. 2005) was found on braces and insoles and 20 additional RCTs (Baker et al. 2007; Berry 1992; Brouwer et al. 2006; Chan and Smith 2005; Cushnaghan et al. 1994; Hinman et al. 2003a, 2003b; Huang et al. 2006; Nigg et al. 2006; Pham et al. 2004; Quilty et al. 2003; Richards 2005; Toda et al. 2004, 2005; Toda and Tsukimura 2004a, 2004b, 2006; Wajon et al. 2005; Weiss and Ada 2000, 2004) were found on shoes, insoles, canes, braces, strapping, splinting and taping. Two of these studies (Toda and Tsukimura 2004, 2006) were reports of the same RCT, showing mid-study results (Toda 2004) and end-of-study results (Toda and Tsukimura 2006). One study (Pham et al. 2004) reports the long-term results of an RCT (Maillefert and Hudry 2001) (mid-study results) that was included in the Cochrane systematic review. Five RCTs (Berry 1992; Hinman et al. 2003; Huang et al. 2006; Richards 2005; Weiss 2004) were excluded due to methodological limitations. Therefore overall 12 RCTs were found in addition to the Cochrane review.

The Cochrane MA (Brouwer et al. 2005) included four RCTs (with N=444 participants) on insoles and braces in people with knee osteoarthritis. Studies were all randomised, parallel-group design but were inadequately blinded (single blind or blinding not mentioned). The RCTs included in the analysis differed with respect to:

- interventions and comparisons
- trial size, length, follow-up and quality.

The Cochrane meta-analysis assessed the RCTs for quality and pooled together all data for the outcomes of symptoms and function. However, the outcome of quality of life was not reported because quality of life was not assessed by the individual RCTs included in this systematic review.

The 13 RCTs not included in the Cochrane systematic review differed with respect to:

- osteoarthritis site (11 RCTs knee 2 RCTs thumb)
- interventions and comparisons
- trial size, blinding, length and follow-up.

▷ Assistive devices

We looked for studies that investigated the efficacy and safety of assistive devices vs no devices with respect to symptoms, function and quality of life in adults with osteoarthritis. One RCT (Stamm et al. 2002) was found on assistive devices and assessed the outcomes of pain and function. Four additional observational studies (Mann et al. 1995; Tallon et al. 2000; Sutton et al. 2002; Veitiene and Tamulaitiene 2005) were found on usage and assessment of the effectiveness of assistive devices.

The included RCT was a randomised, single-blind parallel group study.

The four observational studies differed with respect to osteoarthritis site, study design, sample size and outcomes measured.

6.5.3 Evidence statements: footwear, bracing and walking aids

Table 6.65 Symptoms: pain

Pain outcome	Reference	Intervention	Assessment time	Outcome/effect size
Knee				
Brace				
Pain on function (6 minute walk test, 30 second stair-climb test).	1 MA (Brouwer et al. 2005) 1 RCT, N=119	Knee brace vs neoprene sleeve	6 months	Knee brace better
Pain on function (6 minute walk test, 30 second stair-climb test)	1 MA (Brouwer et al. 2005) 1 RCT, N=119	Knee brace vs medical treatment	6 months	Knee brace better
Pain on function (6 minute walk test, 30 second stair-climb test)	1 MA (Brouwer et al. 2005) 1 RCT, N=119	Neoprene sleeve vs medical treatment	6 months	Neoprene sleeve better

continued

Table 6.65 Symptoms: pain – *continued*

Pain outcome	Reference	Intervention	Assessment time	Outcome/effect size
Knee				
Brace – *continued*				
Pain severity (VAS)	1 RCT (Brouwer et al. 2006) (N-=118)	Knee brace + conservative treatment vs control (conservative treatment)	3 months, 6 months 12 months or overall	NS
Insoles				
WOMAC pain	1 MA (Brouwer et al. 2005) 1 RCT, N=147	Laterally wedged insole vs neutrally wedged insole	1 month, 3 months and 6 months follow-up	NS
WOMAC pain; overall pain (VAS); clinical improvement in WOMAC pain (score ≥50 points); Pain improvement in patients with KL grade 4 compared with KL grade <4; pain improvement in patients with BMI <30 kg/m^2 compared with patients with BMI ≥30 kg/m^2	1 RCT (Baker et al. 2007) (N=90)	Laterally wedged insole vs neutrally wedged insole	6 weeks (end of treatment)	NS
Pain (VAS)	1 MA (Brouwer et al. 2005) 1 RCT, N=90	Subtalar strapped insole vs inserted insole	8 weeks	NS
WOMAC pain (change from baseline)	1 RCT (Pham et al. 2004) (N=156)	Laterally wedged insole vs neutrally wedged insole	2 years (end of treatment)	NS
Taping				
Daily pain, VAS	1 RCT (Cushnaghan et al. 1994) (N=14)	Medial taping vs neutral taping	4 days, end of treatment	p<0.05 Favours medial taping
Patient's change scores (number of patients 'better')	1 RCT (Cushnaghan et al. 1994) (N=14)	Medial taping vs neutral taping	4 days, end of treatment	p<0.05 Favours medial taping
Pain on standing, VAS (change from baseline)	1 RCT (Cushnaghan et al. 1994) (N=14)	Medial taping vs neutral taping	6 months, end of treatment	−1.2 (medial) and −0.3 (neutral) Medial taping better
Daily pain, VAS	1 RCT (Cushnaghan et al. 1994) (N=14)	Medial taping vs lateral taping	4 days, end of treatment	p<0.05 Favours medial taping

continued

Table 6.65 Symptoms: pain – *continued*

Pain outcome	Reference	Intervention	Assessment time	Outcome/effect size
Knee				
Taping – *continued*				
Patient's change scores (number of patients 'better')	1 RCT (Cushnaghan et al. 1994) (N=14)	Medial taping vs lateral taping	4 days, end of treatment	p<0.05 Favours medial taping
Pain on standing, VAS (change from baseline)	1 RCT (Cushnaghan et al. 1994) (N=14)	Medial taping vs lateral taping	6 months, end of treatment	–1.2 (medial) and –0.3 (neutral) Medial taping better
Pain on movement, VAS (change from baseline)	1 RCT (Hinman et al. 2003) (N=87)	Therapeutic tape vs control tape	3 weeks, end of treatment and 3 weeks post-treatment	3 weeks: –2.1 (therapeutic) and –0.7 (neutral) 3 weeks post-treatment –1.9 (therapeutic) and –1.1 (control) Therapeutic tape better
Pain on worst activity, VAS (change from baseline)	1 RCT (Hinman et al. 2003) (N=87)	Therapeutic tape vs control tape	3 weeks, end of treatment and 3 weeks post-treatment	3 weeks: –2.5 (therapeutic) and –1.1 (neutral) 3 weeks post-treatment –2.8 (therapeutic) and –1.4 (control) Therapeutic tape better
WOMAC pain (change from baseline)	1 RCT (Hinman et al. 2003) (N=87)	Therapeutic tape vs control tape	3 weeks, end of treatment	3 weeks: –1.8 (therapeutic) and –1.6 (neutral) Therapeutic tape better
Knee Pain Scale, KPS, Severity (change from baseline)	1 RCT (Hinman et al. 2003) (N=87)	Therapeutic tape vs control tape	3 weeks, end of treatment	3 weeks: –2.7 (therapeutic) and –1.9 (neutral) Therapeutic tape better
Knee Pain Scale, KPS, Frequency (change from baseline)	1 RCT (Hinman et al. 2003) (N=87)	Therapeutic tape vs control tape	3 weeks, end of treatment	3 weeks: –2.6 (therapeutic) and –2.4 (neutral) Therapeutic tape better
WOMAC pain (change from baseline)	1 RCT (Hinman et al. 2003) (N=87)	Therapeutic tape vs control tape	3 weeks, end of treatment	3 weeks: –1.7 (therapeutic) and –2.0 (neutral) Control tape better
Knee Pain Scale, KPS, severity (change from baseline)	1 RCT (Hinman et al. 2003) (N=87)	Therapeutic tape vs control tape	3 weeks, end of treatment	3 weeks: –2.3 (therapeutic) and –2.9 (neutral) Control tape better

continued

Table 6.65 Symptoms: pain – *continued*

Pain outcome	Reference	Intervention	Assessment time	Outcome/effect size
Knee				
Taping – *continued*				
Knee Pain Scale, KPS, Frequency (change from baseline)	1 RCT (Hinman et al. 2003) (N=87)	Therapeutic tape vs control tape	3 weeks, end of treatment	3 weeks: –2.7 (therapeutic) and –3.3 (neutral) Control tape better
Pain on movement, VAS (change from baseline)	1 RCT (Hinman et al. 2003) (N=87)	Therapeutic tape vs no tape	3 weeks, end of treatment and 3 weeks post-treatment	3 weeks: –2.1 (therapeutic) and +0.1 (no tape) 3 weeks post-treatment –1.9 (therapeutic) and –0.1 (none) Therapeutic tape better
Pain on worst activity, VAS (change from baseline)	1 RCT (Hinman et al. 2003) (N=87)	Therapeutic tape vs no tape	3 weeks, end of treatment and 3 weeks post-treatment	3 weeks: –2.5 (therapeutic) and –0.4 (no tape) 3 weeks post-treatment –2.8 (therapeutic) and –0.4 (none) Therapeutic tape better
WOMAC pain (change from baseline)	1 RCT (Hinman et al. 2003) (N=87)	Therapeutic tape vs no tape	3 weeks, end of treatment and 3 weeks post-treatment	3 weeks: –1.8 (therapeutic) and –0.1 (no tape) 3 weeks post-treatment –1.7 (therapeutic) and +0.4 (none) Therapeutic tape better
Knee Pain Scale, KPS, Severity (change from baseline)	1 RCT (Hinman et al. 2003) (N=87)	Therapeutic tape vs no tape	3 weeks, end of treatment and 3 weeks post-treatment	3 weeks: –2.7 (therapeutic) and 0.0 (no tape) 3 weeks post-treatment –2.6 (therapeutic) and +0.5 (none) Therapeutic tape better
Knee Pain Scale, KPS, Frequency (change from baseline)	1 RCT (Hinman et al. 2003) (N=87)	Therapeutic tape vs no tape	3 weeks, end of treatment and 3 weeks post-treatment	3 weeks: –2.6 (therapeutic) and –0.1 (no tape) 3 weeks post-treatment –2.7 (therapeutic) and –0.1 (none) Therapeutic tape better

continued

Table 6.65 Symptoms: pain – *continued*

Pain outcome	Reference	Intervention	Assessment time	Outcome/effect size
Knee				
Shoes				
WOMAC pain total (change from baseline)	1 RCT (Nigg et al. 2006) (N=125)	Masai barefoot technology (MBT) shoe vs high-end walking shoe	12 weeks (end of treatment)	NS
WOMAC pain walking (change from baseline)	1 RCT (Nigg et al. 2006) (N=125)	MBT shoe vs high-end walking shoe	12 weeks (end of treatment)	NS
WOMAC pain stairs (change from baseline)	1 RCT (Nigg et al. 2006) (N=125)	MBT shoe vs high-end walking shoe	12 weeks (end of treatment)	NS
Mixed				
Pain, VAS (change from baseline)	1 RCT (Quilty et al. 2003) (N=87)	Taping + exercises + posture correction + education vs standard treatment (no experimental intervention)	5 months (3 months post-treatment) and at 12 months (10 months post-treatment).	NS
Pain, VAS (change from baseline)	1 RCT (Toda and Tsukimura 2004) (N=66)	Urethane insole + strapping + NSAID vs rubber insole + NSAID	3 months, mid-study and at 6 months, mid-study	3 months: −16.4 (urethane insole) and −2.8 (rubber insole) 6 months: −17.3 (urethane insole) and −3.6 (rubber insole) Urethane insole + strapping + NSAID better
Hand (thumb – CMC joint)				
Pain, VAS (change from baseline)	1 RCT (Wajon and Ada 2005) (N=40)	Thumb strap splint + abduction exercises vs control (short opponens splint + pinch exercises	2 weeks (mid-treatment) and at 6 weeks (end of treatment	NS
Pain, VAS (change from baseline); Splint/pinch Pain, VAS (change from baseline)	1 RCT (Weiss 2000) (N=26)	Short opponens splint vs long opponens splint	1 week (end of treatment)	NS

Table 6.66 Symptoms: stiffness

Stiffness outcome	Reference	Intervention	Assessment time	Outcome/effect size
Knee				
Insoles				
WOMAC stiffness	1 MA (Brouwer et al. 2005) 1 RCT, N=147	Laterally wedged insole vs neutrally wedged insole	1 month, 3 months and 6 months follow-up	NS
WOMAC stiffness	1 RCT (Pham et al. 2004) (N=156)	Laterally wedged insole vs neutrally wedged insole	2 years (end of treatment)	NS
Shoes				
WOMAC stiffness (change from baseline)	1 RCT (Nigg et al. 2006) (N=125)	MBT shoe vs high-end walking shoe	12 weeks (end of treatment)	NS

Table 6.67 Symptoms: function

Function outcome	Reference	Intervention	Assessment time	Outcome/effect size
Knee				
Brace				
WOMAC score	1 MA (Brouwer et al. 2005) 1 RCT, N=119	Knee brace vs neoprene sleeve	6 months	Knee brace better
WOMAC score; MACTAR score	1 MA (Brouwer et al. 2005) 1 RCT, N=119	Knee brace vs medical treatment	6 months	Knee brace better
WOMAC score	1 MA (Brouwer et al. 2005) 1 RCT, N=119	Neoprene sleeve vs medical treatment	6 months	Neoprene sleeve better
Walking distance	1 RCT (Brouwer et al. 2006) (N-=118)	Knee brace + conservative treatment vs control (conservative treatment)	3 months 12 months and overall	3 months (effect size 0.3; p=0.03) 12 months (effect size 0.4; p=0.04) Overall (effect size 0.4; p=0.02) Favours knee brace
Walking distance	1 RCT (Brouwer et al. 2006) (N-=118)	Knee brace + conservative treatment vs control (conservative treatment)	6 months	NS
Knee function (HSS)	1 RCT (Brouwer et al. 2006) (N-=118)	Knee brace + conservative treatment vs control (conservative treatment)	3 months, 6 months 12 months or overall	NS

continued

Table 6.67 Symptoms: function – *continued*

Function outcome	Reference	Intervention	Assessment time	Outcome/effect size
Knee				
Insoles				
WOMAC physical function	1 MA (Brouwer et al. 2005) 1 RCT, N=147	Laterally wedged insole vs neutrally wedged insole	1 month, 3 months and 6 months follow-up	NS
WOMAC disability; 50-foot walk time; 5 chair stand time	1 RCT (Baker et al. 2007) (N=90)	Laterally wedged insole vs neutrally wedged insole	6 weeks (end of treatment)	NS
Lequesne's Index; femoro-tibial angle (FTA), talocalcaneal angle and talar tilt angle	1 MA (Brouwer et al. 2005) 1 RCT, N=90	Subtalar strapped insole vs inserted insole	8 weeks	NS
FTA angle and talar tilt angle	1 MA (Brouwer et al. 2005) 1 RCT, N=90	Subtalar strapped insole vs no insole	8 weeks	P<0.05 Favours strapped insole
FTA angle; aggregate score	1 MA (Brouwer et al. 2005) 1 RCT, N=88	Subtalar strapped insole vs sock-type insole	8 weeks	NS
WOMAC function (change from baseline)	1 RCT (Pham et al. 2004) (N=156)	Laterally wedged insole vs neutrally wedged insole	2 years (end of treatment)	NS
Taping				
Restriction of activity, VAS (change from baseline)	1 RCT (Hinman et al. 2003) (N=87)	Therapeutic tape vs control tape	3 weeks, end of treatment	3 weeks: −1.5 (therapeutic) and −1.4 (control) Therapeutic tape better
WOMAC physical function (change from baseline)	1 RCT (Hinman et al. 2003) (N=87)	Therapeutic tape vs control tape	3 weeks, end of treatment	3 weeks: −4.0 (therapeutic) and −3.1 (control) Therapeutic tape better
Restriction of activity, VAS (change from baseline)	1 RCT (Hinman et al. 2003) (N=87)	Therapeutic tape vs control tape	3 weeks, end of treatment	3 weeks: −1.0 (therapeutic) and −1.2 (control) 3 weeks post-treatment: −3.4 (therapeutic) and −6.0 (control) Control tape better
Restriction of activity, VAS (change from baseline)	1 RCT (Hinman et al. 2003) (N=87)	Therapeutic tape vs no tape	3 weeks, end of treatment and 3 weeks post-treatment	3 weeks: −1.0 (therapeutic) and +0.2 (no tape) 3 weeks post-treatment −1.5 (therapeutic) and +0.1 (none) Therapeutic tape better

continued

Table 6.67 Symptoms: function – *continued*

Function outcome	Reference	Intervention	Assessment time	Outcome/effect size
Knee				
Taping – *continued*				
WOMAC physical function (change from baseline)	1 RCT (Hinman et al. 2003) (N=87)	Therapeutic tape vs no tape	3 weeks, end of treatment and 3 weeks post-treatment	3 weeks: −4.0 (therapeutic) and +1.7 (no tape) 3 weeks post-treatment −3.4 (therapeutic) and +1.9 (none) Therapeutic tape better
Shoes				
WOMAC total (change from baseline); WOMAC physical function (change from baseline); ROM extension, degrees (change from baseline); ROM flexion, degrees (change from baseline)	1 RCT (Nigg et al. 2006) (N=125)	MBT shoe vs high-end walking shoe	12 weeks (end of treatment)	NS
Cane				
Walking speed, m/s	1 RCT (Chan and Smith 2005) (N=14)	Ipsilateral cane vs no cane (unaided walking)	Immediate	p=0.00 Favours cane
Cadence, steps/ minute	1 RCT (Chan and Smith 2005) (N=14)	Ipsilateral cane vs no cane (unaided walking)	Immediate	p<0.001 Favours cane
Stride length	1 RCT (Chan and Smith 2005) (N=14)	Ipsilateral cane vs no cane (unaided walking)	Immediate	NS
Walking speed, m/s	1 RCT (Chan and Smith 2005) (N=14)	Contralateral cane vs no cane (unaided walking)	Immediate	p=0.00 Favours cane
Cadence, steps/ minute	1 RCT (Chan and Smith 2005) (N=14)	Contralateral cane vs no cane (unaided walking)	Immediate	P<0.001 Favours cane
Mixed				
WOMAC function (change from baseline)	1 RCT (Quilty et al. 2003) (N=87)	Taping + exercises + posture correction + education vs standard treatment (no experimental intervention)	5 months (3 months post-treatment) and at 12 months (10 months post-treatment)	NS

continued

Table 6.67 Symptoms: function – *continued*

Function outcome	Reference	Intervention	Assessment time	Outcome/effect size
Knee				
Mixed – *continued*				
Lequesne's Index of Disease Severity, % remission	1 RCT (Toda et al. 2004) (N=84)	Urethane insoles + strapping + NSAID vs rubber insoles + strapping + NSAID	4 weeks, end of treatment	p=0.001 Favours urethane insole + strapping + NSAID
Lequesne's Index of disease severity, % remission	1 RCT (Toda et al. 2005) (N=81)	Urethane insoles + strapping + NSAID worn for the medium length of time (5–10 hrs/day) vs short-length (<5 hrs/day)	2 weeks, end of treatment	p=0.001
Lequesne's Index of disease severity, % remission	1 RCT (Toda et al. 2005) (N=81)	Urethane insoles + strapping + NSAID worn for the medium length of time (5-10 hrs/day) vs long length (>10 hrs/day)	2 weeks, end of treatment	p=0.001
Lequesne's index of disease severity (change from baseline)	1 RCT (Toda et al. 2004) (N=62)	Insoles + strapping + NSAID – insoles at different elevations (8 mm vs 12 mm vs 16 mm)	2 weeks, end of treatment	NS
Lequesne's index of disease severity, % remission	1 RCT (Toda et al. 2004) (N=62)	12mm insole + strapping + NSAID vs 16 mm insole	2 weeks, end of treatment	p=0.029
Lequesne's index of disease severity (change from baseline)	1 RCT (Toda and Tsukimura 2004b, Toda and Tsukimura 2006) (N=66)	Urethane insole + strapping + NSAID vs rubber insole + NSAID	3 months and 6 months (mid-study) and at 2 years, end of study.	3 months: –2.1 (urethane) and –0.7 (rubber) 6 months: –2.2 (urethane) and –0.9 (rubber) 2 years: –2.4 (urethane) and –0.3 (rubber) Urethane insole better
Progression of Kellgren-Lawrence grade	1 RCT (Toda and Tsukimura 2006) (N=66)	Urethane insole + strapping + NSAID vs rubber insole + NSAID	2 years, end of study	NS
Hand (thumb – carpometacarpal (CMC) joint)				
Tip pinch, kg (change from baseline); hand function, Sollerman Test, ADL (change from baseline)	1 RCT (Wajon and Ada 2005) (N=40)	Thumb strap splint + abduction exercises vs control (short opponens splint + pinch exercises	2 weeks (mid-treatment) and at 6 weeks (end of treatment).	NS

continued

Table 6.67 Symptoms: function – *continued*

Function outcome	Reference	Intervention	Assessment time	Outcome/effect size
Hand (thumb – carpometacarpal (CMC) joint) – *continued*				
Tip pinch strength, kg, (change from baseline) at 1 week (end of treatment)	1 RCT (Weiss 2000) (N=26)	Short opponens splint vs long opponens splint	1 week (end of treatment)	NS
ADL, % same or easier at 1 week (end of treatment)	1 RCT (Weiss 2000) (N=26)	Short opponens splint vs long opponens splint	1 week (end of treatment)	Both groups similar

Table 6.68 Global assessment

Global assessment outcome	Reference	Intervention	Assessment time	Outcome/effect size
Knee				
Insoles				
Patient's overall assessment	1 MA (Brouwer et al. 2005) 1 RCT, N=147	Laterally wedged insole vs neutrally wedged insole	1 month, 3 months and 6 months	NS
Patient's global assessment (change from baseline)	1 RCT (Pham et al. 2004) (N=156)	Laterally wedged insole vs neutrally wedged insole	2 years (end of treatment)	NS
Taping				
Patient's preference	1 RCT (Cushnaghan et al. 1994) (N=14)	Medial taping vs neutral taping	4 days (end of treatment)	p<0.05 Favours medial taping
Patient's preference	1 RCT (Cushnaghan et al. 1994) (N=14)	Medial taping vs lateral taping	4 days (end of treatment)	NS

Table 6.69 Quality of life

QoL outcome	Reference	Intervention	Assessment time	Outcome/effect size
Knee				
Brace				
QoL measurements (EuroQoL-5D)	1 RCT (Brouwer et al. 2006) (N-=118)	Knee brace + conservative treatment vs control (conservative treatment)	3 months, 6 months 12 months or overall	NS
Taping				
SF-36 bodily pain (change from baseline)	1 RCT (Hinman et al. 2003) (N=87)	Therapeutic tape vs control tape	3 weeks end of treatment and at 3 weeks post-treatment	3 weeks: +10.0 (therapeutic) and +5.5 (control) 3 weeks post-treatment: +7.9 (therapeutic) and +2.0 (control) Therapeutic tape better

continued

Table 6.69 Quality of life – *continued*

QoL outcome	Reference	Intervention	Assessment time	Outcome/effect size
Knee				
Taping – *continued*				
SF-36 physical function (change from baseline)	1 RCT (Hinman et al. 2003) (N=87)	Therapeutic tape vs control tape	3 weeks end of treatment	3 weeks: +2.1 (therapeutic) and +2.0 (control) Therapeutic tape better
SF-36 physical role (change from baseline)	1 RCT (Hinman et al. 2003) (N=87)	Therapeutic tape vs control tape	3 weeks end of treatment	3 weeks: +4.3 (therapeutic) and 0.0 (control) Therapeutic tape better
SF-36 physical function (change from baseline)	1 RCT (Hinman et al. 2003) (N=87)	Therapeutic tape vs control tape	3 weeks post-treatment	+2.1 (therapeutic) and +4.4 (control) Control tape better
SF-36 physical role (change from baseline)	1 RCT (Hinman et al. 2003) (N=87)	Therapeutic tape vs control tape	3 weeks post-treatment	+2.6 (therapeutic) and +13.0 (control) Control tape better
SF-36 bodily pain (change from baseline)	1 RCT (Hinman et al. 2003) (N=87)	Therapeutic tape vs no tape	3 weeks end of treatment and at 3 weeks post-treatment	3 weeks: +10.0 (therapeutic) and −3.7 (control) 3 weeks post-treatment: +7.9 (therapeutic) and −2.0 (control) Therapeutic tape better
SF-36 physical function (change from baseline) at 3 weeks end of treatment (+2.1 and 0.0 respectively) and at 3 weeks post-treatment (+2.1 and −1.3 respectively)	1 RCT (Hinman et al. 2003) (N=87)	Therapeutic tape vs no tape	3 weeks end of treatment and at 3 weeks post-treatment	3 weeks: +10.0 (therapeutic) and −3.7 (control) 3 weeks post-treatment: +7.9 (therapeutic) and −2.0 (control) Therapeutic tape better
SF-36 physical role (change from baseline)	1 RCT (Hinman et al. 2003) (N=87)	Therapeutic tape vs no tape	3 weeks end of treatment and at 3 weeks post-treatment	3 weeks: +4.3 (therapeutic) and +2.9 (control) 3 weeks post-treatment: +2.6 (therapeutic) and −1.0 (control) Therapeutic tape better

Table 6.70 Adverse events

AEs outcome	Reference	Intervention	Assessment time	Outcome/effect size
Knee				
Insoles				
AEs (popliteal pain, low back pain and foot sole pain)	1 MA (Brouwer et al. 2005) 1 RCT, N=90	Subtalar strapped insole vs inserted insole	8 weeks	NS
Number of AEs	1 RCT (Toda et al. 2004) (N=62)	8 mm insole + strapping + NSAID vs 12 mm insole + strapping + NSAID	2 weeks (end of treatment)	p=0.003 Favours 8 mm insole
Number of AEs	1 RCT (Toda et al. 2004) (N=62)	12 mm insole + strapping + NSAID vs 16 mm insole + strapping + NSAID	2 weeks (end of treatment)	p=0.005 Favours 12 mm insole
Total number of AEs	1 RCT (Toda and Tsukimura 2004 547) (N=84)	Urethane insoles + strapping + NSAID vs rubber insoles + strapping + NSAID	4 weeks (end of treatment)	p=0.028 Favours urethane insoles
Taping				
Number of patients with AEs, skin irritation	1 RCT (Hinman et al. 2003) (N=87)	Therapeutic tape vs control tape	3 weeks (end of treatment)	28% (therapeutic) and 1% (control) Control tape better
Number of patients with AEs, skin irritation	1 RCT (Hinman et al. 2003) (N=87)	Therapeutic tape vs no tape	3 weeks (end of treatment)	28% (therapeutic tape) and 0% (no tape) No tape better
Mixed				
Number of patients with AEs (16% and 0% respectively)	1 RCT (Quilty et al. 2003) (N=87)	Taping + exercises + posture correction + education vs standard treatment (no experimental intervention)	10 weeks (end of treatment)	16% (taping) and 0% (no intervention) No intervention better

Table 6.71 Analgesic use

Analgesic use outcome	Reference	Intervention	Assessment time	Outcome/effect size
Knee				
Insoles				
Analgesic or NSAID use	1 MA (Brouwer et al. 2005) 1 RCT, N=147	Laterally wedged insole vs neutrally wedged insole	Over 3 months	NS
Number of days receiving rescue medication	1 RCT (Baker et al. (2007) (N=90)	Laterally wedged insole vs neutrally wedged insole	Over 6 weeks (end of treatment)	NS

continued

Table 6.71 Analgesic use – *continued*

Analgesic use outcome	Reference	Intervention	Assessment time	Outcome/effect size
Knee				
Insoles – *continued*				
NSAID usage, number of days with NSAID intake	1 RCT (Pham et al. 2004) (N=156)	Laterally wedged insole vs neutrally wedged insole	Over 2 years (end of treatment)	71 (lateral) and 168 (neutral), p=0.003 Favours lateral wedge
Analgesic usage, number of days with analgesic intake; intra-articular Injection, mean number of injections/patient	1 RCT (Pham et al. 2004) (N=156)	Laterally wedged insole vs neutrally wedged insole	Over 2 years (end of treatment)	NS
Taping				
Analgesic usage, number of patients	1 RCT (Hinman et al. 2003) (N=87)	Therapeutic tape vs control tape	Over 3 weeks (end of treatment)	NS
Analgesic usage, number of patients	1 RCT (Hinman et al. 2003) (N=87)	Therapeutic tape vs no tape	Over 3 weeks (end of treatment)	NS
Mixed				
Number of days with NSAID intake	1 RCT (Toda and Tsukimura 2004b, Toda and Tsukimura 2006) (N=66)	Urethane insole + strapping + NSAID vs rubber insole + NSAID	Over the 2 years	36.1% (urethane) and 42.2% (rubber) Urethane better
Number of patients who discontinued NSAIDs due to pain relief	1 RCT (Toda and Tsukimura 2004b, Toda and Tsukimura 2006) (N=66)	Urethane insole + strapping + NSAID vs rubber insole + NSAID	Over the 6 months (mid-study	N=1, 4.8% (urethane) and N=2 (rubber) 9.5% Urethane better
Number of patients who discontinued NSAIDs due to GI (stomach ache) AEs	1 RCT (Toda and Tsukimura 2004b, Toda and Tsukimura 2006) (N=66)	Urethane insole + strapping + NSAID vs rubber insole + NSAID	Over the 6 months (mid-study)	N=1, 4.8% (urethane) and N=2 (rubber) 9.5% Urethane better
Number of patients who discontinued NSAIDs due to AEs	1 RCT (Toda and Tsukimura 2004b, Toda and Tsukimura 2006) (N=66)	Urethane insole + strapping + NSAID vs rubber insole + NSAID	Over the 6 months (mid-study)	3.4% (urethane) and 3.1% (rubber)

Table 6.72 Withdrawals

Withdrawals outcome	Reference	Intervention	Assessment time	Outcome/effect size
Knee				
Brace				
Number of patients stopped treatment number of patients stopped treatment due to strong reduction in symptoms (N=3 and N=0 respectively)	1 RCT (Brouwer et al. 2006) (N-=118)	Knee brace + conservative treatment vs control (conservative treatment)	3 months, 6 months 12 months or overall	N=25 (brace) and N=14 (conservative) Knee brace worse
Number of patients stopped treatment due to strong reduction in symptoms	1 RCT (Brouwer et al. 2006) (N-=118)	Knee brace + conservative treatment vs control (conservative treatment)	3 months, 6 months 12 months or overall	N=3 (brace) and N=0 (conservative) Knee brace worse
Number of patients who stopped treatment due to lack of efficacy	1 RCT (Brouwer et al. 2006) (N-=118)	Knee brace + conservative treatment vs control (conservative treatment)	3 months, 6 months 12 months or overall	N=15 (brace) and N=14 (conservative) Knee brace worse
Insoles				
Total number of withdrawals	1 MA (Brouwer et al. 2005) 1 RCT, N=147	Laterally wedged insole vs neutrally wedged insole	Not mentioned	33% (lateral) and 31% (neutral) Both groups similar
Taping				
Total number of withdrawals	1 RCT (Hinman et al. 2003) (N=87)	Therapeutic tape vs control tape	3 weeks post-treatment	Both: 0% Both groups same
Total number of withdrawals	1 RCT (Hinman et al. 2003) (N=87)	Therapeutic tape vs no tape	3 weeks post-treatment	0% (therapeutic) and 3% (no tape) Both groups similar
Shoes				
Total number of withdrawals	1 RCT (Nigg et al. 2006) (N=125)	Masai barefoot technology (MBT) shoe vs high-end walking shoe	12 weeks (end of treatment)	1.8% (MBT shoe) and 1.5% (walking shoe) Both groups similar
Mixed				
Study withdrawals	1 RCT (Quilty et al. 2003) (N=87)	Taping + exercises + posture correction + education vs standard treatment (no experimental intervention)	5 months (3 months post-treatment) and at 12 months (10 months post-treatment)	N=3, 7% (taping) and N=1 2% (standard treatment) Both groups similar

continued

Table 6.72 Withdrawals – *continued*

Withdrawals outcome	Reference	Intervention	Assessment time	Outcome/effect size
Knee				
Mixed – *continued*				
Number of study withdrawals	1 RCT (Toda and Tsukimara 2004) (N=66)	Urethane insole + strapping + NSAID vs rubber insole + NSAID	3 months and 6 months (mid-study) and at 2 years (end of study).	NS
Hand (Thumb – CMC joint)				
Total withdrawals	1 RCT (Wajon and Ada 2005) (N=40)	Thumb strap splint + abduction exercises vs control (short opponens splint + pinch exercises	6 weeks (end of treatment)	N=1, 5.2% (thumb strap splint) and N=5 24% (short opponens splint) Thumb splint better
Withdrawals due to AEs	1 RCT (Wajon and Ada 2005) (N=40)	Thumb strap splint + abduction exercises vs control (short opponens splint + pinch exercises	6 weeks (end of treatment)	N=1, 5.2% (thumb strap splint) and N=1, 4.7% (short opponens splint) Both groups similar

Table 6.73 Structural changes

Structural changes outcome	Reference	Intervention	Assessment time	Outcome/effect size
Knee				
Insoles				
Joint spacing width, mean narrowing rate/year, mm	1 RCT (Pham et al. 2004) (N=156)	Laterally wedged insole vs neutrally wedged insole	Rate/year	NS

6.5.4   Evidence statements: assistive devices

Table 6.74 Symptoms: pain

Pain outcome	Reference	Intervention	Assessment time	Outcome/effect size
Hand osteoarthritis				
Pain (VAS), % of patients improved	1 RCT (Stamm et al. 2002) (N=40)	Assistive devices + exercise + education vs jar opening aid + education	6 weeks, end of treatment	65% and 25% respectively, p<0.05 Favours assistive devices

Table 6.75 Symptoms: function

Function outcome	Reference	Intervention	Assessment time	Outcome/effect size
Hand osteoarthritis				
Grip strength in both hands (change from baseline); grip strength % of patients with 10% improvement in both hands	1 RCT (Stamm et al. 2002) (N=40)	Assistive devices + exercise + education vs jar opening aid + education	6 weeks, end of treatment	Both: p<0.05 Favours assistive devices
HAQ score	1 RCT (Stamm et al. 2002) (N=40)	Assistive devices + exercise + education vs jar opening aid + education	6 weeks, end of treatment	NS

Table 6.76 Use of assistive devices

Use of devices outcome	Reference	Intervention	Assessment time	Outcome/effect size
Hip or knee osteoarthritis				
Use of assistive devices (canes, crutches or walker)	1 observational study (Veitiene and Tamulaitiene 2005) (N=27)	Assistive devices	n/a	59.3% of patients used devices
Use of assistive devices	1 observational study (Tallon et al. 2000) (N=88 participants responses)	Assistive devices	n/a	56% of patients used devices and 27% of patients used them often or very often
Site not specified				
Total percentage of patients using at least 1 assistive device	1 observational study (Sutton et al. 2002) (N=248)	Assistive devices	n/a	67.3% (medical devices) and 91.5% (everyday devices)
Use of both medical and everyday devices for personal care/in-home mobility	1 observational study (Sutton et al. 2002) (N=248)	Assistive devices	n/a	59.7% (medical devices) and 85.1% (everyday devices)
Use of both medical and everyday devices for household activities and for community mobility	1 observational study (Sutton et al. 2002) (N=248)	Assistive devices	n/a	21.4% (medical devices) and 66.5% (everyday devices)
Use of both medical and everyday devices for community mobility	1 observational study (Sutton et al. 2002) (N=248)	Assistive devices	n/a	20.6% (medical devices) and 27.0% (everyday devices)
Number of assistive devices (all category types of device) needed by patients	1 observational study (Mann et al. 1995) (N=66)	Assistive devices	n/a	Higher for patients with severe osteoarthritis compared with moderate arthritis (number of devices = 94 and 36 respectively)

Table 6.77 Patient satisfaction/views of devices

Patient satisfaction/ views outcome	Reference	Intervention	Assessment time	Outcome/effect size
Hip or knee osteoarthritis				
Most effective treatments out of different OIA therapies (assistive devices, cold, heat, rest, exercise and joint protection)	1 observational study (Veitiene and Tamulatiene 2005) (N=27)	Assistive devices	n/a	29.6% patients found assistive devices (canes crutches or walker) were 1 of the 3 most effective treatments
Use of canes	1 observational study (Tallon et al. 2000) (N=7 participants)	Assistive devices	n/a	Perceived as useful but some felt their pride would be affected and did not use them
Coping strategies	1 observational study (Tallon et al. 2000) (N=7 participants)	Assistive devices	n/a	Strategies included the use of aids to daily living
Helpfulness of aids and adaptations	1 observational study (Tallon et al. 2000) (N=88 participants)	Assistive devices	n/a	Rated moderately and extremely helpful (29.5%); rated not helpful or slightly helpful (26%)
Site not specified				
Positive attitudes towards assistive devices	1 observational study (Sutton et al. 2002) (N=248)	Assistive devices	n/a	Assistive devices helped people do things they want to do (94.8%), allowed independence (91.5%), were not more bother than they were worth (94.0%)
Negative attitudes towards assistive devices	1 observational study (Sutton et al. 2002) (N=248)	Assistive devices	n/a	Devices were awkward (79%); costs prevented use (58.9%); devices made people feel dependent (48.4%)
Rate of satisfaction with assistive devices	1 observational study (Mann et al. 1995) (N=66)	Assistive devices	n/a	Rate range: 78% to 100% (patients with moderate and severe arthritis), lowest satisfaction was with vision devices

6.5.5   From evidence to recommendations

There is a paucity of well-designed trials in this area, and the GDG considered various additional sources of evidence, including non-controlled studies. Evidence generally showed that aids and devices are well accepted by many people with OA who report high satisfaction with use.

There are limited data for the effectiveness of insoles (either wedged or neutral) in reducing the symptoms of knee OA. However in the absence of well-designed trial data and given the low cost of the intervention, the GDG felt that attention to footware with shock-absorbing properties was worth consideration.

There is some evidence for the effectiveness of walking aids and assistive devices (such as braces) for hip and knee OA. Walking aids (ipsi- or contralateral cane use) can significantly improve stride length and cadence.

There is some evidence for the effectiveness of aids/devices for hand OA. Thumb splints (of any design) can help reduce pain from thumb OA and improve hand function. There are many different designs of thumb CMC splint for OA described in the literature, frequently accompanied by biomechanical rationales for which is most effective. As yet it is unclear which design/s are considered most comfortable to patients, and thus will be worn long term, and what degree of splint rigidity/support is required at what stage of OA in order to effectively improve pain and function. The best study to date (Wajon and Ada 2005) has included exercises within the trial design which confounds identifying whether it was splinting or exercise which was most effective. Clinically, patients are commonly provided with both a splint and exercise regime.

Disability equipment assessment centres have a role in providing expert advice. The MHRA regularly publishes reports on assistive devices.

▷   Referral: hand osteoarthritis

This evidence suggests that those people with hand pain, difficulty and frustration with performing daily activities and work tasks should be referred to occupational therapy for splinting, joint protection training and assistive device provision. This may be combined with hand exercise training. People should be referred early particularly if work abilities are affected.

▷   Referral: lower limb

Provision of rehabilitation and physical therapies is commonly recommended in guidelines. Physiotherapists and occupational therapists may be able to help with provision and fitting of appropriate aids and devices. Insoles are commonly provided by podiatrists and orthotists but may also be provided by physiotherapists and occupational therapists. Referral for, or direct local provision of, footwear advice should always be considered.

RECOMMENDATIONS

R16   Healthcare professionals should offer advice on appropriate footwear (including shock absorbing properties) as part of core treatment for people with lower limb osteoarthritis.

R17   People with osteoarthritis who have biomechanical joint pain or instability should be considered for assessment for bracing/joint supports/insoles as an adjunct to their core treatment.

R18   Assistive devices (for example, walking sticks and tap turners) should be considered as adjuncts to core treatment for people with OA who have specific problems with activities of daily living. Healthcare professionals may need to seek expert advice in this context (for example from occupational therapists or disability equipment assessment centres).

6.6   Nutraceuticals

6.6.1   Clinical introduction

Nutraceuticals is a term used to cover foods or food supplements thought to have health benefits. The most widely used are glucosamine and chondroitin, which are widely sold in various combinations, compounds, strengths and purities over the counter in the UK. Medical quality glucosamine hydrochloride is licensed in the European Union and can be prescribed. These compounds are not licensed by the Food and Drug Administration in the USA, so are marketed there (and on the internet) as health food supplements.

Glucosamine is an amino sugar and an important precursor in the biochemical synthesis of glycosylated proteins, including glycosaminoglycans. The sulfate moiety of glucosamine sulfate is associated with the amino group. Chondroitin sulfate is a sulfated glycosaminoglycan (GAG) dimer, which can be polymerised to the chain of alternating sugars (N-acetylgalactosamine and glucuronic acid) found attached to proteins as part of a proteoglycan. It is hypothesised that substrate availability (of glucosamine, chondroitin or sulfate itself) may be the limiting factor in the synthesis of the GAG component of cartilage, which provides the rationale for oral supplementation of these compounds in osteoarthritis. The mode of action and both in vitro and in vivo effects of these compounds remain highly controversial, although their safety is rarely disputed.

6.6.2   Methodological introduction

We looked for studies that investigated the efficacy and safety of glucosamine and chondroitin alone or in compound form vs placebo with respect to symptoms, function, quality of life and ability to beneficially modify structural changes of OA. Two systematic reviews and meta-analyses (Reichenbach et al. 2007; Towheed et al. 2005) were found on glucosamine or chondroitin sulphate and six additional RCTs (Clegg et al. 2006; Cohen et al. 2003; Das and Hammad 2000; Herrero-Beaumont et al. 2007; Rai et al. 2004) on glucosamine, chondroitin or a combination of the two. Due to the large volume of evidence, trials with a sample size of less than 40 were excluded.

Both of the meta-analyses assessed the RCTs for quality and pooled together all data for the outcomes of symptoms and function. However, the outcomes of quality of life were not reported. Results for quality of life have therefore been taken from the individual RCTs included in these systematic reviews.

▷ Glucosamine

One SR/MA (Towheed et al. 2005) was found that focused on oral glucosamine vs placebo in patients with osteoarthritis (knee, mixed sites or unspecified). The MA included 20 RCTs (with N=2596 participants). All RCTs were high quality, double blind and of parallel group design. Studies included in the analysis differed with respect to:

- osteoarthritis site (16 RCTs knee, two RCTs multiple sites, two RCTs not specify)
- type of glucosamine used (19 RCTs glucosamine sulfate, one RCT glucosamine hydrochloride)
- treatment regimen – method of glucosamine administration (16 RCTs oral route, two RCTs intra-articular route, three RCTs intramuscular route, one RCT intravenous route, two RCTs multiple routes)
- treatment regimen – dose of glucosamine (oral glucosamine 1,500 mg/day, other routes 400 mg once daily or twice weekly)
- trial size and length.

The two RCTs not included in the MA (Clegg et al. 2006; Herrero-Beaumont et al. 2007) were methodologically sound and focused on the outcomes of symptoms, function and AEs in patients with knee OA. The first RCT (Clegg et al. 2006) compared oral glucosamine hydrochloride (GH)+ chondroitin sulfate (CS) with GH and CS alone and with placebo (all given 3 times daily; 1200 mg/day CS 1500 mg/day GH) in N=1,583 patients in a 24-week treatment phase. The second RCT (Herrero-Beaumont 2007) was a parallel group study and treated N=325 patients once a day with glucosamine sulfate (1500 mg/day) vs paracetamol vs placebo in a 6-month treatment phase.

▷ Chondroitin

One SR/MA (Reichenbach et al. 2007) and one RCT (Mazieres et al. 2007) were found that focused on oral chondroitin.

The MA (Reichenbach et al. 2007) included 19 RCTs and one clinical trial (total N=3846 participants) that focused on comparisons between oral chondroitin and placebo or no treatment in patients with knee and/or hip osteoarthritis. The SR assessed the trials for quality and all were methodologically sound. Studies included in the analysis differed with respect to:

- osteoarthritis site (N=17 knee, N=2 knee or hip, N=1 hip)
- study size and length
- dose of chondroitin (N=8 RCTs 800 mg, N=6 RCTs 1200 mg, N=5 RCTs 1000 mg, N=1 RCT 2000 mg).

The one RCT (Mazieres et al. 2007) not included in the systematic review was a parallel group study with outcomes of symptoms, function and AEs in patients with knee osteoarthritis and was methodologically sound. Treatment consisted of chondroitin sulphate (1000 mg/day – taken as 500 mg twice/day) vs placebo in N=153 in a 6-month treatment phase with follow-up at 8 weeks post-treatment.

▷ Mixed (chondoitin + glucosamine)

Four RCTs (Cohen et al. 2003; Clegg et al. 2006; Das and Hammad 2000; Rai et al. 2004) were found on chondroitin + glucosamine vs chiondroitin or glucosamine alone and/or placebo. The four RCTs (Cohen et al. 2003; Clegg et al. 2006; Das and Hammad 2000; Rai et al. 2004) were all methodologically sound (randomised and double blind) parallel studies that focused on the outcomes of symptoms, function, quality of life and adverse events in patients with knee osteoarthritis.

The first RCT (Clegg et al. 2006) compared oral glucosamine hydrochloride (GH)+ chondroitin sulphate (CS) with GH and CS alone and vs placebo (all given three times daily; 1200 mg/day CS 1500 mg/day GH) in N=1583 patients in a 24-week treatment phase. The second RCT (Cohen et al. 2003) compared glucosamine sulphate (GS)+ chondroitin sulphate (CS) vs placebo (all taken as necessary) in N=63 patients in an 8-week treatment phase. The third RCT (Das and Hammad 2000) compared oral glucosamine hyrochloride (GH) and chondroitin sulphate (CS) with placebo (taken twice a day; 1600 mg/day CS 2000 mg/day GH) in N=93 patients in a 6-month treatment phase. The fourth RCT (Rai et al. 2004) compared oral glucosamine sulphate (GS)+ chondroitin sulphate (CS) vs placebo (regimen and dose not mentioned) in N=100 patients in a 1-year treatment phase.

6.6.3 Evidence statements: glucosamine

Table 6.78 Symptoms: pain

Pain outcome	Reference	Intervention	Assessment time	Outcome/effect size
Knee				
Glucosamine hydrochloride (GH)				
20% decrease in WOMAC pain; 50% decrease in WOMAC pain; WOMAC pain score (change from baseline); HAQ pain (change from baseline)	1 RCT (Clegg et al. 2006) (N=1583)	GH vs placebo	24 weeks (end of treatment)	NS
Glucosamine sulphate (GS)				
WOMAC pain (change from baseline)	1 RCT (Herrero-Beaumont et al. 2007) (N=325)	GS vs placebo	6 months (end of treatment) NS	
Mixed (knee or mixed or unspecified sites)				
Glucosamine (general)				
WOMAC pain	1 MÀ (Towheed et al. 2005) 7 RCTs, N=955	Glucosamine vs placebo	Trial length: range 3 weeks to 3 years; follow-up: range immediate to 8 weeks	NS
Pain	1 MA (Towheed et al. 2005) 15 RCTs, N=1481	Glucosamine vs placebo	Trial length: range 3 weeks to 3 years; follow-up: range immediate to 8 weeks	Significant heterogeneity

Table 6.79 Symptoms: stiffness

Stiffness outcome	Reference	Intervention	Assessment time	Outcome/effect size
Knee				
Glucosamine hydrochloride				
WOMAC stiffness score, change from baseline	1 RCT (Clegg et al. 2006) (N=1583)	GH vs placebo	24 weeks (end of treatment)	NS
Mixed (knee or mixed or unspecified sites)				
Glucosamine (general)				
WOMAC stiffness	1 MA (Towheed et al. 2005) 5 RCTs, N=538	Glucosamine vs placebo	Trial length: range 3 weeks to 3 years; follow-up: range immediate to 8 weeks	NS

Table 6.80 Symptoms: function

Function outcome	Reference	Intervention	Assessment time	Outcome/effect size
Knee				
Glucosamine hydrochloride				
WOMAC function score, change from baseline; HAQ disability score, change from baseline; joint swelling, effusion or both on clinical examination	1 RCT (Clegg et al. 2006) (N=1583)	GH vs placebo	24 weeks (end of treatment)	NS
Glucosamine sulphate				
Lequesne's Index (change from baseline)	1 RCT (Herrero-Beaumont et al. 2007) (N=325)	GS vs placebo	6 months (end of treatment)	Mean difference –1.2,% CI –2.3 to –0.8, p=0.032 Favours GS
WOMAC total (change from baseline)	1 RCT (Herrero-Beaumont et al. 2007) (N=325)	GS vs placebo	6 months (end of treatment)	Mean difference –4.7,% CI –9.1 to –0.2, p=0.039 Favours GS
WOMAC physical function (change from baseline)	1 RCT (Herrero-Beaumont et al. 2007) (N=325)	GS vs placebo	6 months (end of treatment)	Mean difference –3.7,% CI –6.9 to –0.5, p=0.022 Favours GS

continued

Table 6.80 Symptoms: function – *continued*

Function outcome	Reference	Intervention	Assessment time	Outcome/effect size
Mixed (knee or mixed or unspecified sites)				
Glucosamine (general)				
Lequesne Index	1 MA (Towheed et al. 2005) 2 RCTs, N=407	Glucosamine vs placebo	Trial length: range 3 weeks to 3 years; follow-up: range immediate to 8 weeks	RR 1.52,% CI 1.20 to 1.91, p=0.0005 Favours glucosamine
Lequesne Index, relative risk	1 MA (Towheed et al. 2005) 4 RCTs, N=741	Glucosamine vs placebo	Trial length: range 3 weeks to 3 years; follow-up: range immediate to 8 weeks	NS
WOMAC function	1 MA (Towheed et al. 2005) 6 RCTs, N=750	Glucosamine vs placebo	Trial length: range 3 weeks to 3 years; follow-up: range immediate to 8 weeks	NS
WOMAC total	1 MA (Towheed et al. 2005) 5 RCTs, N=672	Glucosamine vs placebo	Trial length: range 3 weeks to 3 years; follow-up: range immediate to 8 weeks	NS

Table 6.81 Structure modification

Structure modification outcome	Reference	Intervention	Assessment time	Outcome/effect size
Mixed (knee or mixed or unspecified sites)				
Glucosamine (general)				
Minimum joint space width	1 MA (Towheed et al. 2005) 2 RCTs, N=414	Glucosamine vs placebo	Trial length: range 3 weeks to 3 years; follow-up: range immediate to 8 weeks	SMD 0.24,% CI 0.04 to 0.43, p=0.02 Favours glucosamine
Mean joint space width	1 MA (Towheed et al. 2005) 1 RCT, N=212	Glucosamine vs placebo	Trial length: range 3 weeks to 3 years; follow-up: range immediate to 8 weeks	NS

Table 6.82 Global assessment

Global assessment outcome	Reference	Intervention	Assessment time	Outcome/effect size
Knee				
Glucosamine hydrochloride				
Patient's global assessment of response to therapy; patient's global assessment of disease status	1 RCT (Clegg et al. 2006) (N=1583)	GH vs placebo	24 weeks (end of treatment)	NS
Physician's global assessment of disease status				

Table 6.83 Quality of life

QoL outcome	Reference	Intervention	Assessment time	Outcome/effect size
Mixed (knee or mixed or unspecified sites)				
Glucosamine (general)				
European Quality of Life questionnaire (EQ-5D) subsets: utility score and VAS	1 MA (Towheed et al. 2005) 1 RCT, (Cibere et al. 2004) N=137	Glucosamine vs placebo	6 months (end of treatment) or disease flare (whichever occurred first)	NS

Table 6.84 Adverse events

AEs outcome	Reference	Intervention	Assessment time	Outcome/effect size
Knee				
Glucosamine sulphate				
Withdrawals due to AEs	1 RCT (Herrero-Beaumont et al. 2007) (N=325)	GS vs placebo treatment)	6 months (end of (placebo)	N=4 (GS) and N=9 GS better
Number of patients with AEs; number of patients with GI AEs	1 RCT (Herrero-Beaumont et al. 2007) (N=325)	GS vs placebo	6 months (end of treatment)	NS
Mixed (knee or mixed or unspecified sites)				
Glucosamine (general)				
Number of patients reporting AEs	1 MA (Towheed et al. 2005) 14 RCTs, N=1685	Glucosamine vs placebo	Trial length: range 3 weeks to 3 years; follow-up: range immediate to 8 weeks	NS
Number of withdrawals due to AEs	1 MA (Towheed et al. 2005) 17 RCTs, N=1908	Glucosamine vs placebo	Trial length: range 3 weeks to 3 years; follow-up: range immediate to 8 weeks	NS

Table 6.85 Study withdrawals

Withdrawals outcome	Reference	Intervention	Assessment time	Outcome/effect size
Knee				
Glucosamine hydrochloride				
Total number of withdrawals; withdrawals due to AE; withdrawals due to lack of efficacy	1 RCT (Clegg et al. 2006) (N=1583)	GH vs placebo	24 weeks (end of treatment)	NS
Glucosamine sulphate				
Withdrawals due to lack of efficacy (N=7 and N=8 respectively)	1 RCT (Herrero-Beaumont et al. 2007) (N=325)	GS vs placebo	6 months (end of treatment)	N=7 (GH) and N=8 (placebo) Both groups similar

Table 6.86 Rescue medication

Rescue medication outcome	Reference	Intervention	Assessment time	Outcome/effect size
Knee				
Glucosamine hydrochloride				
Rescue paracetamol, No. of tablets taken	1 RCT (Clegg et al. 2006) (N=1583)	GH vs placebo	24 weeks (end of treatment)	NS
Glucosamine sulphate				
Use of rescue analgesia, % completers not using rescue medication	1 RCT (Herrero-Beaumont et al. 2007) (N=325)	GS vs placebo	over 6 months (end of study)	22% and 9% respectively, p=0.027 Favours GS

6.6.4 Evidence statements: chondroitin

Table 6.87 Symptoms: pain

Pain outcome	Reference	Intervention	Assessment time	Outcome/effect size
Knee				
Chondroitin sulphate				
Pain during activity, VAS (change from baseline)	1 RCT (Mazieres et al. 2007) (N=307)	CS vs placebo	6 months (end of treatment)	41% (CS) and –32% (placebo) respectively, p=0.029 Favours CS
Pain at rest, VAS (change from baseline)	1 RCT (Mazieres et al. 2007) (N=307)	CS vs placebo	6 months (end of treatment)	NS
Knee or hip				
Chondroitin (general)				
Pain-related outcomes	1 MA (Reichenbach et al. 2007) 20 RCTs, N=3846	Chondroitin vs placebo/ no treatment	Trial length range: 6 to 132 weeks	Significant heterogeneity
Pain-related outcomes (subgroup analysis of methodologically sound trials)	1 MA (Reichenbach et al. 2007) 3 RCTs, N=1553	Chondroitin vs placebo/ no treatment	Trial length range: 6 to 132 weeks	NS

Table 6.88 Symptoms: function

Function outcome	Reference	Intervention	Assessment time	Outcome/effect size
Knee				
Chondroitin sulphate (CS)				
Joint swelling, effusion or both on clinical examination	1 RCT (Clegg et al. 2006) (N=1583)	CS vs placebo	End of treatment (24 weeks	CS significantly better
Lequesne's Index (change from baseline)	1 RCT (Mazieres et al. 2007) (N=307)	CS vs placebo	6 months (end of treatment)	NS

Table 6.89 Structure modification

Structure modification outcome	Reference	Intervention	Assessment time	Outcome/effect size
Knee or hip				
Chondroitin (general)				
Minimum joint space width	1 MA (Reichenbach et al. 2007) 5 RCTs, (N=1192)	Chondroitin vs placebo/no treatment	Trial length range: 6 to 132 weeks	Effect size mean difference 0.16mm,% CI 0.08 to 0.24 Favours chondroitin
Mean joint space width	1 MA (Reichenbach et al. 2007) 5 RCTs, (N=1192)	Chondroitin vs placebo/no treatment	Trial length range: 6 to 132 weeks	Effect size mean difference 0.23mm,% CI 0.09 to 0.37 Favours chondroitin

Table 6.90 Global assessment

Global assessment outcome	Reference	Intervention	Assessment time	Outcome/effect size
Knee				
Chondroitin sulphate				
Investigators global assessment of clinical improvement	1 RCT (Mazieres et al. 2007) (N=307)	CS vs placebo	6 months (end of treatment)	3.1 (CS) and 2.5 (placebo), p=0.044 Favours CS
Patients global assessment of clinical improvement	1 RCT (Mazieres et al. 2007) (N=307)	CS vs placebo	6 months (end of treatment)	NS

Table 6.91 Quality of life

Global assessment outcome	Reference	Intervention	Assessment time	Outcome/effect size
Knee				
Chondroitin sulphate				
SF-12 physical component (change from baseline)	1 RCT (Mazieres et al. 2007) (N=307)	CS vs placebo	6 months (end of treatment)	5.8 (CS) and 3.8 (placebo), p=0.021 Favours CS
SF-12 mental component	1 RCT (Mazieres et al. 2007) (N=307)	CS vs placebo	6 months (end of treatment)	NS

Table 6.92 Withdrawals

Global assessment outcome	Reference	Intervention	Assessment time	Outcome/effect size
Knee				
Chondroitin sulphate				
Number of withdrawals due to AEs	1 RCT (Mazieres et al. 2007) (N=307)	CS vs placebo	6 months (end of treatment) N=13 (CS) and N=8 (placebo)	Placebo better

Table 6.93 Adverse events

AEs outcome	Reference	Intervention	Assessment time	Outcome/effect size
Knee				
Chondroitin sulphate				
Number of patients with at least one treatment-related AEs	1 RCT (Mazieres et al. 2007) (N=307)	CS vs placebo	24 weeks (end of treatment)	NS
Total number of AEs	1 RCT (Mazieres et al. 2007) (N=307)	CS vs placebo	24 weeks (end of treatment)	N=18 (CS) and N=20 (placebo) Both groups similar
Knee or hip				
Chondroitin (general)				
Patients experiencing AEs	1 MA (Reichenbach et al. 2007) 12 RCTs (N=1929)	Chondroitin vs placebo/ no treatment	Trial length range: 6 to 132 weeks	NS
Withdrawals due to AEs	1 MA (Reichenbach et al. 2007) 9 RCTs (N=1781)	Chondroitin vs placebo/ no treatment	Trial length range: 6 to 132 weeks	NS
Patients experiencing SAEs	1 MA (Reichenbach et al. 2007) 2 RCTs (N=217)	Chondroitin vs placebo/ no treatment	Trial length range: 6 to 132 weeks	NS

Table 6.94 Withdrawals

Rescue medication outcome	Reference	Intervention	Assessment time	Outcome/effect size
Knee				
Chondroitin sulphate				
Use of rescue paracetamol over 6 months (end of treatment)	1 RCT (Mazieres et al. 2007) (N=307)	CS vs placebo	Over 6 months (end of treatment)	NS

6.6.5   Evidence statements: glucosamine + chondroitin

Table 6.95 Symptoms: pain

Pain outcome	Reference	Intervention	Assessment time	Outcome/effect size
Knee				
CS + GS				
Pain, VAS (change from baseline)	1 RCT (Cohen et al. 2003) (N=63)	CS + GS vs placebo	4 weeks (mid-treatment) and 8 weeks, end of treatment	p=0.03 and 0.002 Favours CS + GS
CS + GH				
20% decrease in WOMAC pain; 50% decrease in WOMAC pain; WOMAC pain score, change from baseline; HAQ pain, change from baseline.	1 RCT (Clegg et al. 2006) (N=1583)	CS + GS vs placebo	24 weeks	NS

Table 6.96 Symptoms: stiffness

Pain outcome	Reference	Intervention	Assessment time	Outcome/effect size
Knee				
CS + GH				
WOMAC stiffness score, change from baseline, change from baseline.	1 RCT (Clegg et al. 2006) (N=1583)	CS + GS vs placebo	24 weeks	NS

Table 6.97 Symptoms: function

Function outcome	Reference	Intervention	Assessment time	Outcome/effect size
Knee				
CS + GS				
Lequesne Index (change from baseline)	1 RCT (Rai et al. 2004) (N=100)	CS + GS vs placebo	1 year, end of treatment	p<0.01 Favours CS + GS
WOMAC score (change from baseline)	1 RCT (Rai et al. 2004) (N=100)	CS + GS vs placebo	Week 8 (end of treatment).	NS

continued

Table 6.97 Symptoms: function – *continued*

Function outcome	Reference	Intervention	Assessment time	Outcome/effect size
Knee				
CS + GH				
Lequesne ISK (mild/moderate osteoarthritis patients)	1 RCT (Das and Hammad 2000) (N=93)	CS + GH vs placebo	4 months (mid-treatment) and 6 months (end of treatment)	4 months: p=0.003 6 months: p=0.04 Favours CS + GH
Lequesne ISK > 25% improvement (mild/moderate osteoarthritis patients)	1 RCT (Das and Hammad 2000) (N=93)	CS + GH vs placebo	6 months (end of treatment)	p=0.04 Favours CS + GH
WOMAC function score, change from baseline; HAQ disability score, change from baseline; Joint swelling, effusion or both on clinical examination	1 RCT (Clegg et al. 2006) (N=1583)	CS + GH vs placebo	End of treatment (24 weeks)	NS
Lequesne ISK (severe osteoarthritis patients); WOMAC score (mild/moderate osteoarthritis patients); WOMAC score (severe osteoarthritis patients)	1 RCT (Das and Hammad 2000) (N=93)	CS + GH vs placebo	2 and 4 months (mid-treatments) and 6 months (end of treatment)	NS
Lequesne ISK (mild/moderate osteoarthritis patients)	1 RCT (Das and Hammad 2000) (N=93)	CS + GH vs placebo	2 months (mid-treatment)	NS
Lequesne ISK > 25% improvement (severe osteoarthritis patients); WOMAC > 25% improvement (mild/moderate osteoarthritis patients); WOMAC > 25% improvement (severe osteoarthritis patients)	1 RCT (Das and Hammad 2000) (N=93)	CS + GH vs placebo	6 months (end of treatment)	NS

Table 6.98 Structure modification

Structure modification outcome	Reference	Intervention	Assessment time	Outcome/effect size
Knee				
CS + GS				
Mean joint space width (change from baseline)	1 RCT (Rai et al. 2004) (N=100)	CS + GS vs placebo	1 year, end of treatment	p<0.01 Favours placebo

Table 6.99 Global assessment

Global assessment outcome	Reference	Intervention	Assessment time	Outcome/effect size
Knee				
CS + GH				
Patient's global assessment > 25% improvement (mild/moderate osteoarthritis patients)	1 RCT (Das and Hammad 2000) (N=93)	CS + GH vs placebo	6 months (end of treatment)	p=0.04 Favours CS + GH
Patient's global assessment (severe osteoarthritis patients); patient's global assessment (mild/moderate osteoarthritis patients)	1 RCT (Das and Hammad 2000) (N=93)	CS + GH vs placebo	2 and 4 months (mid-treatments) and 6 months (end of treatment)	NS
Patient's global assessment > 25% improvement (severe osteoarthritis patients)	1 RCT (Das and (Hammad 2000) (N=93)	CS + GH vs placebo	6 months (end of treatment)	NS
Patient's global assessment of response to therapy; patient's global assessment of disease status; physician's global assessment of disease status.	1 RCT (Clegg et al. 2006) (N=1583)	CS + GH vs placebo	End of treatment (24 weeks)	NS

Table 6.100 Quality of life

QoL outcome	Reference	Intervention	Assessment time	Outcome/effect size
Knee				
CS + GH				
SF-36 mental health (change from baseline)	1 RCT (Cohen et al. 2003) (N=63)	CS + GH vs placebo	8 weeks, end of treatment	p=0.04 Favours CS + GH
SF-36 physical health (change from baseline)	1 RCT (Cohen et al. 2003) (N=63)	CS + GH vs placebo	8 weeks, end of treatment	NS

Table 6.101 Study withdrawals

Withdrawals outcome	Reference	Intervention	Assessment time	Outcome/effect size
Knee				
CS + GS				
Total number of withdrawals; withdrawals due to AEs	1 RCT (Cohen et al. 2003) (N=63)	CS + GS vs placebo	8 weeks (end of treatment)	NS
CS + GH				
Total number of withdrawals; withdrawals due to AEs	1 RCT (Das and Hammad 2000) (N=93)	CS + GH vs placebo	6 months (end of treatment)	Total withdrawals: both N=2 Due to AEs: N=1 (CS+GH) and N=3 (placebo) Both groups similar
Total number of withdrawals; withdrawals due to AE; withdrawals due to lack of efficacy	1 RCT (Clegg et al. 2006) (N=1583	CS + GH vs placebo	24 weeks (end of treatment)	NS

Table 6.102 Adverse events

AEs outcome	Reference	Intervention	Assessment time	Outcome/effect size
Knee				
CS + GS				
Number of patients with AEs	1 RCT (Cohen et al. 2003) (N=63)	CS + GS vs placebo	8 weeks (end of treatment)	N=15, 46.9% (CS+GS) and N=11, 35.5% (placebo) Placebo better
CS + GH				
Number of patients with AEs	1 RCT (Das and Hammad 2000) (N=93)	CS + GH vs placebo	6 months (end of treatment)	N=8 17% (CS+GS) and N=9 19% (placebo) Both groups similar

Table 6.103 Rescue medication

Rescue medication outcome	Reference	Intervention	Assessment time	Outcome/effect size
Knee				
CS + GH				
Rescue paracetamol consumption for severe osteoarthritis patients and for mild/moderate osteoarthritis patients	1 RCT (Das and Hammad 2000) (N=93)	CS + GH vs placebo	6 months (end of treatment)	NS
Rescue paracetamol (no. of tablets taken)	1 RCT (Clegg et al. 2006) (N=1583)	CS + GH vs placebo	24 weeks (end of treatment)	NS

6.6.6   From evidence to recommendations

The evidence from these studies is often difficult to compare due to differences between the products employed (and their bioavailability), between the study populations, patient BMI, and the use of analgesia at the time of pain and function assessment in the trials. Overall, those trials which used glucosamine sulfate as a single dose of 1500 mg, rather than hydrochloride 500 mg tds, showed a small benefit over placebo for treatment of knee OA. However, at the time of writing, the hydrochloride preparation has been granted a European Medicines Evaluatory Agency licence, while the sulfate has not. The evidence for efficacy of chondroitin was less convincing.

Evidence to support the efficacy of glucosamine hydrochloride as a symptom modifier is poor. For the non-licensed product (glucosamine sulfate), the evidence is not strong enough to warrant recommending that it should be prescribed on the NHS. Notwithstanding some evidence of benefit and very little evidence of harm in clinical practice, and despite the extra scrutiny these agents have received, the economic cost-consequence table (see Appendix C, online at www.rcplondon.ac.uk/pubs/brochure.aspx?e=242) shows that only glucosamine sulfate is potentially cost effective out of the interventions considered in this section. There are a wide range of incremental cost-effectiveness ratios (ICERs) reported and the poorest estimates of efficacy would take it beyond the threshold of affordability in the NHS. Because only one glucosamine hydrochloride product is licensed, it would not be cost effective to prescribe glucosamine on the NHS.

In assessing the outcomes given in the evidence base, the GDG regarded measurement of joint space narrowing as of questionable value in assessing any potential beneficial structural modification, and convincing evidence of improvement in patient-centred outcomes consequent on any structural modification is still lacking. There is therefore no positive recommendation regarding structure modification.

Many people with osteoarthritis take over-the-counter nutriceutical products and may benefit from clear, evidence-based information. This is reinforced in the recommendation in section 5.1. In particular, the GDG felt that it would be beneficial to advise people who wanted to trial over-the-counter glucosamine that the only potential benefits identified in early research are purely related to a reduction of pain (to some people, and to only mild or modest degree) with glucosamine sulfate 1500 mg daily. They could also benefit from advice on how to perform their own trial of therapy, that is, to evaluate their pain before starting glucosamine and ensure they review the benefits of glucosamine after three months.

RECOMMENDATION

R19   The use of glucosamine or chondroitin products is not recommended for the treatment of osteoarthritis.

6.7   Invasive treatments for knee osteoarthritis

6.7.1   Clinical introduction

In clinical practice, arthroscopic lavage, debridement and tidal irrigation are invasive procedures offered to patients who are failing medical management, predominantly for knee osteoarthritis. There is no general consensus on which patients should be offered these procedures.

Arthroscopy usually involves a day-stay hospital admission with general anaesthesia and the insertion of a fibre-optic instrument into the knee, allowing thorough inspection of pathology. The joint is irrigated with a sizable volume of fluid, a process known as lavage, which may remove microscopic and macroscopic debris resulting from cartilage breakdown, as well as removing the pro-inflammatory effects of this material. This procedure may be associated with debridement, the surgical 'neatening' of obviously frayed cartilage or meniscal surfaces.

Tidal irrigation refers to the process of irrigating the joint and does not require general anaesthesia – rather a needle is inserted in the knee under local anaesthesia and a large volume of fluid run into the knee and then allowed to drain out. The rationale is the same as for arthroscopic lavage.

Evaluating these therapies is difficult due to the lack of standardised referral criteria, the absence of many randomised trials and the lack of standardisation of co-therapies including exercises.

6.7.2 Methodological introduction

We looked for studies that investigated the efficacy and safety of arthroscopic lavage (with or without debridement) compared with tidal irrigation and placebo (sham procedure) with respect to symptoms, function, and quality of life in adults with osteoarthritis. Ten RCTs (Bradley et al. 2002; Chang and Falconer 1993; Dawes et al. 1987; Gibson et al. 1992; Hubbard 1996; Ike et al. 1992; Kalunian et al. 2000; Merchan and Galindo 1993; Moseley et al. 2002; Ravaud et al. 1999) were found on the outcomes of symptoms, function and quality of life; no data for adverse events were reported. No relevant cohort or case-control studies were found. Two RCTs (Hubbard 1996, Merchan 1993) were excluded as evidence due to methodological limitations.

The eight included RCTs were methodologically sound and were similar in terms of:

- osteoarthritis site (all looked at knee osteoarthritis)
- osteoarthritis diagnosis (radiologically)
- trial design (parallel group).

However, they differed with respect to:

- interventions and comparisons
- trial size and length.

6.7.3 Evidence statements

Table 6.104 Symptoms: pain

Pain outcome	Reference	Intervention	Assessment time	Outcome/effect size
Knee				
Lavage				
KSPS (knee specific pain scale, 0–100)	1 RCT (Moseley et al. 2002), N=180	Lavage vs placebo (sham procedure)	1 year or 2 years post-intervention	NS
Arthritis pain (0–100)	1 RCT (Moseley 2002), N=180	Lavage vs placebo (sham procedure)	2 weeks, 6 weeks, 3 months, 6 months 1 year 18 months and 2 years post-intervention	NS
KSPS (knee specific pain scale, 0–100)	1 RCT (Moseley et al. 2002), N=180	Lavage + debridement vs placebo (sham procedure)	1 year or 2 years post-intervention	NS
Arthritis pain (0–100)	1 RCT (Moseley et al. 2002), N=180	Lavage + debridement vs placebo (sham procedure)	2 weeks, 6 weeks, 3 months, 6 months 1 year 18 months and 2 years post-intervention	NS
AIMS pain score; AIMS pain (Improvement of ≥1 cm)	1 RCT (Chang and Falconer 1993), N=34	Lavage + debridement vs tidal irrigation	3 months and 1 year post-intervention	NS

continued

Table 6.104 Symptoms: pain – *continued*

Pain outcome	Reference	Intervention	Assessment time	Outcome/effect size
Knee				
Lavage – continued				
Pain at rest, VAS (change from baseline)	1 RCT (Dawes et al. 1987), N=20	Lavage vs control (saline injection)	12 weeks post-intervention	−0.55 (lavage) and −2.1 (saline) Saline better
Pain walking, VAS (change from baseline)	1 RCT (Dawes et al. 1987), N=20	Lavage vs control (saline injection)	12 weeks post-intervention	−2.85 (lavage) and −3.3 (saline) Saline better
Pain at night, VAS (change from baseline)	1 RCT (Dawes et al. 1987), N=20	Lavage vs control (saline injection)	12 weeks post-intervention	−1.2 (lavage) and −5.0 (saline) Saline better
Pain (relative change)	1 RCT (Ravaud et al. 1992), N=98	Lavage vs placebo	24 weeks post-treatment	p=0.02 Favours lavage
Clinical improvement in pain (% patients with at least 30% pain reduction from baseline)	1 RCT (Ravaud et al. 1992), N=98	Lavage vs placebo	1 week, 4 weeks 12 weeks and 24 weeks post-treatment	1 week: 48% (lavage) and 25% (placebo) 4 weeks: 48% (lavage) and 29% (placebo) 12 weeks: 48% (lavage) and 29% (placebo) 24 weeks: 48% (lavage) and 22% (placebo). Lavage better
Irrigation				
WOMAC pain (change from baseline, % of improvement)	1 RCT (Bradley et al. 2002), N=180	Tidal irrigation vs sham irrigation	12 weeks post-intervention	21% (tidal) and 23% (sham) Both groups similar
WOMAC pain (change from baseline)	1 RCT (Bradley et al. 2002), N=180	Tidal irrigation vs sham irrigation	12 weeks, 24 weeks and 52 weeks post-intervention	12 weeks: −2.8 (tidal) and -3.3 (sham) 24 weeks: −2.1 (tidal) and −2.7 (sham) 52 weeks -2.8 (tidal) and −2.6 (sham)
Knee tenderness (change from baseline)	1 RCT (Bradley et al. 2002), N=180	Tidal irrigation vs sham irrigation	12 weeks, 24 weeks and 52 weeks post-intervention	12 weeks: −0.10 (tidal) and -0.17 (sham) 24 weeks: −0.04 (tidal) and −0.07 (sham) 52 weeks +0.06 (tidal) and −0.11 (sham)
Pain in the previous 24 hours (VAS)	1 RCT (Ike et al. 1992), N=77	Tidal irrigation + medical management vs medical management:	Over 12 weeks	p=0.02 Favours tidal irrigation

continued

Table 6.104 Symptoms: pain – *continued*

Pain outcome	Reference	Intervention	Assessment time	Outcome/effect size
Knee				
Irrigation – continued				
Pain after walking 50-feet (VAS)	1 RCT (Ike et al. 1992), N=77	Tidal irrigation + medical management vs medical management:	Over 12 weeks	p=0.03 Favours tidal irrigation
Pain after climbing 4 stairs (VAS)	1 RCT (Ike et al. 1992), N=77	Tidal irrigation + medical management vs medical management:	Over 12 weeks	P<0.01 Favours tidal irrigation
Pain, VAS (change from baseline)	1 RCT (Kalunian et al. 2000), N=90	Full irrigation vs minimal irrigation	12 weeks post-intervention	Favours full irrigation
Pain, VAS (change from baseline – analysis of covariance with irrigation group as independent variable, baseline score and swelling as covariates)	1 RCT (Kalunian et al. 2000), N=90	Full irrigation vs minimal irrigation	12 weeks post-intervention	1.47,% CI –1.2 to 4.1 (full) and 0.12,%CI 0 to 0.3 (minimal); p=0.02 Favours full irrigation
WOMAC pain (change from base-line – analysis of covariance with irrigation group as independent variable, baseline score and swelling as covariates)	1 RCT (Kalunian et al. 2000), N=90	Full irrigation vs minimal irrigation	12 weeks post-intervention	4.2,% CI –0.9 to 9.4 (full) and 2.3,% CI –0.1 to 4.7 (minimal); p=0.04 Favours full irrigation
WOMAC pain (change from baseline)	1 RCT (Kalunian et al. 2000), N=90	Full irrigation vs minimal irrigation	12 weeks post-intervention	NS

Table 6.105 Symptoms: stiffness

Stiffness outcome	Reference	Intervention	Assessment time	Outcome/effect size
Knee				
Lavage				
Immobility stiffness, mins (change from baseline)	1 RCT (Dawes et al. 1987), N=20	Lavage vs control (saline injection)	12 weeks post-intervention	–9.5 (lavage) and +7.5 (placebo) Lavage better
Morning stiffness, mins (change from baseline)	1 RCT (Dawes et al. 1987), N=20	Lavage vs control (saline injection)	12 weeks post-intervention	–6.0 (lavage) and –3.8 (saline) Saline better

continued

Table 6.105 Symptoms: stiffness – *continued*

Stiffness outcome	Reference	Intervention	Assessment time	Outcome/effect size
Knee				
Irrigation				
WOMAC stiffness (change from baseline)	1 RCT (Bradley et al. 2002), N=180	Tidal irrigation vs sham irrigation	12 weeks, 24 weeks and 52 weeks post-intervention.	12 weeks: –0.7 (tidal) and –1.2 (sham) 24 weeks: –0.6 (tidal) and –0.9 (sham) 52 weeks: –0.7 (tidal) and –0.9 (sham) Both groups similar
Knee stiffness, number of days/week	1 RCT (Ike et al. 1992), N=77	Tidal irrigation + medical management vs medical management	12 weeks post-intervention	p=0.03 Favours tidal
Stiffness with inactivity	1 RCT (Ike et al. 1992), N=77	Tidal irrigation + medical management vs medical management	12 weeks post-intervention	p=0.01 Favours tidal
WOMAC stiffness (change from baseline); WOMAC stiffness (change from baseline – analysis of covariance with irrigation group as independent variable, baseline score and swelling as covariates)	1 RCT (Kalunian et al. 2000), N=90	Full irrigation vs minimal irrigation	12 weeks post-intervention	NS

Table 6.106 Symptoms: function

Function outcome	Reference	Intervention	Assessment time	Outcome/effect size
Knee				
Lavage				
Self-reported ability to walk and bend (AIMS2-WB score)	1 RCT (Moseley et al. 2002), N=180	Lavage vs placebo (sham procedure)	1 year or 2 years post-intervention	NS
Physical functioning scale (30-minute walk time and stair climb time, minutes)	1 RCT (Moseley et al. 2002), N=180	Lavage vs placebo (sham procedure)	2 weeks, 6 weeks, 3 months, 6 months 1 year 18 months and 2 years post-intervention	NS
Physical functioning scale (30-minute walk time and stair climb time, seconds)	1 RCT (Moseley et al. 2002), N=180	Lavage + debridement vs placebo (sham procedure)	1 year or 2 years post-intervention	2 weeks: 56.0 (lavage) and 48.3 (sham); p=0.02 1 year 52.5 (lavage) and 45.6 (sham); p=0.04 Favours sham

continued

Function outcome	Reference	Intervention	Assessment time	Outcome/effect size

Table 6.106 Symptoms: function – *continued*

Knee

Lavage – *continued*

Function outcome	Reference	Intervention	Assessment time	Outcome/effect size
Self-reported ability to walk and bend (AIMS2-WB score)	1 RCT (Moseley et al. 2002), N=180	Lavage + debridement vs placebo (sham procedure)	1 year or 2 years post-intervention	NS
Physical functioning scale (30-metre walk time and stair climb time, seconds)	1 RCT (Moseley et al. 2002), N=180	Lavage + debridement vs placebo (sham procedure)	2 weeks, 6 weeks, 3 months, 6 months 1 year 18 months and 2 years post-intervention	NS
AIMS physical activity; AIMS physical function; active range of motion (degrees); 50-foot walk time (seconds)	1 RCT (Chang and Falconer 1993), N=34	Lavage + debridement vs tidal irrigation	3 months and 1 year post-intervention	NS
25 yard walk time, seconds (change from baseline)	1 RCT (Dawes et al. 1987), N=20	Lavage vs control (saline injection)	12 weeks post-intervention	–23.0 (lavage) and –6.0 (saline) Saline better
Knee flexion, degrees (change from baseline)	1 RCT (Dawes et al. 1987), N=20	Lavage vs control (saline injection)	12 weeks post-intervention	+4.0 (lavage) and +9.0 (saline) Saline better
Lequesne's functional index	1 RCT (Ravaud et al. 1992) N=98	Lavage vs placebo	24 weeks post-treatment	NS

Irrigation

Function outcome	Reference	Intervention	Assessment time	Outcome/effect size
WOMAC physical functioning (change from baseline)	1 RCT (Bradley et al. 2002), N=180	Tidal irrigation vs sham irrigation	12 weeks post-intervention	17% (tidal) and 21% (sham) Both groups similar
WOMAC function (change from baseline	1 RCT (Bradley et al. 2002), N=180	Tidal irrigation vs sham irrigation	12 weeks, 24 weeks and 52 weeks post-intervention	12 weeks: –7.7 (tidal) and –10.8 (sham) 24 weeks: –6.5 (tidal) and –8.7 (sham) 52 weeks –7.7 (tidal) and –9.6 (sham)
50-foot walk time (change from baseline)	1 RCT (Bradley et al. 2002), N=180	Tidal irrigation vs sham irrigation	12 weeks, 24 weeks and 52 weeks post-intervention	12 weeks: –0.4 (tidal) and –0.6 (sham) 24 weeks: –0.4 (tidal) and –0.7 (sham) 52 weeks –0.5 (tidal) and –0.4 (sham)

continued

Table 6.106 Symptoms: function – *continued*

Function outcome	Reference	Intervention	Assessment time	Outcome/effect size
Knee				
Irrigation – *continued*				
50-foot walk time; 4-stair climb time; passive and active range of motion	1 RCT (Ike et al. 1992), N=77	Tidal irrigation + medical management vs medical management	Over 12 weeks	NS
WOMAC total (change from baseline); WOMAC total (change from baseline – analysis of covariance with irrigation group as independent variable, baseline score and swelling as covariates); WOMAC function (change from baseline); WOMAC function (change from baseline – analysis of covariance with irrigation group as independent variable, baseline score and swelling as covariates)	1 RCT (Kalunian et al. 2000), N=90	Full irrigation vs minimal irrigation	12 weeks post-intervention	NS

Table 107 Global assessment

Global assessment outcome	Reference	Intervention	Assessment time	Outcome/effect size
Knee				
Lavage				
Physicians global assessment (% improved)	1 RCT (Chang and Falconer 1993), N=34	Lavage + debridement vs tidal irrigation	1 year post-intervention	41% (lavage) and 23% (tidal), p<0.05 Favours lavage
Physicians global assessment (% improved)	1 RCT (Chang and Falconer 1993), N=34	Lavage + debridement vs tidal irrigation	3 months post-intervention	NS

continued

Table 107 Global assessment – *continued*

Global assessment outcome	Reference	Intervention	Assessment time	Outcome/effect size
Knee				
Lavage – *continued*				
Patients global assessment (VAS); Patients global assessment (Improvement of ≥1 cm)	1 RCT (Chang and Falconer 1993), N=34	Lavage + debridement vs tidal irrigation	3 months and 1 year post-intervention	NS
Global status	1 RCT (Ravaud et al. 1992), N=98	Lavage vs placebo	24 weeks post-treatment	NS
Irrigation				
Physician's assessment of arthritis global activity (number of patients 'severe', change from baseline)	1 RCT (Bradley et al. 2002), N=180	Tidal irrigation vs sham irrigation	12 weeks, 24 weeks and 52 weeks post-intervention	12 weeks: –8 (tidal) and –9 (sham) 24 weeks: –9 (tidal) and –13 (sham) 52 weeks –9 (tidal) and –13 (sham)
Physician's assessment of arthritis global activity (number of patients 'mild', change from baseline) at 12 weeks post-intervention (+19 and +29 respectively), at 24 weeks post-intervention (+15 and +19 respectively) and at 52 weeks post-intervention (+15 and +21 respectively)	1 RCT (Bradley et al. 2002), N=180	Tidal irrigation vs sham irrigation	12 weeks, 24 weeks and 52 weeks post-intervention	12 weeks: –+19 (tidal) and +29 (sham) 24 weeks: +15 (tidal) and +19 (sham) 52 weeks +15 (tidal) and +21.4 (sham)
Patients assessment of treatment efficacy	1 RCT (Ike et al. 1992), N=77	Tidal irrigation + medical management vs medical management:	Over 12 weeks	p<0.01 at all time periods Favours tidal
Patients assessment of treatment as somewhat or very effective at relieving pain	1 RCT (Ike et al. 1992), N=77	Tidal irrigation + medical management vs medical management	Over 12 weeks	N=17/29 (tidal) and N=11/28 (medical) Favours tidal
Physician's assessment of treatment as somewhat or very effective at relieving pain.	1 RCT (Ike et al. 1992), N=77	Tidal irrigation + medical management vs medical management	Over 12 weeks	P=0.02 at all time periods Favours tidal

Table 6.108 Quality of life

QoL outcome	Reference	Intervention	Assessment time	Outcome/effect size
Knee				
Lavage				
AIMS social activity score; AIMS depression score; AIMS anxiety score	1 RCT (Chang and Falconer 1993), N=34	Lavage + debridement vs tidal irrigation	3 months and 1 year post-intervention	NS
Irrigation				
QWB score (change from baseline)	1 RCT (Bradley et al. 2002), N=180	Tidal irrigation vs sham irrigation	24 weeks and 52 weeks post-intervention	Both: 0.02 (tidal) and 0.0 (sham) Both groups similar

Table 6.109 Use of rescue medication/analgesia

Rescue medication outcome	Reference	Intervention	Assessment time	Outcome/effect size
Knee				
Irrigation				
Use of medication (NSAIDs, narcotic analgesia, muscle relaxants, anti-depressants, glucosamine or chondroitin sulphate)	1 RCT (Bradley et al. 2002), N=180	Tidal irrigation vs sham irrigation	12 weeks post-intervention	N=18 (tidal) and N=32 (sham) Tidal better
Use of medication (NSAIDs, narcotic analgesia, muscle relaxants, anti-depressants, glucosamine or chondroitin sulphate)	1 RCT (Bradley et al. 2002), N=180	Tidal irrigation vs sham irrigation	24 weeks and 52 weeks post-intervention	24 weeks: both N=29 52 weeks: N=36 (tidal) and N=32 (sham) Both groups similar
Paracetamol use (change from baseline, mean number of tablets/day)	1 RCT (Bradley et al. 2002), N=180	Tidal irrigation vs sham irrigation	12 weeks 24 weeks and 52 weeks post-intervention	12 weeks: +1.1 (tidal) and +0.1 (sham) 24 weeks: +1.4 (tidal) and +0.6 (sham) 52 weeks: +0.8 (tidal) and +0.1 (sham) Both groups similar

Table 6.110 Other				
Other outcome	**Reference**	**Intervention**	**Assessment time**	**Outcome/effect size**
Knee				
Irrigation				
Clinical scores for symptoms and mobility	1 RCT (Gibson et al. 1992), N=20	Lavage vs Lavage + debridement	6 and 12 weeks post-intervention	6 weeks: 33.7 (lavage) and 32.7 (lavage + debridement) 12 weeks: 33.9 (lavage) and 33.0 (lavage + debridement) No improvement in either group

6.7.4 From evidence to recommendations

Arthroscopic lavage and debridement are surgical procedures that have become widely used. Tidal irrigation, through large bore needles, has been practised by physicians to a limited degree. These procedures have limited risks, though arthroscopy usually involves a general anaesthetic. These procedures are offered to patients when usual medical care is failing or has failed and the next option, knee arthroplasty, appears too severe, for a variety of reasons, for either the patient or the medical adviser.

Arthroscopy may be indicated for true locking, caused by meniscal lesions or loose bodies in the knee joint. These situations are uncommon in patients with osteoarthritis of the knee.

Many procedures in medicine have a large placebo effect and when assessing minimalistic surgical procedures it can be very difficult to separate this placebo effect from the surgical procedure itself.

RECOMMENDATION

R20   Referral for arthroscopic lavage and debridement* should not be offered as part of treatment for osteoarthritis, unless the person has knee osteoarthritis with a clear history of mechanical locking (not gelling, 'giving way' or x-ray evidence of loose bodies).

---

* This recommendation is a refinement of the indication in 'Arthroscopic knee washout, with or without debridement, for the treatment of osteoarthritis' (NICE interventional procedure guidance 230). This guideline has reviewed the clinical and cost-effectiveness evidence, which has led to this more specific recommendation on the indication for which arthroscopic lavage and debridement is judged to be clinically and cost effective.

7 Pharmacological management of osteoarthritis

7.1 Oral analgesics

7.1.1 Clinical introduction

Appropriate pharmacological analgesia forms one of the key platforms for treating osteoarthritis when non-pharmacological therapy on its own is insufficient. The use of such analgesia may be aimed at different aspects of the patient's pain, including night pain or exercise-associated pain. Oral analgesics, especially paracetamol, have been used for many years, with increasing use of opioid analgesics in recent years, partly fuelled by fears over the safety of NSAIDs. The exact mechanism of action of paracetamol is unclear, although it may work in part by inhibiting prostaglandin synthesis; its action seems to work via the central nervous system rather than through peripheral effects. Opioid analgesics work by action on endogenous opioid receptors in the central nervous system.

There is still surprisingly little data on how patients use these therapies, which may influence their efficacy (for example, intermittent usage only at times of increased pain versus regular daily dosing). There are also many assumptions made on the effectiveness of these therapies in osteoarthritis, based on concepts such as 'analgesic ladders' which are not well supported in osteoarthritis cohorts.

It should be noted that this section includes the use of tricyclic agents as analgesics in osteo-arthritis. This refers to the concept of low-dose usage of these agents, rather than antidepressant doses; it has been suggested that such low-dose usage may result in significant antinociceptive effects. However, it is important to note that depression may be associated with any chronic painful condition such as osteoarthritis and may require treatment in its own right. Readers should refer to the NICE depression guidelines (National Institute for Health and Clinical Excellence 2007)

7.1.2 Methodological introduction: paracetamol versus NSAIDs including COX-2 inhibitors

We looked at studies on the efficacy and safety of paracetamol compared with oral NSAIDs or selective COX-2 inhibitors for symptomatic relief from pain in adults with osteoarthritis. We found one Cochrane meta-analysis (Towheed et al. 2006) of randomised controlled trials that addressed the topic. In addition, one RCT (Temple et al. 2006), four relevant N-of-1 trials (March et al. 1994; Nikles et al. 2005; Wegman et al. 2003; Yelland et al. 2007) and one cohort study (Fries and Bruce 2003) were identified. All studies were found to be methodologically sound and were included as evidence.

The meta-analysis included ten RCTs with comparisons between paracetamol and NSAIDs (celecoxib, diclofenac, ibuprofen, naproxen and rofecoxib). The analysis did not provide separate results for non-selective and COX-2 selective NSAIDs on pain outcomes, but did for gastrointestinal adverse events. Studies included in the analysis differed with respect to:

- paracetamol dosage
- site of disease
- osteoarthritis diagnosis
- trial design
- funding sources
- study site location.

To avoid double counting of participants receiving paracetamol, the analysis was stratified into three comparator groups involving paracetamol and:

- ibuprofen 2400 mg, diclofenac, Arthrotec (diclofenac with misoprostol) , celecoxib, naproxen (comparator 1)
- ibuprofen 1200 mg, Arthrotec, rofecoxib 25 mg, naproxen (comparator 2)
- ibuprofen 1200 mg, Arthrotec, rofecoxib 12.5 mg, naproxen (comparator 3).

The four N-of-1 trials reported on courses of paracetamol and NSAIDs given in random order to blinded participants acting as their own controls. There were high numbers of non-completers across all studies. One cohort study retrospectively examined the prevalence of serious gastrointestinal adverse events in participants taking paracetamol or ibuprofen.

The RCT (Temple et al. 2006) looked at paracetamol (4 g/day) versus naproxen (750 mg/day) in N=581 patients with knee or hip osteoarthritis in a 12-month or 6-month treatment phase.

7.1.3 Methodological introduction: paracetamol versus opioids, and paracetamol-opioid combinations

We looked at studies that investigated the efficacy and safety of i) paracetamol compared with opioids or opioid-paracetamol compounds, and ii) NSAIDs compared with opioid-paracetamol compounds to relieve pain in adult patients with osteoarthritis. One Cochrane systematic review and meta-analysis (Cepeda et al. 2006), six RCTs (Bianchi et al. 2003; Boureau et al. 1990; Irani 1980; Kjaersgaard et al. 1990; McIntyre et al. 1981; Parr et al. 1989) and one prospective cohort study (Mitchell 1984) were found on paracetamol versus opioids, paracetamol versus paracetamol-opioids, NSAIDs versus paracetamol-opioids and opioids versus NSAIDs. The cohort study had a mixed arthritis population, did not stratify the study findings in terms of diagnostic category, and had multiple methodological limitations: it was excluded.

The Cochrane meta-analysis only included one RCT comparing the opioid tramadol (up to 300 mg/day) with the NSAID diclofenac (up to 150 mg/day) for 28 days of treatment in N=108 patients with hip or knee osteoarthritis. The RCT was assessed for quality and found to be methodologically sound.

The included RCTs addressing individual questions were as follows:

- paracetamol versus opioids (Bianchi et al. 2003; Boureau et al. 1990; Kjaersgaard et al. 1990)
- paracetamol-opioid combinations (Irani 1980; McIntyre et al. 1981; Parr et al. 1989).

Studies differed with respect to the anatomical site of osteoarthritis, and treatment regimens (doses and treatment length). All studies included as evidence had methodological issues, including:

- small sample sizes
- inadequate blinding
- no washout period for previous analgesic medication
- ITT analysis was rarely performed.

7.1.4 Methodological introduction: opioids

We looked at studies that investigated the efficacy and safety of low-dose opioids with or without paracetamol compared with higher-strength opioids with respect to symptoms, function and quality of life in adults with osteoarthritis. Two systematic reviews and meta-analyses (Bjordal et al. 2007; Cepeda et al. 2006) and four RCTs (Andrews et al. 1976; Bird et al. 1995; Gana 2006; Jensen and Ginsberg 1994) were found that addressed the question. One RCT (Andrews 1976) was excluded due to methodological limitations.

The Cochrane systematic review (Cepeda et al. 2006) included three RCTs (N=467 patients) comparing tramadol (opioid) with placebo and two RCTs (N=615 patients) comparing tramadol vs paracetamol vs placebo and tramadol vs diclofenac.

▷ Opioid versus placebo

The three RCTs included in the MA were similar in terms of trial design (parallel-group studies), blinding (double blind) and study quality. However, trials varied in terms of:
- osteoarthritis site (two RCTs knee, one RCT hip or knee)
- treatment regimen – dose of tramadol one RCT 200 mg/day, two RCTs up to 400 mg/day)
- trial size and length.

▷ Opioid–paracetamol combinations versus placebo

The two RCTs included in the MA were similar in terms of trial design (parallel-group studies), blinding (double blind) and study quality. However, trials varied in terms of:
- trial size and length
- dose of tramadol 37.5 mg/day, paracetamol 325 mg/day (increased to 4 or 8 tablets/day further into the trial).

The second systematic review (Bjordal et al. 2007) included 63 RCTs (of which N=6 RCTs compared opioids with placebo, N=1057 patients) and assessed the outcome of pain. Trials were similar in terms of osteoarthritis site (knee osteoarthritis) and study quality. However, trials varied in terms of:
- trial size and length
- treatment – type of opioid used (N=2 RCTs tramadol, N=2 RCTs oxymorphone, N=1 RCT oxycodone, N=1 RCT codeine, N=1 RCT morphine sulphate).

Note: the Bjordal MA (Bjordal et al. 2007) includes two RCTs that were also included in the Cepeda MA (Cepeda et al. 2006). However, both MAs included a number of different additional studies and thus both MAs were included as evidence.

The three included RCTs were methodologically sound and assessed patients with knee and/or hip osteoarthritis. The first RCT (Bird et al. 1995) was a cross-over study and compared low dose tramadol with pentazocine in N=40 patients for a 2-week treatment period. The second RCT (Jensen and Ginsberg 1994) used parallel group design and compared dextropropoxyphene with high dose tramadol in N=264 patients for a 2-week treatment period. The third RCT (Gana et al. 2006) compared tramadol (at increasing doses 100, 200, 300 and 400 mg/day) with placebo for a 12-week treatment period.

The cross-over study (Bird et al. 1995) did not include a wash-out period between treatment periods. However, in an attempt to reduce the influence of any carry-over effects, the final 7 days of each treatment period were used to compare the treatments. This study also had a high withdrawal rate (48%), but was otherwise fairly well conducted. The parallel group study (Jensen and Ginsberg 1994) was methodologically sound.

7.1.5 Methodological introduction: paracetamol versus placebo

We looked at studies that investigated the efficacy and safety of paracetamol compared with placebo with respect to symptoms, function, and quality of life in adults with osteoarthritis. We found one Cochrane systematic review and meta-analysis (Towheed et al. 2006) and two RCTs (Altman et al. 2007; Herrero-Beaumont et al. 2007) on paracetamol versus placebo.

The Cochrane meta-analysis assessed the RCTs for quality and pooled together all data for the outcomes of symptoms, function and AEs. However, the outcomes of quality of life and GI AEs were not reported. The results for these outcomes have been taken from the individual RCTs included in the systematic review. No relevant RCTs, cohort or case-control studies were found.

Outcomes in the RCTs of the MA were analysed by a number of different assessment tools, using either categorical or quantitative data. For continuous outcome data, the MA has used SMD (standardised mean difference) to pool across RCTs. For dichotomous outcome data, the MA has calculated RR.

The meta-analysis included seven RCTs (with N=2491 participants) that focused on comparisons between paracetamol and placebo. Studies included in the analysis differed with respect to:

- paracetamol dosage (five RCTs 1000 mg daily, two RCTs 4000 mg daily)
- site of disease (five RCTs knee two RCTs knee or hip)
- osteoarthritis diagnosis (five RCTs radiological one RCT clinical and radiological one RCT Lequesne criteria)
- trial length and design (four RCTs were parallel group design, three RCTs cross-over design)
- funding sources (three RCTs had involvement of a pharmaceutical company).

The two RCTs (Altman et al. 2007; Herrero-Beaumont et al. 2007) not included in the systematic review were parallel studies that focused on the outcomes of symptoms, function and AEs. The first RCT (Altman et al. 2007) was methodologically sound (randomised and double-blind) and compared paracetamol extended release (ER) (3900 mg/day) versus paracetamol ER (1950 mg/day) versus placebo in N=483 patients with knee or hip osteo-arthritis in a 12-week treatment phase. The second RCT (Herrero-Beaumont et al. 2007) was methodologically sound (randomised and double-blind) and compared paracetamol ER (3000 mg/day) versus placebo or glucosamine sulfate in N=325 patients with knee osteoarthritis in a 6-months treatment phase. The results for the glucosamine arm are not presented here.

7.1.6 Methodological introduction: tricyclics, SSRIs and SNRIs

We looked for studies that investigated the efficacy and safety of tricyclics/SSRI/SNRI drugs compared with placebo with respect to symptoms, function, and quality of life in adults with osteoarthritis. One RCT (Scott 1969) was found that on the outcomes of symptoms and function. No relevant cohort or case-control studies were found.

The RCT (Scott 1969) (N=24) used a cross-over design and involved a mixed population of osteoarthritis (N=7), RA (N=14) or ankylosing spondylitis (N=1) patients who were randomised to treatment with the tricyclic antidepressant imipramine or placebo. Results for osteoarthritis patients only are reported here. The study length was 6 weeks (3 weeks for each treatment). The results for each patient were reported separately and therefore the osteoarthritis data have been extracted. The anatomical site of osteoarthritis was not mentioned and AEs were not reported for the separate osteoarthritis subgroup. Overall, the study was fairly well conducted (although it did not include a wash-out period between treatments) and is therefore included as evidence.

7.1.7 Evidence statements: paracetamol vs NSAIDs including COX-2 inhibitors

Table 7.1 Symptoms: pain

Pain outcome	Reference	Intervention	Assessment time	Outcome/effect size
Rest pain	1 MA (Towheed et al. 2006), 3 RCTs	NSAIDs (ibuprofen 2400 mg, diclofenac, arthrotec, celecoxib, naproxen) versus paracetamol	Mean duration 13.1 weeks (range 1–104 weeks)	SMD –0.20, 95% CI–0.36 to –0.03, p<0.05 Favours NSAIDs
Rest pain	1 MA (Towheed et al. 2006), 4 RCTs	NSAIDs (ibuprofen 1200 mg, arthrotec, rofecoxib 25 mg, naproxen) versus paracetamol	Mean duration 13.1 weeks (range 1–104 weeks)	SMD –0.19, 95% CI –0.35 to –0.03, p<0.05 Favours NSAIDs
Overall pain	1 MA (Towheed et al. 2006), 8 RCTs	NSAIDs (ibuprofen 2400 mg, diclofenac, arthrotec, celecoxib, naproxen) versus paracetamol	Mean duration 13.1 weeks (range 1–104 weeks)	SMD –0.25, 95% CI –0.33 to –0.17, p<0.05 Favours NSAIDs
Overall pain	1 MA (Towheed et al. 2006), 7 RCTs	NSAIDs (ibuprofen 1200 mg, arthrotec, rofecoxib 25 mg, naproxen) versus paracetamol	Mean duration 13.1 weeks (range 1–104 weeks)	SMD –0.31, 95% CI –0.40 to –0.21, p<0.05 Favours NSAIDs
Pain on motion	1 MA (Towheed et al. 2006)	NSAIDs versus paracetamol	Mean duration 13.1 weeks (range 1–104 weeks)	NS
WOMAC pain	1 MA (Towheed et al. 2006) 2 RCTs	NSAIDs (ibuprofen 2400 mg, diclofenac, arthrotec, celecoxib, naproxen) versus paracetamol	Mean duration 13.1 weeks (range 1–104 weeks)	SMD –0.24, 95% CI –0.38 to –0.09, p<0.05 Favours NSAIDs
WOMAC pain	1 MA (Towheed et al. 2006) 2 RCTs	NSAIDs (ibuprofen 1200 mg, arthrotec, rofecoxib 25 mg, naproxen) versus paracetamol	Mean duration 13.1 weeks (range 1–104 weeks)	SMD –0.37, 95% CI –0.50 to –0.24, p<0.05 Favours NSAIDs

continued

Table 7.1 Symptoms: pain – *continued*

Pain outcome	Reference	Intervention	Assessment time	Outcome/effect size
WOMAC pain	1 MA (Towheed et al. 2006) 1 RCT	NSAIDs (ibuprofen 1200 mg, arthrotec, rofecoxib 12.5 mg, naproxen) versus paracetamol	Mean duration 13.1 weeks (range 1–104 weeks)	SMD – 0.31, 95% CI –0.48 to –0.13, p<0.05 Favours NSAIDs
Lequesne Pain	1 MA (Towheed et al. 2006)	NSAIDs versus paracetamol	Mean duration 13.1 weeks (range 1–104 weeks)	NS
Symptom control/ pain relief	1 N-of-1 trial (March et al. 1994) (N=25)	NSAIDs versus paracetamol	n/a	NS (53% of patients), 33% preferred NSAIDs
Pain relief	1 N-of-1 trial (Nikles et al. 2005) (N=116)	NSAIDs versus paracetamol	n/a	20% preferred NSAIDs, 4% preferred paracetamol NSAIDs better
Pain (VAS), differences in mean scores	1 N-of-1 study (Yelland et al. 2007) (N=59)	Celecoxib versus paracetamol	n/a	Effect size 0.2 Celecoxib better
Overall symptom relief	1 N-of-1 study (Yelland et al. 2007) (N=59)	Celecoxib versus paracetamol	n/a	NS for 80% of patients Remaining patients – Celecoxib better
WOMAC pain	1 RCT (Temple et al. 2006) (N=581)	Naproxen vs paracetamol	6 months (end of treatment)	NS

Table 7.2 Symptoms: stiffness

Stiffness outcome	Reference	Intervention	Assessment time	Outcome/effect size
WOMAC stiffness	1 MA (Towheed et al. 2006), 3 RCTs	NSAIDs (ibuprofen 2400 mg, diclofenac, arthrotec, celecoxib, naproxen) vs paracetamol	Mean duration 13.1 weeks (range 1–104 weeks)	SMD –0.20, 95% CI –0.34 to –0.05, p<0.05 Favours NSAIDs
WOMAC stiffness	1 MA (Towheed et al. 2006), 4 RCTs	NSAIDs (ibuprofen 1200 mg, arthrotec, rofecoxib 25 mg, naproxen) vs paracetamol	Mean duration 13.1 weeks (range 1–104 weeks)	Significant heterogeneity
WOMAC stiffness	1 MA (Towheed et al. 2006), 8 RCTs	NSAIDs (ibuprofen 1200 mg, arthrotec, rofecoxib 12.5 mg, naproxen) vs paracetamol	Mean duration 13.1 weeks (range 1–104 weeks)	SMD –0.26, CI 95% –0.43 to –0.08, p<0.05 Favours NSAIDs
Stiffness relief (patients preference)	1 N of 1 trial (Nikles et al. 2005) (N=116)	NSAIDs vs paracetamol	n/a	More patients (13%) preferred NSAIDs to paracetamol although for most there was no clear preference between the two treatments. 2% preferred paracetamol.

continued

Table 7.2 Symptoms: stiffness – *continued*

Stiffness outcome	Reference	Intervention	Assessment time	Outcome/effect size
Stiffness (VAS), differences in mean scores	1 N-of-1 study (Yelland et al. 2007) (N=59)	Celecoxib vs paracetamol	n/a	Effect size 0.3. Celecoxib better
WOMAC stiffness	1 RCT (Temple et al. 2006) (N=581)	Naproxen vs paracetamol	6 months (end of treatment)	Both groups similar

Table 7.3 Symptoms: function

Function outcome	Reference	Intervention	Assessment time	Outcome/effect size
Function (patient-specific functional scale), differences in mean scores	1 N-of-1 study (Yelland et al. 2007) (N=59)	Celecoxib vs paracetamol	n/a	Effect size 0.3 Celecoxib better
Functional limitation	1 N-of-1 study (Yelland et al. 2007) (N=59)	Celecoxib vs paracetamol	n/a	2/42 completers Celecoxib better
WOMAC function	1 RCT (Temple et al. 2006) (N=581)	Naproxen vs paracetamol	6 months (end of treatment)	Both groups similar

Table 7.4 Global efficacy

Global efficacy outcome	Reference	Intervention	Assessment time	Outcome/effect size
WOMAC total	1 MA (Towheed et al. 2006), 3 RCTs	NSAIDs (ibuprofen 2400 mg, diclofenac, arthrotec, celecoxib, naproxen) vs paracetamol	Mean duration 13.1 weeks (range 1–104 weeks)	SMD –0.25, 95% CI–0.39 to –0.11, p<0.05 Favours NSAIDs
WOMAC total	1 MA(Towheed et al. 2006) 1 RCT	NSAIDs (ibuprofen 1200 mg, arthrotec, rofecoxib 25 mg, naproxen) vs paracetamol	Mean duration 13.1 weeks (range 1–104 weeks)	SMD –0.46, 95% CI –0.73 to –0.19, p<0.05 Favours NSAIDs
Patient global assessment of overall efficacy	1 MA(Towheed et al. 2006) 2 RCTs	NSAIDs (ibuprofen 2400 mg, diclofenac, arthrotec, celecoxib, naproxen) vs paracetamol	Mean duration 13.1 weeks (range 1–104 weeks)	NS
Patient global assessment of overall efficacy	1 MA(Towheed et al. 2006) 2 RCTs	NSAIDs (ibuprofen 2400 mg, diclofenac, arthrotec, celecoxib, naproxen) vs paracetamol	Mean duration 13.1 weeks (range 1–104 weeks)	RR 1.23, 95% CI 1.06 to 1.43, p<0.05 Favours NSAIDs
Patient global assessment of overall efficacy	1 MA(Towheed et al. 2006), 3 RCTs	NSAIDs (ibuprofen 1200 mg, arthrotec, rofecoxib 25 mg, naproxen) vs paracetamol	Mean duration 13.1 weeks (range 1–104 weeks)	RR 1.50, 95% CI 1.27 to 1.76, p<0.05 Favours NSAIDs

continued

Table 7.4 Global efficacy – *continued*

Global efficacy outcome	Reference	Intervention	Assessment time	Outcome/effect size
Patient global assessment of overall efficacy	1 MA (Towheed et al. 2006), 3 RCTs	NSAIDs (ibuprofen 1200 mg, arthrotec, rofecoxib 12.5 mg, naproxen) vs paracetamol	Mean duration 13.1 weeks (range 1–104 weeks)	Significant heterogeneity
Physician global assessment of overall efficacy	1 MA (Towheed et al. 2006)	NSAIDs vs paracetamol	Mean duration 13.1 weeks (range 1–104 weeks)	NS
Patient preference (for pain and stiffness)	1 RCT (Nikles et al. 2005), N=116	NSAIDs vs paracetamol	n/a	5% favoured NSAIDs, and 2% favoured paracetamol Both groups similar
Patient preference (for general efficacy)	1 N-of-1 trial (Wegman et al. 2003), N=13	NSAIDs vs paracetamol	n/a	71% = no preference participants 29% = preferred NSAIDs

Table 7.5 General adverse events (AEs)

AEs outcome	Reference	Intervention	Assessment time	Outcome/effect size
Total number of patients with AEs	1 MA (Towheed et al. 2006)	NSAIDs vs paracetamol	Mean duration 13.1 weeks (range 1–104 weeks)	NS
Frequency of AEs	1 N-of-1 trial (March et al. 1041–45), N=25	NSAIDs vs paracetamol	n/a	NS
Frequency of AEs	1 N-of-1 trial (Wegman et al. 2003), N=13	NSAIDs vs paracetamol	n/a	NS
Number of AEs	1 N-of-1 trial (Nikles et al. 2005), N=116	NSAIDs vs paracetamol	n/a	41% = more AEs with NSAIDs and 31% same in both groups and 28% = more AEs with paracetamol NSAIDs worse
Number of patients with AEs	1 N-of-1 study (Yelland et al. 2007) (N=59)	Celecoxib vs SR paracetamol	n/a	N=5 – celecoxib worse N=9 – pracetamol worse N=25 – NS difference Both groups similar
Number of patients with ≥1 AE	1 RCT (Temple et al. 2006) (N=581)	Naproxen vs paracetamol	6 months (end of treatment)	NS
Number of patients with SAEs	1 RCT (Temple et al. 2006) (N=581)	NSAIDs vs paracetamol	6 months (end of treatment)	3.5% (naproxen) and 2.5% (paracetamol) Both groups similar

Table 7.6 Gastro-intestinal adverse events (AEs)

GI AEs outcome	Reference	Intervention	Assessment time	Outcome/effect size
Number of GI AEs	1 MA (Towheed et al. 2006), 5 RCTs	Non-selective NSAIDs vs paracetamol	Mean duration 13.1 weeks (range 1–104 weeks)	Significant heterogeneity RR 1.47, 95% CI 1.08 to 2.00, p<0.05. Favours paracetamol
Number of GI AEs	1 MA (Towheed et al. 2006)	NSAIDs vs paracetamol	Mean duration 13.1 weeks (range 1–104 weeks)	NS
Number of GI AEs	1 MA (Towheed et al. 2006)	COX-2 vs paracetamol	Mean duration 13.1 weeks (range 1–104 weeks)	NS
Number of patients with initial GI AEs	1 cohort study (Fries and Bruce 2003) N=3124	Ibuprofen vs paracetamol	Not mentioned	0.2% (paracetamol) and 0.3% (ibuprofen) Both groups similar
GI AE rates per 1000 patient years	1 cohort study (Fries and Bruce 2003) N+3124	Ibuprofen vs paracetamol	Not mentioned	Rates: 2.1 (paracetamol) and 2.4 (ibuprofen) Both groups similar
GI AE rates per 1000 patient years	1 cohort study (Fries and Bruce 2003) N=3124	Ibuprofen vs paracetamol (Both drugs at doses of 101–1100 mg, >2000 mg and at 1301–2600 mg)	Not mentioned	101–1100 mg rates: 0 (paracetamol) and 3.2 (ibuprofen) = Ibuprofen worse >2000 mg rates: 0 (paracetamol) and 9.1 (ibuprofen) = Ibuprofen worse 1301–2600 mg rates: 8.97 (paracetamol) and 0 (ibuprofen) = paracetamol worse
Number of patients with stomach pain and vomiting	1 N-of-1 study (Yelland et al. 2007)) (N=59)	Celecoxib vs SR paracetamol	n/a	Stomach pain: 27% (paracetamol) and 15% (celecoxib) Vomiting: 7% (paracetamol) and 2% (celecoxib) Celecoxib better
Number of GI AEs (constipation and peripheral oedema)	1 RCT (Temple et al. 2006) (N=581)	NSAIDs vs paracetamol	6 months (end of treatment)	Constipation: p<0.002 Peripheral oedema: p<0.033 Favours paracetamol

Table 7.7 Withdrawals

Withdrawals outcome	Reference	Intervention	Assessment time	Outcome/effect size
Total number of withdrawals due to AEs	1 MA (Towheed et al. 2006), 5 RCTs	Non-selective NSAIDs vs paracetamol	Mean duration 13.1 weeks (range 1–104 weeks)	NS
Total number of withdrawals due to AEs	1 MA (Towheed et al. 2006)	NSAIDs vs paracetamol	Mean duration 13.1 weeks (range 1–104 weeks)	RR 2.00, 95% CI 1.05 to 3.81, p<0.05. Favours paracetamol
Number of withdrawals due to AEs	1 RCT (Temple et al. 2006) (N=581)	NSAIDs vs paracetamol	6 months (end of treatment)	NS

Table 7.8 Rescue medication

Rescue medication use as outcome	Reference	Intervention	Assessment time	Outcome/effect size
Overall use of escape analgesia (median number of tablets/week)	1 N-of-1 trial (March et al. 1041–5), N=25	NSAIDs vs paracetamol	n/a	7.5 (paracetamol) versus 1.0 (NSAIDs), p=0.013 Favours NSAIDs

7.1.8 Evidence statements: paracetamol vs opioids, and paracetamol-opioid combinations

Table 7.9 Symptoms: pain

Pain outcome	Reference	Intervention	Assessment time	Outcome/effect size
Paracetamol vs opioids				
Reduction in knee pain, VAS (change from baseline)	1 RCT (Bianchi et al. 2003) N=20	Paracetamol vs tramadol	120 mins post-intervention	–35.0 (paracetamol) and –14.0 (tramadol) Paracetamol better
Paracetamol vs paracetamol-opioids				
Pain reduction (patient diary scores)	1 RCT (Boureau et al. 1990) N=234	Paracetamol vs codeine-paracetamol	3 days	NS
Pain reduction (VAS)	1 RCT (Kjaersgaard et al. 1990) N=161	Paracetamol vs codeine-paracetamol	4 weeks	NS
Paracetamol-opioids vs nsaids				
Pain, VAS	1 RCT (Parr et al. 1989) N=755	Dextropropoxyphene-paracetamol vs slow-release diclofenac	4 weeks	p < 0.05 Favours NSAID

continued

Table 7.9 Symptoms: pain – *continued*

Pain outcome	Reference	Intervention	Assessment time	Outcome/effect size
Paracetamol-opioids vs nsaids – *continued*				
Pain (NHP scale)	1 RCT (Parr et al. 1989) N=755	Dextropropoxyphene-paracetamol vs slow-release diclofenac	4 weeks	NS
Reduced weight-bearing pain and reduced night-time pain	1 RCT (Irani 1980) N=22 indomethacin or sulindac	Dextropropoxyphene-paracetamol (distalgesic) vs	4 weeks	p<0.05 Favours NSAIDs
Day-time pain	1 RCT (Irani 1980) N=22	Dextropropoxyphene-paracetamol (distalgesic) vs indomethacin or sulindac	4 weeks	NS

Table 7.10 Symptoms: function

Function outcome	Reference	Intervention	Assessment time	Outcome/effect size
Paracetamol-opioids vs NSAIDs				
Increased functional activity	1 RCT (Irani 1980) N=22	Dextropropoxyphene-paracetamol (distalgesic) vs indomethacin or sulindac	4 weeks	Indomethacin:100% (p<0.02) Sulindac: 100% (p<0.01) Distalgesic: 11% Favours NSAIDs
Reduced knee joint size	1 RCT (Irani 1980) N=22	Dextropropoxyphene-paracetamol (distalgesic) vs indomethacin or sulindac	4 weeks	Indomethacin: p<0.05 Sulindac p<0.01 Favours NSAIDs
Physical mobility (NHP scale)	1 RCT (Parr et al. 1989) N=755	Dextropropoxyphene-paracetamol vs slow-release diclofenac	4 weeks	p<0.01 Favours NSAID
Opioids vs NSAIDs				
Improvement in WOMAC total score	1 MA (Cepeda et al. 2006) 1 RCT, N=108	Tramadol vs diclofenac	28 days (end of treatment)	3.9 (tramadol) and 4.0 (diclofenac) Both groups similar

Table 7.11 Symptoms: stiffness

Stiffness outcome	Reference	Intervention	Assessment time	Outcome/effect size
Paracetamol-opioids vs NSAIDs				
Morning stiffness	1 RCT (Irani 1980) N=22	Dextropropoxyphene-paracetamol (distalgesic) vs indomethacin or sulindac	4 weeks	NS

Table 7.12 Global assessment

Global assessment outcome	Reference	Intervention	Assessment time	Outcome/effect size
Opioids vs NSAIDs				
Number of patients with at least moderate improvement in global assessment	1 MA (Cepeda et al. 2006) 1 RCT, N=108	Tramadol vs diclofenac	28 days (end of treatment)	NS

Table 7.13 Adverse events

AEs outcome	Reference	Intervention	Assessment time	Outcome/effect size
Paracetamol vs opioids				
Number of patients with AEs, nausea and vomiting	1 RCT (Bianchi et al. 2003) N=20	Paracetamol vs tramadol	1 week	0% (paracetamol) and 20% (tramadol) Paracetamol better
Paracetamol vs paracetamol-opioids				
GI AEs	1 RCT (Boureau et al. 1990) N=234	Paracetamol vs codeine-paracetamol	3 days	NS
Number of AEs	1 RCT (Kjaersgaard et al. 1990) N=161	Paracetamol vs codeine-paracetamol	4 weeks	27.6% (paracetamol) vs 52.3% (codeine-para); p<0.01
Paracetamol-opioids vs NSAIDs				
Number of patients with AEs	1 RCT (Irani 1980) N=22	Dextropropoxyphene-paracetamol (distalgesic) vs indomethacin or sulindac	4 weeks	22% (distalgesic) and both NSAIDs 0% NSAIDs better
New cases of dyspepsia or gastritis	1 RCT (Irani 1980) N=22	Dextropropoxyphene-paracetamol (distalgesic) vs sulindac	4 weeks	N=8 (distalgesic) and N=1 (sulindac) NSAIDs better
New cases of dyspepsia or gastritis	1 RCT (Irani 1980) N=22	Dextropropoxyphene-paracetamol (distalgesic) vs indomethacin	4 weeks	N=8 (distalgesic) and N=6 (indomethacin) Both groups similar
Number of study completers with AEs diarrhoea (0.5% vs 38%) and indigestion/epigastric pain (5% vs 11%; p < 0.01)	1 RCT (Parr et al. 1989) N=755	Dextropropoxyphene-paracetamol vs slow-release diclofenac	4 weeks	24% (dextro-para) and 13% (diclofenac); <0.01 Favours dextro-para
Number of study completers with diarrhoea	1 RCT (Parr et al. 1989) N=755	Dextropropoxyphene-paracetamol vs slow-release diclofenac	4 weeks	0.5% (dextro-para) and 38% (diclofenac); <0.01 Favours dextro-para

continued

Table 7.13 Adverse events – *continued*

AEs outcome	Reference	Intervention	Assessment time	Outcome/effect size
Paracetamol-opioids vs NSAIDs – *continued*				
Number of study completers with indigestion/epigastric pain	1 RCT (Parr et al. 1989) N=755	Dextropropoxyphene-paracetamol vs slow-release diclofenac	4 weeks	5% (dextro-para) and 11% (diclofenac); <0.01 Favours dextro-para
Dizziness/light-headedness	1 RCT (Parr et al. 1989) N=755	Dextropropoxyphene-paracetamol vs slow-release diclofenac	4 weeks	8% (dextro-para) and 4% (diclofenac); <0.05 Favours NSAID
Sleep disturbance/ tiredness	1 RCT (Parr et al. 1989) N=755	Dextropropoxyphene-paracetamol vs slow-release diclofenac	4 weeks	13% (dextro-para) and 6% (diclofenac); <0.01 Favours NSAID
Gastric AEs; mean overall chronic gastritis index; mean overall acute gastritis grading	1 RCT (McIntyre et al. 1981) N=32	Dextropropoxyphene-paracetamol vs indomethacin or sulindac	4 weeks	All groups similar
Opioids vs NSAIDs				
Proportion of patients with major AEs	1 MA (Cepeda et al. 2006) 1 RCT, N=108	Tramadol vs dclofenac	28 days (end of treatment)	NS
Proportion of patients with minor AEs	1 MA (Cepeda et al. 2006) 1 RCT, N=108	Tramadol vs dclofenac	28 days (end of treatment)	RR 6.0, 95% CI 1.41 to 25.5 NSAIDs better

Table 7.14 Withdrawals

Withdrawals outcome	Reference	Intervention	Assessment time	Outcome/effect size
Paracetamol vs opioids				
Number of withdrawals	1 RCT (Bianchi et al. 2003) N=20	Paracetamol vs tramadol	1 week	0% (paracetamol) and 20% (tramadol) Paracetamol better
Paracetamol vs paracetamol-opioids				
Withdrawals due to study drug AEs in the group	1 RCT (Kjaersgaard et al. 1990) N=161	Paracetamol vs codeine-paracetamol	4 weeks	13.5% (paracetamol) and 50% (tramadol); p<0.01 Paracetamol better
Paracetamol-opioids vs nsaids				
Withdrawals due to GI AEs	1 RCT (Parr et al. 1989) N=755	Dextropropoxyphene-paracetamol vs slow-release diclofenac	4 weeks	34% (dextro-para) and 44% (diclofenac) Dextro-para better

continued

Table 7.14 Withdrawals – *continued*

Withdrawals outcome	Reference	Intervention	Assessment time	Outcome/effect size
Paracetamol-opioids vs nsaids – *continued*				
Withdrawals due to respiratory AEs	1 RCT (Parr et al. 1989) N=755	Dextropropoxyphene-paracetamol vs slow-release diclofenac	4 weeks	1.5% (dextro-para) and 3.5% (diclofenac) Dextro-para better
Withdrawals due to CNS AEs	1 RCT (Parr et al. 1989) N=755	Dextropropoxyphene-paracetamol vs slow-release diclofenac	4 weeks	42% (dextro-para) and 23% (diclofenac) NSAID better
Total number of withdrawals	1 RCT (Parr et al. 1989) N=755	Dextropropoxyphene-paracetamol vs slow-release diclofenac	4 weeks	17% (dextro-para) and 15% (diclofenac) Both groups similar

7.1.9   Evidence statements: opioids

Table 7.15 Symptoms: pain

Pain outcome	Reference	Intervention	Assessment time	Outcome/effect size
Knee				
Opioid vs placebo				
Pain relief (VAS)	1 MA (Bjordal et al. 2007) 6 RCTs, N=1057	Opioids vs placebo	2–4 weeks	Mean difference 10.5, 95% CI 7.4 to 13.7 Favours opioids
Knee and/or hip				
Opioid vs placebo				
Improvement in pain (verbal rating scale) during daily activities	1 RCT (Jensen and Ginsberg 1994) N=264	Tramadol vs placebo	2 weeks	p=0.01 Favours tramadol
Improvement in pain (verbal rating scale) during walking	1 RCT (Jensen and Ginsberg 1994) N=264	Tramadol vs placebo	2 weeks	p=0.006 Favours tramadol
Improvement in pain (verbal rating scale) during sleep	1 RCT (Jensen and Ginsberg 1994) N=264	Tramadol vs placebo	2 weeks	p=0.04 Favours tramadol
Pain relief (VAS)	1 RCT (Jensen and Ginsberg 1994) N=264	Tramadol vs placebo	2 weeks	NS
Opioid-paraceatmol vs placebo				
Pain intensity	1 MA (Cepeda et al. 2006) 3 RCTs	Tramadol/tramadol-paracetamol vs placebo	Range 14–91 days	Mean difference –8.47, 95% CI –12.1 to –4.9, p<0.00001 Favours opiod/opioid-paracetamol

continued

Table 7.15 Symptoms: pain – *continued*

Pain outcome	Reference	Intervention	Assessment time	Outcome/effect size
Knee and/or hip				
Opiodis: low strength vs high strength				
Total daily pain score (VAS)	1 RCT (Bird et al. 1995) N=40, cohort 1 (patients who took at least 1 dose in each period and had pain scores for at least 4 days Cohort 2 (patients who took at least 1 dose in each period and recorded pain scores on less than 4 days unless they withdrew due to lack of efficacy)	Low dose tramadol vs pentazocine	2 weeks (end of treatment)	Cohort 1: NS Cohort 2: tramadol SS better
WOMAC pain, change from baseline	1 RCT (Gana et al. 2006) (N=1020)	Tramadol 100 mg vs placebo	12 weeks (end of treatment)	107.2 (tramadol) and 74.2 (placebo), p<0.01 Favours tramadol
Arthritis pain intensity in the index joint, change from baseline	1 RCT (Gana et al. 2006) (N=1020)	Tramadol 100 mg vs placebo	12 weeks (end of treatment)	27.8 (tramadol) and 20.2 (placebo) Favours tramadol
WOMAC pain on walking on a flat surface, change from baseline; Arthritis pain intensity in the non-index joint, change from baseline	1 RCT (Gana et al. 2006) (N=1020)	Tramadol 100 mg vs placebo	12 weeks (end of treatment)	NS
WOMAC pain, change from baseline	1 RCT (Gana et al. 2006) (N=1020)	Tramadol 200 mg vs placebo	12 weeks (end of treatment)	111.5 (tramadol) and 74.2 (placebo), p<0.01 Favours tramadol
WOMAC pain on walking on a flat surface, change from baseline	1 RCT (Gana et al. 2006) (N=1020)	Tramadol 200 mg vs placebo	12 weeks (end of treatment)	20.5 (tramadol) and 13.6 (placebo), p<0.01 Favours tramadol
Arthritis pain intensity in the index joint, change from baseline	1 RCT (Gana et al. 2006) (N=1020)	Tramadol 200 mg vs placebo	12 weeks (end of treatment)	29.9 (tramadol) and 20.2 (placebo), p<0.01 Favours tramadol
Arthritis pain intensity in the non-index joint, change from baseline	1 RCT (Gana et al. 2006) (N=1020)	Tramadol 200 mg vs placebo	12 weeks (end of treatment)	23.3 (tramadol) and 14.5 (placebo), p<0.01 Favours tramadol

continued

Table 7.15 Symptoms: pain – *continued*

Pain outcome	Reference	Intervention	Assessment time	Outcome/effect size
Knee and/or hip				
Opiodis: low strength vs high strength – *continued*				
WOMAC pain, change from baseline	1 RCT (Gana et al. 2006) (N=1020)	Tramadol 300 mg vs placebo	12 weeks (end of treatment)	103.9 (tramadol) and 74.2 (placebo), p<0.05 Favours tramadol
WOMAC pain on walking on a flat surface, change from baseline	1 RCT (Gana et al. 2006) (N=1020)	Tramadol 300 mg vs placebo	12 weeks (end of treatment)	19.4 (tramadol) and 13.6 (placebo), p<0.05 Favours tramadol
Arthritis pain intensity in the index joint, change from baseline	1 RCT (Gana et al. 2006) (N=1020)	Tramadol 300 mg vs placebo	12 weeks (end of treatment)	30.2 (tramadol) and 20.2 (placebo), p<0.01 Favours tramadol
Arthritis pain intensity in the non-index joint, change from baseline	1 RCT (Gana et al. 2006) (N=1020)	Tramadol 300 mg vs placebo	12 weeks (end of treatment)	23.5 (tramadol) and 14.5 (placebo), p<0.01 Favours tramadol
WOMAC pain, change from baseline	1 RCT (Gana et al. 2006) (N=1020)	Tramadol 400 mg vs placebo	12 weeks (end of treatment)	107.8 (tramadol) and 74.2 (placebo), p<0.01 Favours tramadol
WOMAC pain on walking on a flat surface, change from baseline	1 RCT (Gana et al. 2006) (N=1020)	Tramadol 400 mg vs placebo	12 weeks (end of treatment)	19.7 (tramadol) and 13.6 (placebo), p<0.05 Favours tramadol
Arthritis pain intensity in the index joint, change from baseline	1 RCT (Gana et al. 2006) (N=1020)	Tramadol 400 mg vs placebo	12 weeks (end of treatment)	28.0 (tramadol) and 20.2 (placebo), p<0.01 Favours tramadol
Arthritis pain intensity in the non-index joint, change from baseline	1 RCT (Gana et al. 2006) (N=1020)	Tramadol 400 mg vs placebo	12 weeks (end of treatment)	21.3 (tramadol) and 14.5 (placebo), p<0.05 Favours tramadol

Table 7.16 Symptoms: stiffness

Stiffness outcome	Reference	Intervention	Assessment time	Outcome/effect size
Knee and/or hip				
Opioids vs placebo				
WOMAC stiffness, change from baseline	1 RCT (Gana et al. 2006) (N=1020)	Tramadol 100 mg vs placebo	12 weeks (end of treatment)	43.0 (tramadol) and 32.2 (placebo), p<0.05 Favours tramadol
WOMAC stiffness, change from baseline	1 RCT (Gana et al. 2006) (N=1020)	Tramadol 200 mg vs placebo	12 weeks (end of treatment)	46.8 (tramadol) and 32.2 (placebo), p<0.01 Favours tramadol

continued

Table 7.16 Symptoms: stiffness – *continued*

Stiffness outcome	Reference	Intervention	Assessment time	Outcome/effect size
Knee and/or hip				
Opioids vs placebo – *continued*				
WOMAC stiffness, change from baseline	1 RCT (Gana et al. 2006) (N=1020)	Tramadol 300 mg vs placebo	12 weeks (end of treatment)	48.0 (tramadol) and 32.2 (placebo), p<0.01 Favours tramadol
WOMAC stiffness, change from baseline	1 RCT (Gana et al. 2006) (N=1020)	Tramadol 400 mg vs placebo	12 weeks (end of treatment)	45.0 (tramadol) and 32.2 (placebo), p<0.05 Favours tramadol
Opioids: Low strength vs high strength				
Morning stiffness duration	1 RCT (Bird et al. 1995) N=40.	Low dose tramadol vs pentazocine	2 weeks (end of treatment)	p=0.034 Favours tramadol
Morning stiffness severity score.	1 RCT (Bird et al. 1995) N=40.	Low dose tramadol vs pentazocine	2 weeks (end of treatment)	NS

Table 7.17 Symptoms: function

Function outcome	Reference	Intervention	Assessment time	Outcome/effect size
Knee and/or hip				
Opioids vs placebo				
Patient ratings of good or better in their overall assessment of treatment	1 RCT (Jensen and Ginsberg 1994) N=264	Tramadol vs placebo	2 weeks	p=0.022 Favours tramadol
Observers ratings of good or better in their overall assessment of treatment	1 RCT (Jensen and Ginsberg 1994) N=264	Tramadol vs placebo	2 weeks	p=0.017 Favours tramadol
Number of patients reporting improvementin: climbing stairs, getting out of bed and rising from a chair	1 RCT (Jensen and Ginsberg 1994) N=264	Tramadol vs placebo	2 weeks	NS
WOMAC physical function, change from baseline (331.7 and 234.3)	1 RCT(Gana et al. 2006) (N=1020)	Tramadol 100 mg vs placebo	12 weeks (end of treatment)	331.7 (tramadol) and 234.3 (placebo), p<0.05 Favours tramadol
WOMAC total, change from baseline	1 RCT(Gana et al. 2006) (N=1020)	Tramadol 100 mg vs placebo	12 weeks (end of treatment)	481.5 (tramadol) and 340.5 (placebo), p<0.01 Favours tramadol

continued

Table 7.17 Symptoms: function

Function outcome	Reference	Intervention	Assessment time	Outcome/effect size
Knee and/or hip				
Opioids vs placebo – continued				
WOMAC physical function, change from baseline	1 RCT(Gana et al. 2006) (N=1020)	Tramadol 200 mg vs placebo	12 weeks (end of treatment)	350.2 (tramadol) and 234.3 (placebo), p<0.01 Favours tramadol
WOMAC total, change from baseline	1 RCT(Gana et al. 2006) (N=1020)	Tramadol 200 mg vs placebo	12 weeks (end of treatment)	510.0 (tramadol) and 340.5 (placebo), p<0.01 Favours tramadol
WOMAC physical function, change from baseline	1 RCT (Gana et al. 2006) (N=1020)	Tramadol 300 mg vs placebo	12 weeks (end of treatment)	336.1 (tramadol) and 234.3 (placebo), p<0.01 Favours tramadol
WOMAC total, change from baseline	1 RCT (Gana et al. 2006) (N=1020)	Tramadol 300 mg vs placebo	12 weeks (end of treatment)	486.4 (tramadol) and 340.5 (placebo), p<0.01 Favours tramadol
WOMAC physical function, change from baseline	1 RCT (Gana et al. 2006) (N=1020)	Tramadol 400 mg vs placebo	12 weeks (end of treatment)	329.8 (tramadol) and 234.3 (placebo), p<0.05 Favours tramadol
WOMAC total, change from baseline	1 RCT (Gana et al. 2006) (N=1020)	Tramadol 400 mg vs placebo	12 weeks (end of treatment)	479.2 (tramadol) and 340.5 (placebo), p<0.05 Favours tramadol
Opioids/opioid-paracetamol vs placebo				
At least moderate improvement in global assessment	1 MA (Cepeda et al. 2006) 4 RCTs, N=793	Tramadol/ tramadol-paracetamol vs placebo	Range 14–91 days	RR 1.4, 95% CI 1.2 to 1.6, p<0.00001 Favours tramadol
Opioids: Low strength vs high strength				
Patient's overall assessment of treatment	1 RCT (Bird et al. 1995) N=40.	Low dose tramadol vs pentazocine	2 weeks (end of treatment)	p=0.003 Favours tramadol

Table 7.18 Global assessment

Global assessment outcome	Reference	Intervention	Assessment time	Outcome/effect size
Knee and/or hip				
Opioids vs placebo				
Physician's global assessment of disease activity, change from baseline	1 RCT (Gana et al. 2006) (N=1020)	Tramadol 100 mg vs placebo	12 weeks (end of treatment)	22.9 (tramadol) and 17.2 (placebo), p<0.05 Favours tramadol

continued

Table 7.18 Global assessment – *continued*

Global assessment outcome	Reference	Intervention	Assessment time	Outcome/effect size
Knee and/or hip				
Opioids vs placebo – *continued*				
Patient's global assessment of disease activity	1 RCT (Gana et al. 2006) (N=1020)	Tramadol 100 mg vs placebo	12 weeks (end of treatment)	NS
Physician's global assessment of disease activity, change from baseline	1 RCT (Gana et al. 2006) (N=1020)	Tramadol 200 mg vs placebo	12 weeks (end of treatment)	22.4 (tramadol) and 17.2 (placebo), p<0.01 Favours tramadol
Patient's global assessment of disease activity	1 RCT (Gana et al. 2006) (N=1020)	Tramadol 200 mg vs placebo	12 weeks (end of treatment)	21.8 (tramadol) and 16.2 (placebo), p<0.01 Favours tramadol
Physician's global assessment of disease activity, change from baseline	1 RCT (Gana et al. 2006) (N=1020)	Tramadol 300 mg vs placebo	12 weeks (end of treatment)	23.8 (tramadol) and 17.2 (placebo), p<0.01 Favours tramadol
Patient's global assessment of disease activity	1 RCT (Gana et al. 2006) (N=1020)	Tramadol 300 mg vs placebo	12 weeks (end of treatment)	23.5 (tramadol) and 16.2 (placebo), p<0.01 Favours tramadol
Physician's global assessment of disease activity, change from baseline	1 RCT (Gana et al. 2006) (N=1020)	Tramadol 400 mg vs placebo	12 weeks (end of treatment)	22.9 (tramadol) and 17.2 (placebo), p<0.05 Favours tramadol
Patient's global assessment of disease activity	1 RCT (Gana et al. 2006) (N=1020)	Tramadol 400 mg vs placebo	12 weeks (end of treatment)	NS
Opioids/opioid-paracetamol vs palcebo				
At least moderate improvement in global assessment	1 MA (Cepeda et al. 2006) 4 RCTs, N=793	Tramadol/tramadol-paracetamol vs placebo	Range 14–91 days	RR 1.4, 95% CI 1.2 to 1.6, p<0. Favours tramadol

Table 7.19 Quality of life

QoL outcome	Reference	Intervention	Assessment time	Outcome/effect size
Knee and/or hip				
Opioids vs placebo				
Sleep quality, trouble falling asleep, awakened by pain in the night and in the morning, the need for sleep medication	1 RCT (Gana et al. 2006) (N=1020)	Tramadol 100 mg vs placebo	12 weeks (end of treatment)	All p<0.05 Favours tramadol
SF-36 physical and mental components, change from baseline	1 RCT (Gana et al. 2006) (N=1020)	Tramadol 100 mg vs placebo	12 weeks (end of treatment)	NS
Sleep quality, trouble falling asleep, awakened by pain in the night and in the morning	1 RCT (Gana et al. 2006) (N=1020)	Tramadol 200 mg vs placebo	12 weeks (end of treatment)	All p<0.05 Favours tramadol
SF-36 physical and mental components; The need for sleep medication, change from baseline	1 RCT (Gana et al. 2006) (N=1020)	Tramadol 200 mg vs placebo	12 weeks (end of treatment)	NS
Sleep quality, trouble falling asleep, awakened by pain in the night and in the morning	1 RCT (Gana et al. 2006) (N=1020)	Tramadol 300 mg vs placebo	12 weeks (end of treatment)	All p<0.05 Favours tramadol
SF-36 physical and mental components; The need for sleep medication, change from baseline	1 RCT (Gana et al. 2006) (N=1020)	Tramadol 300 mg vs placebo	12 weeks (end of treatment)	NS
Sleep quality, trouble falling asleep, awakened by pain in the night	1 RCT (Gana et al. 2006) (N=1020)	Tramadol 400 mg vs placebo	12 weeks (end of treatment)	All p<0.05 Favours tramadol
SF-36 physical and mental component; Being awakened by pain in the morning; The need for sleep medication, change from baseline	1 RCT (Gana et al. 2006) (N=1020)	Tramadol 400 mg vs placebo	12 weeks (end of treatment)	NS

Table 7.20 Adverse events and withdrawals

Adverse events and withdrawals as outcome	Reference	Intervention	Assessment time	Outcome/effect size
Knee and/or hip				
Opioids vs placebo				
Withdrawal rate	1 MA (Bjordal et al. 2007)	Opiodis vs placebo	Not mentioned	Opioids had high withdrawal rates (20–50%)
Withdrawals due to AEs	1 RCT (Gana et al. 2006) (N=1020)	Tramadol 100 mg vs placebo	12 weeks (end of treatment)	14% (tramadol) and 10% (placebo) Favours placebo
Number of patients reporting at least 1 AE	1 RCT (Gana et al. 2006) (N=1020)	Tramadol 100 mg vs placebo	12 weeks (end of treatment)	71% (tramadol) and 56% (placebo) Favours placebo
Number of patients reporting at least 1 SAE	1 RCT (Gana et al. 2006) (N=1020)	Tramadol 100 mg vs placebo	12 weeks (end of treatment)	1.5% (tramadol) and 1% (placebo) Favours placebo
Withdrawals due to AEs	1 RCT (Gana et al. 2006) (N=1020)	Tramadol 200 mg vs placebo	12 weeks (end of treatment)	20% (tramadol) and 10% (placebo) Favours placebo
Number of patients reporting at least 1 AE	1 RCT (Gana et al. 2006) (N=1020)	Tramadol 200 mg vs placebo	12 weeks (end of treatment)	73% (tramadol) and 56% (placebo) Favours placebo
Number of patients reporting at least 1 SAE	1 RCT (Gana et al. 2006) (N=1020)	Tramadol 200 mg vs placebo	12 weeks (end of treatment)	2% (tramadol) and 1% (placebo) Favours placebo
Withdrawals due to AEs	1 RCT (Gana et al. 2006) (N=1020)	Tramadol 300 mg vs placebo	12 weeks (end of treatment)	26% (tramadol) and 10% (placebo) Favours placebo
Number of patients reporting at least 1 AE	1 RCT (Gana et al. 2006) (N=1020)	Tramadol 300 mg vs placebo	12 weeks (end of treatment)	76% (tramadol) and 56% (placebo) Favours placebo
Number of patients reporting at least 1 SAE	1 RCT (Gana et al. 2006) (N=1020)	Tramadol 300 mg vs placebo	12 weeks (end of treatment)	1.5% (tramadol) and 1% (placebo) Favours placebo
Withdrawals due to AEs	1 RCT (Gana et al. 2006) (N=1020)	Tramadol 400 mg vs placebo	12 weeks (end of treatment)	29% (tramadol) and 10% (placebo) Favours placebo
Number of patients reporting at least 1 AE	1 RCT (Gana et al. 2006) (N=1020)	Tramadol 400 mg vs placebo	12 weeks (end of treatment)	84% (tramadol) and 56% (placebo) Favours placebo
Number of patients reporting at least 1 SAE	1 RCT (Gana et al. 2006) (N=1020)	Tramadol 400 mg vs placebo	12 weeks (end of treatment)	3% (tramadol) and 1% (placebo) Favours placebo

continued

Table 7.20 Adverse events and withdrawals – *continued*

Adverse events and withdrawals as outcome	Reference	Intervention	Assessment time	Outcome/effect size
Knee and/or hip				
Opioids/opioid-paracetamol vs placebo				
Minor AEs	1 MA (Cepeda et al. 2006) 4 RCTs, N=953	Tramadol/tramadol-paracetamol vs placebo	Range 14–91 days	Mean difference 2.17, 95% CI 1.8 to 2.7, p<0.00001 Favours placebo
Opioids: low strength vs high strength				
Percentage of patients experiencing AEs, nausea, vomiting and the percentage of withdrawals due to AEs	1 RCT (Jensen and Ginsberg 1994) N=264	High dose tramadol vs dextropropoxyphene	2 weeks (end of study)	All p≤0.001 Favours dextropropoxyphene
Percentage of patients experiencing constipation	1 RCT (Jensen and Ginsberg 1994) N=265	High dose tramadol vs dextropropoxyphene	2 weeks (end of study)	NS
Numbers of patients with AEs and nausea, patient withdrawals due to AEs and treatment failure	1 RCT (Bird et al. 1995) N=40	Low dose tramadol vs pentazocine	2 weeks (end of treatment)	No p-values given Favours tramadol
Number of patients who experienced vomiting and diarrhoea	1 RCT (Bird et al. 1995) N=40	Low dose tramadol vs pentazocine	2 weeks (end of treatment)	No p-values given Favours pentazocine

Table 7.21 Rescue medication

Rescue medication outcome	Reference	Intervention	Assessment time	Outcome/effect size
Knee and/or hip				
Opioids vs placebo				
Rescue medication use	1 RCT (Gana et al. 2006) (N=1020)	Tramadol 100 mg vs placebo	12 weeks (end of treatment)	3% (tramadol) and 7% (placebo) Favours tramadol
Rescue medication use	1 RCT (Gana et al. 2006) (N=1020)	Tramadol 200 mg vs placebo	12 weeks (end of treatment)	3% (tramadol) and 7% (placebo) Favours placebo
Rescue medication use	1 RCT (Gana et al. 2006) (N=1020)	Tramadol 300 mg vs placebo	12 weeks (end of treatment)	1.5% (tramadol) and 7% (placebo); p<0.05 Favours placebo
Rescue medication use	1 RCT (Gana et al. 2006) (N=1020)	Tramadol 400 mg vs placebo	12 weeks (end of treatment)	2.5% (tramadol) and 7% (placebo); p<0.05 Favours placebo

7.1.10 Evidence statements: paracetamol vs placebo

Table 7.22 Symptoms: pain

Pain outcome	Reference	Intervention	Assessment time	Outcome/effect size
Knee				
WOMAC Pain (change from baseline)	1 RCT (Herrero-Beaumont et al. 2007) (N=325)	Paracetamol vs placebo	6 months (end of treatment)	NS
Knee or hip				
Pain response	1 MA (Towheed et al. 2006), 1 RCT	Paracetamol vs placebo	Range: 7 days to 12 weeks	RR 8.0, 95% CI 2.08 to 30.73, p=0.002 Favours paracetamol
Pain response	1 MA (Towheed et al. 2006), 3 RCTs	Paracetamol vs placebo	Range: 7 days to 12 weeks	SMD –0.11, 95% CI –0.22 to –0.01, p=0.03 Favours paracetamol
Pain on motion	1 MA (Towheed et al. 2006), 1 RCT	Paracetamol vs placebo	Range: 7 days to 12 weeks	RR 3.75, 95% CI 1.48 to 9.52, p=0.005 Favours paracetamol
Day pain	1 MA (Towheed et al. 2006), 1 RCT	Paracetamol vs placebo	Range: 7 days to 12 weeks	SMD –0.29, 95% CI –0.52 to –0.06, p=0.01 Favours paracetamol
Night pain	1 MA (Towheed et al. 2006), 1 RCT	Paracetamol vs placebo	Range: 7 days to 12 weeks	SMD –0.28, 95% CI –0.51 to –0.05, p=0.02 Favours paracetamol
MDHAQ VAS pain	1 MA (Towheed et al. 2006), 2 RCTs	Paracetamol vs placebo	Range: 7 days to 12 weeks	SMD –0.18, 95% CI –0.33 to –0.03, p=0.02 Favours paracetamol
Overall pain	1 MA (Towheed et al. 2006), 5 RCTs	Paracetamol vs placebo	Range: 7 days to 12 weeks	SMD –0.13, 95% CI –0.22 to –0.04, p=0.005 Favours paracetamol
WOMAC pain; Lequesne pain; pain at rest; pain on passive motion	1 MA (Towheed et al. 2006) 1 RCT	Paracetamol vs placebo	Range: 7 days to 12 weeks	NS
WOMAC pain (average change from baseline)	1 RCT (Altman et al. 2007) (N=483)	Paracetamol ER 1950 mg/day vs placebo	Over 12 weeks, end of treatment	–26.5 and –19.6 respectively, p=0.012 Favours paracetamol
WOMAC pain (average change from baseline)	1 RCT (Altman et al. 2007) (N=483)	Paracetamol ER 3900 mg/day vs placebo	Over 12 weeks, end of treatment	NS

Table 7.23 Symptoms: stiffness

Stiffness outcome	Reference	Intervention	Assessment time	Outcome/effect size
Knee or hip				
WOMAC stiffness; stiffness at rest	1 MA (Towheed et al. 2006), 1 RCT	Paracetamol vs placebo	Range: 7 days to 12 weeks	NS
WOMAC stiffness	1 RCT (Altman et al. 2007) (N=483)	Paracetamol ER 1950 mg/day vs placebo	Over 12 weeks, end of treatment	NS
WOMAC stiffness	1 RCT (Altman et al. 2007) (N=483)	Paracetamol ER 3900 mg/day vs placebo	Over 12 weeks, end of treatment	NS

Table 7.24 Symptoms: function

Function outcome	Reference	Intervention	Assessment time	Outcome/effect size
Knee				
Lequesne's Index (change from baseline); WOMAC total (change from baseline); WOMAC physical function (change from baseline); OARSI-A responders	1 RCT (Herrero-Beaumont et al. 2007) (N=325)	Paracetamol vs placebo	6 months (end of treatment)	NS
Knee or hip				
Physician's global assessment of therapeutic response	1 MA (Towheed et al. 2006), 1 RCT	Paracetamol vs placebo	Range: 7 days to 12 weeks	RR 20.0, 95% CI 2.95 to 135.75, p=0.002 Favours paracetamol
Patient's global assessment of therapeutic response	1 MA (Towheed et al. 2006), 1 RCT	Paracetamol vs placebo	Range: 7 days to 12 weeks	RR 18.0, 95% CI 2.66 to 121.63, p=0.003 Favours paracetamol
WOMAC function,	1 MA (Towheed et al. 2006), 2 RCT	Paracetamol vs placebo	Range: 7 days to 12 weeks	NS
WOMAC total	1 MA (Towheed et al. 2006), 3 RCTs	Paracetamol vs placebo	Range: 7 days to 12 weeks	NS
Lequesne function; Lequesne total; Lequesne subset of walking; 50-foot walk time	1 MA (Towheed et al. 2006), 1 RCT	Paracetamol vs placebo	Range: 7 days to 12 weeks	NS
WOMAC total (average change from baseline)	1 RCT (Altman et al. 2007) (N=483)	Paracetamol ER 3900 mg/day vs placebo	Over 12 weeks, end of treatment	24.5 (paracetamol) and −18.6 (placebo), p<0.05 Favours paracetamol

continued

Table 7.24 Symptoms: function – *continued*

Function outcome	Reference	Intervention	Assessment time	Outcome/effect size
Knee or hip – *continued*				
WOMAC physical function (average change from baseline)	1 RCT (Altman et al. 2007) (N=483)	Paracetamol ER 3900 mg/day vs placebo	Over 12 weeks, end of treatment	–24.9 (paracetamol) and –17.8 (placebo), p=0.016 Favours paracetamol
WOMAC total (average change from baseline); WOMAC physical function (average change from baseline)	1 RCT (Altman et al. 2007) (N=483)	Paracetamol ER 1950 mg/day vs placebo	Over 12 weeks, end of treatment	NS

Table 7.25 Global assessment

Global assessment outcome	Reference	Intervention	Assessment time	Outcome/effect size
Knee or hip				
Patient's global assessment of Knee osteoarthritis in the last 24 hours	1 MA (Towheed et al. 2006) 1 RCT	Paracetamol vs placebo	Range: 7 days to 12 weeks	NS
Patient global assessment of response to therapy (average change from baseline)	1 RCT (Altman et al. 2007) (N=483)	Paracetamol ER 1950 mg/day vs placebo	Over 12 weeks, end of treatment	p=0.015 Favours paracetamol
Patient global assessment of response to therapy (average change from baseline)	1 RCT (Altman et al. 2007) (N=483)	Paracetamol ER 1950 mg/day vs placebo	Over 12 weeks, end of treatment	p=0.024 Favours paracetamol

Table 7.26 Quality of life

QoL outcome	Reference	Intervention	Assessment time	Outcome/effect size
Knee or hip				
Modified version of the AIMS-2 questionnaire: subsets of mobility level, household tasks, walking and bending	1 RCT (Golden et al. 2004)	Paracetamol vs placebo	Range: 7 days to 12 weeks	All p<0.05
Modified version of the AIMS-2 questionnaire: all other subsets	1 RCT (Golden et al. 2004)	Paracetamol vs placebo		NS

Table 7.27 Adverse events

AEs outcome	Reference	Intervention	Assessment time	Outcome/effect size
Knee				
Number of patients with AEs; number of patients with GI AEs	1 RCT (Herrero-Beaumont et al. 2007) (N=325)	Paracetamol vs placebo	6 months (end of treatment).	Both groups similar
Knee or hip				
Total number of patients reporting any AE; total number of withdrawals due to toxicity	1 MA (Towheed et al. 2006), 6 RCTs	Paracetamol vs placebo	Range: 7 days to 12 weeks	NS
Number of patients with AEs and SAEs	1 RCT (Altman et al. 2007) (N=483)	Paracetamol ER 3900 mg/day vs placebo	Over 12 weeks, end of treatment	NS
Number of patients with AEs and SAEs	1 RCT (Altman et al. 2007) (N=483)	Paracetamol ER 1950 mg/day vs placebo	Over 12 weeks, end of treatment	NS
GI AEs	3 RCTs (Amadio and Cummings 1983) (Miceli-Richard 2004) (Pincus 2004) in the SR (Towheed 2006)	Paracetamol vs placebo	Range: 7 days to 12 weeks	NS
GI AEs	1 RCT (Golden et al. 2004)	Paracetamol vs placebo	Range: 7 days to 12 weeks	20.9% (paracetamol) and 17.4% (placebo) Both groups similar

Table 7.28 Rescue medication

Rescue medication outcome Outcome/effect size	Reference	Intervention	Assessment time
Knee			
Use of rescue analgesia, % completers not using rescue medication	1 RCT (Herrero-Beaumont et al. 2007) (N=325)	Paracetamol vs placebo	Over 6 months (end of treatment). 21% (paracetamol) and 9% (placebo), p=0.045 over 6 months (end of study) Favours paracetamol
Knee or hip			
Rescue medication (number of capsules taken)	1 RCT (Altman et al. 2007) (N=483)	Paracetamol ER 3900 mg/day vs placebo	Over 12 weeks, end of treatment NS
Rescue medication (number of capsules taken)	1 RCT (Altman et al. 2007) (N=483)	Paracetamol ER 1950 mg/day vs placebo	Over 12 weeks, end of treatment NS

Table 7.29 Withdrawals

Withdrawals outcome	Reference	Intervention	Assessment time	Outcome/effect size
Knee				
Withdrawals due to lack of efficacy (N=5 and N=8 respectively)	1 RCT (Herrero-Beaumont et al. 2007) (N=325)	Paracetamol vs placebo	Over 6 months (end of treatment)	N=5 (paracetamol) and N=8 (placebo) Both groups similar
Withdrawals due to AEs	1 RCT (Herrero-Beaumont et al. 2007) (N=325)	Paracetamol vs placebo	Over 6 months (end of treatment)	N=12 (paracetamol) and N=9 (placebo) Both groups similar
Knee or hip				
Total number of withdrawals due to toxicity.	1 MA (Towheed et al. 2006), 6 RCTs	Paracetamol vs placebo	Range: 7 days to 12 weeks	NS

7.1.11 Evidence statements: tricyclics, SSRIs and SNRIs

▷ Symptoms: pain

1 RCT (Scott 1969) (N=7) found that when imipramine was given as the first treatment, the pain severity score (measured change from baseline) improved when measured after imipramine treatment (–0.8) but stayed the same when measured after placebo. (1+)

The same RCT (Scott 1969) (N=7) found that when placebo was given as the first treatment, the pain score stayed the same when measured after imipramine treatment and after placebo. (1+)

▷ Symptoms: function

One RCT (Scott 1969) (N=7) found that when imipramine was given as the first treatment, function score and grip strength (measured change from baseline) improved when measured after imipramine treatment (–0.4 and +19 mmHg respectively) but stayed the same when measured after placebo. (1+)

The same RCT (Scott 1969) (N=7) found that when placebo was given as the first treatment, function score stayed the same when measured after imipramine treatment and after placebo. However, grip strength increased after treatment with imipramine and after placebo, the increase being greater after imipramine (+42.5 and +12.5 mmHg respectively). (1+)

▷ Global assessment

One RCT (Scott 1969) (N=7) found that when imipramine was given as the first treatment, most of the patients and physicians preferred imipramine to placebo (three out of four patients for both). (1+)

The same RCT (Scott 1969) (N=7) found that when placebo was given as the first treatment, no patients preferred imipramine to placebo. (1+)

7.1.12 From evidence to recommendations

There is a good amount of evidence from RCTs on the efficacy of paracetamol in knee osteo-arthritis, with less evidence supporting its use in osteoarthritis of other sites. The long-term safety data on paracetamol from observational studies are reassuring. The GDG noted that patients commonly use infrequent dosing of paracetamol which may lead to reduced efficacy. There are limited data on the efficacy of paracetamol used in combination with other pharmacological therapies, and most such data are drawn from studies where paracetamol is used as 'escape' analgesia.

The evidence supporting the use of opioid analgesia in osteoarthritis is poor, and it must be noted there are virtually no good studies using these agents in peripheral joint osteoarthritis patients. There is little evidence to suggest that dose escalation of these agents is effective. There are also few data comparing different opioid formulations or routes of administration. Toxicity remains a concern with opioid use, especially in the elderly. Constipation, nausea, itchiness, drowsiness and confusion remain important side effects to be considered.

There is no good evidence to support the use of low dose tricyclic agents for osteoarthritis pain. However, consideration of sleep and mood disturbance is part of the assessment of the osteoarthritis patient and appropriate pharmacological therapy may be warranted. The reader is also referred to the NICE depression guideline (National Institute for Health and Clinical Excellence 2007).

RECOMMENDATIONS

R21   Healthcare professionals should consider offering paracetamol for pain relief in addition to core treatment (see Fig 3.2); regular dosing may be required. Paracetamol and/or topical NSAIDs should be considered ahead of oral NSAIDs, COX-2 inhibitors or opioids.

R22   If paracetamol or topical NSAIDs are insufficient for pain relief for people with osteoarthritis, then the addition of opioid analgesics should be considered. Risks and benefits should be considered, particularly in elderly people.

7.2   Topical treatments

7.2.1   Clinical introduction

Topical NSAIDs, capsaicin and rubefacients and are widely used to treat osteoarthritis.

After topical application, therapeutic levels of NSAIDs can be demonstrated in synovial fluid, muscles and fasciae. They may have their pharmacological effects on both intra-and extra-articular structures (Dominkus et al. 1996; Lin et al. 2004; Rolf et al. 1999). It is assumed that their mechanism of action is similar to that of oral NSAIDs. Topical NSAIDs produce a maximal plasma NSAID concentration of only 15% that achieved following oral administration of a similar dose (Dominkus et al. 1996; Heyneman et al. 2000). Thus, it would be expected that topical NSAIDs would have far fewer systemic side effects than oral NSAIDs. Even if their pain relieving effect is less than that of oral NSAIDs, they may be an attractive option for the treatment of osteoarthritis because they will produce fewer NSAID-related adverse effects.

It is possible that the act of rubbing and expectation of benefit may also contribute to any therapeutic effect from topical preparations (Arcury et al. 1999; Vaile and Davis 1998). This may partially account for the continued popularity of rubefacients. Rubefacients produce counter-irritation of the skin that may have some pain relieving effect in musculoskeletal disorders.

Capsaicin is derived from chilli peppers. As well as a counter-irritant effect it depletes neurotransmitters in sensory terminals reducing the transmission of painful stimuli. There may be a delay of some days for the effects of topical capsaicin to be evident, perhaps due to this progressive neurotransmitter depletion.

7.2.2 Methodological introduction

We looked for studies that investigated the efficacy and safety of topical agents (NSAIDs/capsaicin/rubefacients) compared with oral NSAIDs or placebo with respect to symptoms, function and quality of life in adults with osteoarthritis. Two systematic reviews and meta-analyses (Lin et al. 2004; Towheed 2006) were found on topical NSAIDs and 10 additional RCTs (Algozzine et al. 1982; Altman et al. 1994; Deal et al. 1991; McCleane 2000; Niethard et al. 2005; Rothacker et al. 1994, 1998; Schnitzer et al. 1994; Shackel et al. 1997; Trnavsky et al. 2004) on topical NSAIDs, capsaicin and rubefacients.

Both of the meta-analyses assessed the RCTs for quality and pooled together all data for the outcomes of symptoms, function and AEs. However, the outcome of quality of life was not reported. No QoL data were reported by the individual trials in the Towheed MA (Towheed 2006). However, QoL was reported in the individual RCTs included in the Lin MA (Lin et al. 2004). Results for quality of life have therefore been taken from the individual RCTs included in this systematic review.

▷ Topical NSAIDs

Two SRs/MAs (Towheed 2006b; Lin et al. 2004) and two RCTs (Niethard et al. 2005, Trnavsky et al. 2004) were found on topical NSAIDs.

The first MA (Lin et al. 2004) included 13 RCTs (with N=1983 participants) that focused on comparisons between topical NSAIDs versus placebo or oral NSAIDs in patients with osteoarthritis. All RCTs were randomised and double-blind. Studies included in the analysis differed with respect to:

- osteoarthritis site (eight RCTs knee osteoarthritis; three RCTs hand osteoarthritis; one RCT hip, knee and hand osteoarthritis; one RCT hip and knee osteoarthritis)
- type of topical NSAID used
- type of oral NSAID used
- treatment regimen
- trial design (two RCTs cross-over; 11 RCTs parallel group studies), size and length.

The second MA (Towheed 2006b) included four RCTs (with N=1412 participants) that focused on comparisons between topical diclofenac in DMSO carrier versus placebo or oral diclofenac in patients with knee osteoarthritis. All RCTs were randomised, double-blind parallel group studies. Studies included in the analysis differed with respect to:

- treatment regimen (three RCTs vs placebo, 50 drops 4 times daily; one RCT vs oral diclofenac, 50 drops 3 times daily)
- trial size and length.

The two RCTs not included in the systematic review focused on the outcomes of symptoms, function and quality of life in patients with knee osteoarthritis. They were both parallel group studies and were methodologically sound (randomised, double-blind, ITT analysis). However, they differed in terms of study intervention, sample size and study duration.

▷ Topical capsaicin

Four RCTs were found on topical capsaicin versus placebo (given 4 times daily) and focused on the outcomes of symptoms, function and quality of life in patients with osteoarthritis. All trials were parallel group studies and were methodologically sound.

However, they differed in terms of osteoarthritis site, sample size and study duration. One RCT (Altman et al. 1994) looked at 113 patients with knee, ankle, elbow, wrist and shoulder osteoarthritis and treatment lasted for 12 weeks. The second RCT (Deal et al. 1991) looked at 70 patients with knee osteoarthritis and treatment lasted for 4 weeks. The third RCT (McCleane 2000) looked at 200 patients with knee, hip, shoulder and hand osteoarthritis and treatment lasted for 6 weeks. The fourth RCT (Schnitzer et al. 1994) looked at 59 patients with hand osteoarthritis and treatment lasted for 9 weeks.

▷ Topical rubefacients

Four RCTs were found that focused on topical rubefacients versus placebo and focused on the outcomes of symptoms, function and quality of life in patients with osteoarthritis. All trials were methodologically sound (randomised and double-blind; two RCTs also included ITT analysis) (Rothacker et al. 1994; Shackel et al. 1997).

However, they differed in terms of: osteoarthritis site, trial design, sample size, study duration and study intervention. One RCT (Algozzine et al. 1982) compared trolamine salicylate to placebo in 26 patients with knee osteoarthritis and treatment lasted for 7 days. The second RCT (Rothacker et al. 1994) compared trolamine salicylate to placebo in 50 patients with hand osteoarthritis and where treatment was a single application. The third RCT (Rothacker et al. 1998) compared trolamine salicylate to placebo in 86 patients with hand osteoarthritis and where treatment was a single application. The fourth RCT (Shackel et al. 1997) compared copper salicylate to placebo in 116 patients with knee and/or hip osteoarthritis and treatment lasted for 4 weeks. Two of the RCTs were parallel group studies (Rothacker et al. 1998, Shackel et al. 1997) and the other two RCTs (Algozzine et al. 1982; Rothacker et al. 1994) used a cross-over design, both of which included a wash-out period between cross-over treatments.

7.2.3 Evidence statements: topical NSAIDs

Table 7.30 Symptoms: pain

Pain outcome	Reference	Intervention	Assessment time	Outcome/effect size
Knee osteoarthritis				
WOMAC pain	1 MA (Towheed 2006) 3 RCTs (N=697)	Topical diclofenac vs placebo	End of treatment	SMD −0.33, 95% CI −0.48 to −0.18, p<0.0001 Favours topical Pennsaid
WOMAC pain at end of treatment	1 MA (Towheed 2006) 1 RCT (N=622)	Topical diclofenac vs oral diclofenac	End of treatment	NS
Pain on movement, VAS (reduction from baseline)	1 RCT (Niethard et al. 2005) N=238	Topical diclofenac vs placebo	Days 1–14 and days 8–21 (end of treatment)	Day 1–14: p=0.02 Day 8–21: p=0.005
Pain intensity, VAS (reduction from baseline)	1 RCT (Niethard et al. 2005) N=238	Topical diclofenac vs placebo	Weeks 1 2 and 3 (end of treatment)	Week 1: p=0.03 Week 2: p=0.0002 Week 3: p=0.006
WOMAC pain (reduction from baseline)	1 RCT (Niethard et al. 2005) N=238	Topical diclofenac vs placebo	Weeks 2 and 3 (end of treatment)	Week 2: p<0.0001 Week 3: p=0.0002
Pain on movement, VAS (reduction from baseline)	1 RCT (Niethard et al. 2005) N=238	Topical diclofenac vs placebo	Days 1–7;	NS
Spontaneous pain, scale 0–3 (reduction from baseline)	1 RCT (Niethard et al. 2005) N=238	Topical diclofenac vs placebo	Days 1–7 and days 8–21	NS
Pain relief (scale 0–4)	1 RCT (Niethard et al. 2005) N=238	Topical diclofenac vs placebo	Days 1–7 and days 8–21	NS
WOMAC pain (reduction from baseline)	1 RCT (Niethard et al. 2005) N=238	Topical diclofenac vs placebo	Week 1	NS
Pain at rest	1 RCT (Trnavsky et al. 2004) N=50	Topical ibuprofen vs placebo	4 weeks (interim) and 8 weeks (end of treatment)	Topical ibuprofen better than placebo
Pain on motion	1 RCT (Trnavsky et al. 2004) N=50	Topical ibuprofen vs placebo	4 weeks (interim) and 8 weeks (end of treatment)	Topical ibuprofen better than placebo
Overall pain	1 RCT (Trnavsky et al. 2004) N=50	Topical ibuprofen vs placebo	4 weeks (interim) and 8 weeks (end of treatment)	Topical ibuprofen better than placebo

continued

Table 7.30 Symptoms: pain – *continued*

Pain outcome	Reference	Intervention	Assessment time	Outcome/effect size
Knee or hand or mixed sites				
Pain reduction (from baseline)	1 MA (Lin et al. 2004) Week 1: 7 RCTs (N=1000); week 2: 6 RCTs (N=893)	Topical NSAIDs vs placebo	Week 1 and week 2	Week 1: effect size 0.41, 95% CI 0.16 to 0.66, p≤0.05 Week 2: effect size 0.40, 95% CI 0.15 to 0.65, p≤0.05 Favours topical NSAIDs
Pain reduction (from baseline)	1 MA (Lin et al. 2004) Week 3: 2 RCTs (N=442); week 4: 3 RCTs (N=558)	Topical NSAIDs vs placebo	Week 3 and week 4	NS

Table 7.31 Symptoms: stiffness

Stiffness outcome	Reference	Intervention	Assessment time	Outcome/effect size
Knee osteoarthritis				
WOMAC stiffness	1 MA(Towheed 2006) 3 RCTs (N=696)	Topical diclofenac vs placebo	End of treatment	SMD –0.30, 95% CI –0.45 to –0.15, p<0.0001 Favours topical pennsaid
WOMAC stiffness	1 MA(Towheed 2006) 1 RCT (N=622)	Topical diclofenac vs oral diclofenac	End of treatment	NS
Knee or hand or mixed sites				
Stiffness reduction (from baseline)	1 MA (Lin et al. 2004) Week 1: 1 RCT (N=74)	Topical NSAIDs vs placebo	Week 1	Week 1: effect size 0.64, 95% CI 0.19 to 1.09, p≤0.05 Favours topical NSAIDs
Stiffness reduction (from baseline)	1 MA (Lin et al. 2004) Week 2: 1 RCT (N=81)	Topical NSAIDs vs placebo	Week 24	NS

Table 7.32 Symptoms: patient function

Function outcome	Reference	Intervention	Assessment time	Outcome/effect size
Knee osteoarthritis				
WOMAC physical function	1 MA (Towheed 2006) 3 RCTs (N=696)	Topical Pennsaid (diclofenac) vs placebo	End of treatment	SMD −0.35, 95% CI −0.50 to −0.20, p<0.0001 Favours topical Pennsaid
WOMAC physical function	1 MA (Towheed 2006) 1 RCT (N=622)	Topical Pennsaid (diclofenac) vs oral diclofenac	End of treatment	NS
WOMAC physical function (reduction from baseline)	1 RCT (Niethard et al. 2005) N=238	Topical diclofenac vs placebo	Weeks 2 and 3 (end of treatment)	Week 2: p=0.002 Week 3: p=0.0004
WOMAC physical function (reduction from baseline)	1 RCT (Niethard et al. 2005) N=238	Topical diclofenac vs placebo	Week 1	NS
Lequesne Index	1 RCT (Trnavsky et al. 2004) N=50	Topical ibuprofen vs placebo	4 weeks (interim) and 8 weeks (end of treatment)	Topical ibuprofen better than palcebo
Knee or hand or mixed sites				
Improvements in function (from baseline)	1 MA (Lin et al. 2004) Week 1: 4 RCTs (N=556); week 2: 4 RCTs (N=540)	Topical NSAIDs vs placebo	Week 1 and week 2	Week 1: effect size 0.37, 95% CI 0.20 to 0.53, p≤0.05 Week 2: effect size 0.35, 95% CI 0.19 to 0.53, p≤0.05 Favours topical NSAIDs
Improvements in function (from baseline)	1 MA (Lin et al. 2004) Week 3: 1 RCT (N=208); week 4: 1 RCT (N=208)	Topical NSAIDs vs placebo	Week 3 and week 4	NS
Improvements in function (from baseline)	1 MA (Lin et al. 2004) Week 1 and 2 1 RCT (N=208); week 3: 2 RCTs (N=529); week 4: 1 RCT, N=208	Topical NSAIDs vs oral NSAIDs	Weeks 1, 2, 3 and 4	NS

Table 7.33 Global assessment

Global assessment outcome	Reference	Intervention	Assessment time	Outcome/effect size
Knee osteoarthritis				
Patient global assessment	1 MA (Towheed 2006) 3 RCTs (N=689)	Topical Pennsaid (diclofenac) vs placebo	End of treatment	SMD –0.39, 95% CI –0.54 to –0.24, p<0.0001 Favours topical pennsaid
Patient global assessment	1 MA (Towheed 2006) 1 RCT (N=622)	Topical Pennsaid (diclofenac) vs oral diclofenac	End of treatment	NS
Patient's overall global assessment of treatment efficacy	1 RCT (Niethard et al. 2005) N=238	Topical diclofenac vs placebo	Over the 3 weeks treatment	P=0.03
Investigator's global assessment of efficacy (good or very good)	1 RCT (Trnavsky et al. 2004) N=50	Topical ibuprofen vs placebo	4 weeks (interim) and 8 weeks (end of treatment)	Ibuprofen better than placebo
Patients global assessment of efficacy (good or very good)	1 RCT (Trnavsky et al. 2004) N=50	Topical ibuprofen vs placebo	4 weeks (interim) and 8 weeks (end of treatment)	Ibuprofen better than placebo

Table 7.34 Quality of life

QoL outcome	Reference	Intervention	Assessment time	Outcome/effect size
Knee or hand or mixed sites				
SF-36 (all dimensions)	1 RCT (Grace et al. 1999) in the MA (Lin et al. 2004) (N=74)	Topical diclofenac vs placebo	Week 2 (end of treatment)	NS

Table 7.35 Adverse events

AEs outcome	Reference	Intervention	Assessment time	Outcome/effect size
Knee osteoarthritis				
Minor skin dryness	1 MA (Towheed 2006) 3 RCTs	Topical diclofenac vs placebo	Over treatment period	Minor skin dryness RR 1.74, 95% CI 1.37 to 2.22 Favours topical Pennsaid
Paresthsia, rash, any AEs, gastro-intestinal (GI) AEs	1 MA (Towheed 2006) 3 RCTs	Topical diclofenac vs placebo	Over treatment period	NS

continued

Table 7.35 Adverse events – *continued*

AEs outcome	Reference	Intervention	Assessment time	Outcome/effect size
Knee osteoarthritis – *continued*				
GI AEs	1 MA (Towheed 2006) 1 RCT	Topical diclofenac vs oral diclofenac	Over treatment period	RR 0.72, 95% CI 0.59 to 0.87 Favours topical Pennsaid
Severe GI AEs	1 MA (Towheed 2006) 1 RCT	Topical diclofenac vs oral diclofenac	Over treatment period	RR 0.35, 95% CI 0.17 to 0.72 Favours topical Pennsaid
Dry skin reactions	1 MA (Towheed 2006) 1 RCT	Topical diclofenac vs oral diclofenac	Over treatment period	RR 20.8, 95% CI 7.7 to 55.9 Favours oral diclofenac
Rash	1 MA (Towheed 2006) 1 RCT	Topical diclofenac vs oral diclofenac	Over treatment period	RR 7.2, 95% CI 2.9 to 18.1 Favours oral diclofenac
Total number of AEs	1 RCT (Niethard et al. 2005) N=238	Topical diclofenac vs placebo	Over treatment period	Both: 9%
GI AEs	1 RCT (Niethard et al. 2005) N=238	Topical diclofenac vs placebo	Over treatment period	0% (topical) 1.7% (placebo)
Skin AEs	1 RCT (Niethard et al. 2005) N=238	Topical diclofenac vs placebo	Over treatment period	2.9% (topical) 2.5% (placebo)
AEs	1 RCT (Trnavsky et al. 2004) N=50	Topical ibuprofen vs placebo	Over treatment period	None in either group
Knee or hand or mixed sites				
Number of patients with AEs; number of patients with GI AEs; number of patients with CNS AEs; local AEs – skin reactions	1 MA (Lin et al. 2004) (N=1108)	Topical NSAIDs vs placebo	Over treatment period	NS
Local AEs – skin reactions	1 MA (Lin et al. 2004) (N=443)	Topical NSAIDs vs oral NSAIDs	Over treatment period	Rate ratio 5.29, 95% CI 1.14 to 24.51, p≤0.05 Favours oral NSAIDs
Number of patients with AEs or GI AEs	1 MA (Lin et al. 2004) (N=764)	Topical NSAIDs vs oral NSAIDs	Over treatment period	NS
Number of patients with CNS AEs	1 MA (Lin et al. 2004) (N=443)	Topical NSAIDs vs oral NSAIDs	Over treatment period	NS

Table 7.36 Study withdrawals

AEs outcome	Reference	Intervention	Assessment time	Outcome/effect size
Knee osteoarthritis				
Withdrawals due to toxicity	1 MA (Towheed 2006) 3 RCTs	Topical diclofenac vs placebo	Over treatment period	NS
Withdrawals due to lack of efficacy	1 MA (Towheed 2006) 1 RCT	Topical diclofenac vs oral diclofenac	Over treatment period	RR 2.80, 95% CI 1.38 to 5.67
Withdrawals due to toxicity	1 MA (Towheed 2006) 1 RCT	Topical diclofenac vs oral diclofenac	Over treatment period	NS
Total number of withdrawals	1 MA (Towheed 2006) 1 RCT	Topical diclofenac vs oral diclofenac	Over treatment period	NS
Total number of withdrawals	1 RCT (Niethard et al. 2005) N=238	Topical diclofenac vs placebo	Over treatment period	None in either group
Total number of withdrawals	1 RCT (Trnavsky et al. 2004) N=50	Topical Ibuprofen vs placebo	Over treatment period	None in either group
Knee or hand or mixed sites				
Number of patients withdrawn due to AEs	1 MA (Lin et al. 2004) (N=1108)	Topical NSAIDs vs placebo	Over treatment period	NS
Number of patients withdrawn due to AEs	1 MA (Lin et al. 2004) (N=764)	Topical NSAIDs vs oral NSAIDs	Over treatment period	NS

Table 7.37 Other outcomes

Other outcomes	Reference	Intervention	Assessment time	Outcome/effect size
Knee or hand or mixed sites				
Clinical response rate (% of patients reporting at least moderate to excellent or > 50% pain relief or improvement in symptoms)	1 MA (Lin et al. 2004), 2 RCTs (N=149)	Topical NSAIDs vs placebo	Week 1	Rate ratio 1.64, 95% CI 1.26 to 2.13, p≤0.05; NNT 3.3, 95% CI 2.3 to 6.2, p≤0.05
Clinical response rate (% of patients reporting at least moderate to excellent or > 50% pain relief or improvement in symptoms)	1 MA (Lin et al. 2004), 1 RCT (N=152)	Topical NSAIDs vs placebo	Week 2	Rate ratio 1.59, 95% CI 1.30 to 1.95, p≤0.05; NNT 2.9, 95% CI 2.1 to 4.7, p≤0.05
Clinical response rate (% of patients reporting at least moderate to excellent or > 50% pain relief or improvement in symptoms)	1 MA (Lin et al. 2004), 1 RCT (N=114)	Topical NSAIDs vs placebo	Week 4	NS

continued

Table 7.37 Other outcomes – *continued*

Other outcomes	Reference	Intervention	Assessment time	Outcome/effect size
Knee or hand or mixed sites – *continued*				
Clinical response rate (% of patients reporting at least moderate to excellent or > 50% pain relief or improvement in symptoms)	1 MA (Lin et al. 2004), 1 RCT (N=225)	Topical NSAIDs vs Oral NSAIDs	Week 4	NS

7.2.4 Evidence statements: topical capsaicin vs placebo

Table 7.38 Symptoms: pain

Pain outcome	Reference	Intervention	Assessment time	Outcome/effect size
Knee osteoarthritis				
Pain, VAS (% reduction from baseline)	1 RCT (Deal et al. 1991) (N=70)	Topical capsaicin vs placebo	1, 2 and 4 weeks (end of treatment)	Overall p=0.033
Pain severity (scale 0–4, % reduction from baseline)	1 RCT (Deal et al. 1991) (N=70)	Topical capsaicin vs placebo	1, 2 and 4 weeks (end of treatment)	Overall p=0.020
Hand				
Articular tenderness (tenderness units)	1 RCT (Schnitzer et al. 1994) (N=59)	Topical capsaicin vs placebo	Week 3 and week 9	Both: p=0.02
Pain, VAS (% change from baseline)	1 RCT (Schnitzer et al. 1994) (N=59)	Topical capsaicin vs placebo	Week 1, 2, 3, 6 and 9 (end of treatment)	NS
Articular tenderness (tenderness units)	1 RCT (Schnitzer et al. 1994) (N=59)	Topical capsaicin vs placebo	Week 1 and week 6 (mid treatments).	NS
Mixed (knee, ankle, elbow, wrist, shoulder)				
Pain, VAS (% of patients improved)	1 RCT (Altman et al. 1994) (N=113)	Topical capsaicin vs placebo	Weeks 4, 8 and 12 (end of treatment)	Week 4: p=0.003 Week 8: p=0.011 Week 12: p=0.020
Tenderness on passive motion (% of patients improved)	1 RCT (Altman et al. 1994) (N=113)	Topical capsaicin vs placebo	Weeks 8 and 12 (end of treatment)	Both p=0.03
Tenderness on palpation (% of patients improved)	1 RCT (Altman et al. 1994) (N=113)	Topical capsaicin vs placebo	Weeks 4, 8 and 12 (end of treatment)	Week 4: p=0.003 Week 8: p=0.01 Week 12: p=0.01
Pain, VAS (% of patients improved)	1 RCT (Altman et al. 1994) (N=113)	Topical capsaicin vs placebo	Week 1 and week 2	NS
Mixed (knee, hip, shoulder, hand)				
Pain (VAS)	1 RCT (McCleane 2000) (N=200)	Topical capsaicin vs placebo (end of treatment)	Weeks 2, 3, 4, 5 and 6	Topical capsaicin better than placebo

Table 7.39 Symptoms: stiffness

Stiffness outcome	Reference	Intervention	Assessment time	Outcome/effect size
Mixed (knee, ankle, elbow, wrist, shoulder)				
Reduction in morning stiffness	1 RCT (Altman et al. 1994) (N=113)	Topical capsaicin vs placebo	Weeks 4, 8 and 12 (end of treatment)	NS

Table 7.40 Symptoms: patient function

Function outcome	Reference	Intervention	Assessment time	Outcome/effect size
Hand				
Grip strength (% change from baseline)	1 RCT (Schnitzer et al. 1994) (N=59)	Topical capsaicin vs placebo	Week 9 (end of treatment)	p=0.046
Grip strength (% change in baseline)	1 RCT (Schnitzer et al. 1994) (N=59)	Topical capsaicin vs placebo	Week 2 and week 6	Week 2: 30.3 (topical) and 15.6 (placebo) Week 6: 27.0 (topical) and 11.6 (placebo)
Grip strength (% change in baseline)	1 RCT (Schnitzer et al. 1994) (N=59)	Topical capsaicin vs placebo	Week 1	9.1 (topical) and 10.2 (placebo)
Functional assessment (% change in baseline)	1 RCT (Schnitzer et al. 1994) (N=59)	Topical capsaicin vs placebo	Week 9	1.5 (topical) and 0.9 (placebo)

Table 7.41 Global assessment

Global assessment outcome	Reference	Intervention	Assessment time	Outcome/effect size
Knee osteoarthritis				
Physicians' global assessment (% reduction from baseline)	1 RCT (Deal et al. 1991) (N=70)	Topical capsaicin vs placebo	Week 1, 2 and 4 (end of treatment)	Overall p=0.023
Mixed (knee, ankle, elbow, wrist, shoulder)				
Physician's global evaluation (% of patients improved)	1 RCT (Altman et al. 1994) (N=113)	Topical capsaicin vs placebo	Week 4 (mid-treatment) and week 12 (end of treatment)	Week 4: p=0.042 Week 12: p=0.026
Patient's global evaluation (% of patients improved)	1 RCT (Altman et al. 1994) (N=113)	Topical capsaicin vs placebo	Week 4 (mid-treatment) and week 12 (end of treatment)	Week 4: p=0.023 Week 12: p=0.028

continued

Table 7.41 Global assessment – *contnued*

Global assessment outcome	Reference	Intervention	Assessment time	Outcome/effect size
Mixed (knee, ankle, elbow, wrist, shoulder) – *continued*				
Physician's global evaluation (% of patients improved)	1 RCT (Altman et al. 1994) (N=113)	Topical capsaicin vs placebo	Weeks 1, 2 and 8 (mid-treatments)	NS
Patient's global evaluation (% of patients improved)	1 RCT (Altman et al. 1994) (N=113)	Topical capsaicin vs placebo	Weeks 1, 2 and 8 (mid-treatments)	NS

Table 7.42 Quality of life

QoL outcome	Reference	Intervention	Assessment time	Outcome/effect size
Mixed (knee, ankle, elbow, wrist, shoulder)				
Health assessment questionnaire	1 RCT (Altman et al. 1994) (N=113)	Topical capsaicin vs placebo	Weeks 4, 8 and 12 (end of treatment)	NS

Table 7.43 Adverse events

AEs outcome	Reference	Intervention	Assessment time	Outcome/effect size
Hand				
Number of patients with AEs	1 RCT (Schnitzer et al. 1994) (N=59)	Topical capsaicin vs placebo	Over 9 weeks treatment	N=20, 69.0% (topical) and N=9, 30.0% (placebo)

Table 7.44 Study withdrawals

Withdrawals outcome	Reference	Intervention	Assessment time	Outcome/effect size
Knee osteoarthritis				
Number of withdrawals	1 RCT (Deal et al. 1991) (N=70)	Topical capsaicin vs placebo	Over treatment period	N=1 2.9% (topical) and N=5 14.3% (placebo)
Hand				
Number of study withdrawals	1 RCT (Schnitzer et al. 1994) (N=59)	Topical capsaicin vs placebo	Over treatment period	N=4 13.8% (topical) and N=7 23.3% (placebo)
Mixed (knee, ankle, elbow, wrist, shoulder)				
Number of study withdrawals	1 RCT (Altman et al. 1994) (N=113)	Topical capsaicin vs placebo	Over treatment period	N=11 19.3% (topical) and N=6 10.7% (placebo)

continued

Table 7.44 Study withdrawals – *continued*

Withdrawals outcome	Reference	Intervention	Assessment time	Outcome/effect size
Mixed (knee, ankle, elbow, wrist, shoulder) – *continued*				
Withdrawals due to AEs	1 RCT (Altman et al. 1994) (N=113)	Topical capsaicin vs placebo	Over treatment period	N=5, 8.7% (topical) and N=0, 0% (placebo)
Withdrawals due to treatment failure	1 RCT (Altman et al. 1994) (N=113)	Topical capsaicin vs placebo	Over treatment period	N=6 10.5% (topical) and N=4, 7.5% (placebo)
Mixed (knee, hip, shoulder, hand)				
Number of withdrawals	1 RCT (McCleane 2000) (N=200)	Topical capsaicin vs placebo	Over treatment period	Both N=10 20%

Table 7.45 Other outcomes

Withdrawals outcome	Reference	Intervention	Assessment time	Outcome/effect size
Mixed (knee, hip, shoulder, hand)				
Daily use of analgesics	1 RCT (McCleane 2000) (N=200)	Topical capsaicin vs placebo	Over treatment period	Lower use for topical capsaicin patients than placebo
Patients favoured staying on treatment	1 RCT (McCleane 2000) (N=200)	Topical capsaicin vs placebo	Over treatment period	OR 2.4, 95% CI 1.2 to 5.1 Favours topical capsaicin

7.2.5 Evidence statements: topical rubefacients

Table 7.46 Symptoms: pain

Pain outcome	Reference	Intervention	Assessment time	Outcome/effect size
Knee osteoarthritis				
Pain (SDS), mean change after treatment	1 RCT (Algozzine et al. 1982) (N=26)	Trolamine salicylate vs placebo	7 days	NS
Pain (NRS), mean change after treatment	1 RCT (Algozzine et al. 1982) (N=26)	Trolamine salicylate vs placebo	7 days	NS
Hand				
Pain intensity (1–5 scale)	1 RCT (Rothacker et al. 1998) (N=86)	Trolamine salicylate vs placebo	45 minutes post-treatment.	Right hand: p=0.04 Both hands averaged: p=0.026 Dominant hand: p=0.02

continued

Table 7.46 Symptoms: pain – *continued*

Pain outcome	Reference	Intervention	Assessment time	Outcome/effect size
Hand – *continued*				
Pain severity (change from baseline	1 RCT (Rothacker et al. 1994) (N=50)	Trolamine salicylate vs placebo	0, 15, 20, 30, 45 and 120 minutes after treatment	NS
Pain intensity (change from baseline)	1 RCT (Rothacker et al. 1998) (N=86)	Trolamine salicylate vs placebo	Pooled for 30 minutes, 45 minutes and 120 minutes post-intervention	NS
Pain intensity (1–5 scale)	1 RCT (Rothacker et al. 1998) (N=86)	Trolamine salicylate vs placebo	30 minutes and 120 minutes post-intervention	NS
Pain intensity (1–5 scale) in the left hand	1 RCT (Rothacker et al. 1998) (N=86)	Trolamine salicylate vs placebo	45 minutes post-intervention.	NS
Mixed (knee and/or hip)				
Pain at rest, VAS (change from baseline)	One RCT (Shackel et al. 1997) (N=116)	Copper-salicylate vs placebo	End of treatment (4 weeks)	NS
Pain on movement, VAS (change from baseline)	One RCT (Shackel et al. 1997) (N=116)	Copper-salicylate vs placebo	End of treatment (4 weeks)	NS

Table 7.47 Symptoms: stiffness

Stiffness outcome	Reference	Intervention	Assessment time	Outcome/effect size
Hand				
Stiffness intensity (change from baseline)	1 RCT (Rothacker et al. 1998) (N=86)	Trolamine salicylate	Pooled for 30 minutes, 45 minutes and 120 minutes post-intervention	Right hand: p=0.023 Both hands averaged: p=0.028 Dominant hand: p=0.026
Stiffness intensity (1–5 scale)	1 RCT (Rothacker et al. 1998) (N=86)	Trolamine salicylate	45 minutes post intervention	Right hand: p=0.016 Both hands averaged: p=0.024 dominant hand: p=0.004
Stiffness intensity (1–5 scale)	1 RCT (Rothacker et al. 1998) (N=86)	Trolamine salicylate	120 minutes post intervention	Right hand: p=0.026 Both hands averaged: p=0.026 dominant hand: p=0.006
Stiffness intensity (change from baseline) for the left hand	1 RCT (Rothacker et al. 1998) (N=86)	Trolamine salicylate	Pooled for 30 minutes, 45 minutes and 120 minutes post-intervention	NS

continued

Table 7.47 Symptoms: stiffness – *continued*

Stiffness outcome	Reference	Intervention	Assessment time	Outcome/effect size
Hand – *continued*				
Stiffness intensity (1–5 scale) in the left hand	1 RCT (Rothacker et al. 1998) (N=86)	Trolamine salicylate	30 minutes and 45 minutes post-intervention	NS
Stiffness relief (change from baseline)	1 RCT (Rothacker et al. 1994) (N=50)	Trolamine salicylate	0, 15, 20, 30, 45 and 120 minutes after treatment	NS

Table 7.48 Symptoms: function

Function outcome	Reference	Intervention	Assessment time	Outcome/effect size
Knee osteoarthritis				
Degree of swelling (mm), mean change	1 RCT (Algozzine et al. 1982) (N=26)	Trolamine salicylate vs placebo	After treatment (7 days)	1 mm (trolamine) and –8 mm (placebo), p=0.009 Favours placebo
Joint tenderness	1 RCT (Algozzine et al. 1982) (N=26)	Trolamine salicylate vs placebo	After treatment (7 days)	NS
Range of motion (Extension and flexion, degrees)	1 RCT (Algozzine et al. 1982) (N=26)	Trolamine salicylate vs placebo	After treatment (7 days)	NS
Morning stiffness	1 RCT (Algozzine et al. 1982) (N=26)	Trolamine salicylate vs placebo	After treatment (7 days)	NS
Activity (pedometer measurements, km)	1 RCT (Algozzine et al. 1982) (N=26)	Trolamine salicylate vs placebo	After treatment (7 days)	NS

Table 7.49 Global assessment

Global assessment outcome	Reference	Intervention	Assessment time	Outcome/effect size
Knee osteoarthritis				
Patient evaluation of relief	1 RCT (Algozzine et al. 1982) (N=26)	Trolamine salicylate vs placebo	7 days	NS
Examiner evaluation of relief	1 RCT (Algozzine et al. 1982) (N=26)	Trolamine salicylate vs placebo	7 days	NS
Patient preference	1 RCT (Algozzine et al. 1982) (N=26)	Trolamine salicylate vs placebo	7 days	NS

continued

Table 7.49 Global assessment – *continued*

Global assessment outcome	Reference	Intervention	Assessment time	Outcome/effect size
Mixed (Knee and/or hip)				
Patient's global assessment of treatment efficacy, 4-point Likert Scale (change from baseline)	1 RCT (Shackel et al. 1997) (N=116)	Copper-salicylate vs placebo	4 weeks (end of treatment)	NS
Investigator's global assessment of treatment efficacy, 4-point Likert Scale (change from baseline)	1 RCT (Shackel et al. 1997) (N=116)	Copper-salicylate vs placebo	4 weeks (end of treatment)	NS

Table 7.50 Adverse events

AEs outcome	Reference	Intervention	Assessment time	Outcome/effect size
Knee osteoarthritis				
Number of AEs	1 RCT (Algozzine et al. 1982) (N=26)	Trolamine salicylate vs placebo	7 days	None reported for either group
Hand				
Number of AEs	1 RCT (Rothacker et al. 1994) (N=50)	Trolamine salicylate vs placebo	Not mentioned	N=2 (trolamine) N=1 (placebo)
Mixed (knee and/or hip)				
Number of AEs	One RCT (Shackel et al. 1997) (N=116)	Copper-salicylate vs placebo	4 weeks (end of treatment)	N=100 (copper salicylate) N=58 (placebo); p=0.002 Favours placebo

Table 7.51 Study withdrawals

Withdrawal outcomes	Reference	Intervention	Assessment time	Outcome/effect size
Hand				
Number of withdrawals	1 RCT (Rothacker et al. 1994) (N=50)	Trolamine salicylate vs placebo	During treatment	N=1 (trolamine) N=0 (placebo)
Number of withdrawals due to AEs	1 RCT (Rothacker et al. 1994) (N=50)	Trolamine salicylate vs placebo	During treatment	Both: N=0
Number of withdrawals	1 RCT (Rothacker et al. 1998) (N=86)	Trolamine salicylate vs placebo	During treatment	N=2 (trolamine) N=3 (placebo)

continued

Table 7.51 Study withdrawals – *continued*

Withdrawal outcomes	Reference	Intervention	Assessment time	Outcome/effect size
Mixed (Knee and/or hip)				
Number of withdrawals	One RCT (Shackel et al. 1997) (N=116)	Copper-salicylate vs placebo	During 4 weeks treatment	26% (copper-salicylate) 17% (placebo)
Withdrawals due to AEs	One RCT (Shackel et al. 1997) (N=116)	Copper-salicylate vs placebo	During 4 weeks treatment	17% (copper-salicylate) 1.7% (placebo)
Withdrawals due to lack of efficacy	One RCT (Shackel et al. 1997) (N=116)	Copper-salicylate vs placebo	During 4 weeks treatment	5.2 (copper-salicylate) 3.4 (placebo)

Table 7.52 Other outcomes

Withdrawal outcomes	Reference	Intervention	Assessment time	Outcome/effect size
Mixed (knee and/or hip)				
Number of patients taking rescue medication (paracetamol)	One RCT (Shackel et al. 1997) (N=116)	Copper-salicylate vs placebo	During 4 weeks treatment	NS

7.2.6 Health economic evidence

We looked at studies that conducted economic evaluations involving topical NSAIDs, capsaicin or rubefacients. Three papers, two from the UK and one from Australia, relevant to this question were found and included as evidence. After the re-run search one further study was included.

Two UK papers from the early 1990s conducted cost-minimisation analyses rather than full cost effectiveness or cost–utility analysis.

One UK paper compares oral ibuprofen (1200 mg/day) to topical Traxam and oral Arthrotec (diclofenac 50 mg/misoprostol 200 mg one tablet twice daily) (Peacock and Rapier 1993). The study considers the drug cost of each treatment as well as the cost of ulcers caused by the treatment using a simple economic model. It does not include other GI adverse events or CV adverse events. Including these would make the oral NSAID appear more expensive. Ulcer incidence rates are estimated based on findings in the literature, and some simple sensitivity analysis is undertaken around this. In conducting a cost-minimisation analysis the authors have implicitly assumed equal efficacy of the treatments, which may not be appropriate. The duration considered in the study is one month.

Another UK study considers oral ibuprofen (1200 mg/day) and topical piroxicam gel (1g three times daily) (McKell and Stewart 1994). The cost per patient of each treatment is calculated using a decision tree which includes ulcers and dyspepsia as adverse events. CV adverse events are not included. Adverse event rates are estimated using data in the published literature. Importantly, the efficacy of the treatments is assumed to be equal and hence only costs are considered. The duration of the study is three months.

The Australian study considers a number of different treatments for osteoarthritis, one of which is topical capsaicin compared with placebo (Segal et al. 2004). The paper is generally well conducted. Data regarding the effectiveness of capsaicin are taken from the literature (Altman et al. 1994; Deal et al. 1991). The transfer to utility (TTU) technique was used to transform the pain improvement data available in trials into a quality adjusted life year (QALY) gain. The paper assumes that capsaicin does not increase the risk of adverse events over the levels experienced by the general population, and so the only costs included in the study are the specific drugs cost. The study takes a 1-year time period and calculates the incremental cost–effectiveness ratio (ICER) of topical capsaicin compared with placebo.

It is of note that a study protocol for a trial assessing the costs and benefits associated with treating patients with chronic knee pain with topical or ibuprofen was published in November 2005.

One UK study which is yet to be published investigates oral ibuprofen compared with topical ibuprofen in 585 patients with knee pain. The study had an RCT arm and a patient preference arm, and includes 12-month and 24-month data.

7.2.7 Health economic evidence statements

▷ Oral ibuprofen vs topical Traxam or topical piroxicam and Arthrotec

Table 7.53 Cost (1993 £) of treating 1000 patients for 1 month

Ibuprofen (1200 mg/day)	Traxam	Arthrotec
41,408	7,319	17,924

Table 7.54 Cost (1991–1992 £) per patient for 3 months

Ibuprofen (1200 mg/day)	Piroxicam (1g tid)
89.12	54.57

The tables above show the results of the two studies from the UK (McKell and Stewart 1994; Peacock and Rapier 1993). They offer evidence that treatment with topical NSAIDs is likely to be cheaper than treatment with oral NSAIDs. However, it must be noted that the studies are incomplete with regards to the adverse events included (neither include CV adverse events, and not all GI adverse events are included). Including these adverse events would result in topical NSAIDs leading to a higher cost saving compared with oral NSAIDs, providing topical NSAIDs result in fewer of these events than oral NSAIDs. Also the results of the studies are of limited use with regards to cost effectiveness since a health outcome is not included. Equal efficacy is assumed, but if oral NSAIDs are in actuality more effective, then there remains a possibility that they could be considered cost effective despite being more expensive.

In summary, evidence suggests that treatment with topical NSAIDs will result in lower costs than treatment with oral NSAIDs due to the higher prevalence of adverse events with oral

NSAIDs. The cost effectiveness of oral NSAIDs depends on their clinical efficacy compared with topical NSAIDs. If oral NSAIDs are of equal efficacy compared with topical NSAIDs it is likely that topical NSAIDs would be cost effective.

▷ Topical capsaicin vs placebo

Table 7.55 Segal's estimates of cost effectiveness

Program	Mean QALY gain per person	Mean program cost	Cost/QALY best estimate
Non-specific NSAIDs (naproxen, diclofenac)	0.043	Drug: $104/year morbidity: $70/year	$15,000 to infinity
Cox 2s (celecoxib)	0.043	Drug: $391/year morbidity: $70/year	$33,000 to infinity
Topical capsaicin	0.053	$236	$4,453
Glucosamine sulfate	0.052	$180	$3,462

The table above shows the cost effectiveness of a number of drugs as calculated by the Australian study (Segal et al. 2004). NSAIDs, COX-2 inhibitors, and glucosamine sulfate are included to allow some comparison of cost effectiveness between the drugs, although each is only compared with placebo in the analysis, rather than to each other. Where the cost–effectiveness ratio is said to range 'to infinity' this is because the benefits of the drug are not assured.

These results suggest that topical capsaicin brings more QALY gain than NSAIDs or COX-2 inhibitors compared with placebo, while resulting in lower total costs than COX-2 inhibitors (although the total costs are higher than for NSAIDs). Therefore capsaicin appears dominant compared with COX-2 inhibitors. The incremental cost-effectiveness ratio between NSAIDs and topical capsaicin [(236–174)/(0.053–0.043) = $6,200] suggests that topical capsaicin is likely to be cost effective compared with NSAIDs. However, the incremental cost-effectiveness ratio between topical capsaicin and glucosamine sulfate only shows borderline cost effectiveness (236–180)/(0.053–0.052) = $56,000 per QALY. Because the cost of topical capsaicin is relatively low and QALY gains are accrued, the incremental cost-effectiveness ratio of $4,453 stated in Table 7.55 suggests the treatment is cost effective compared with placebo.

Some care has to be taken with these results because of the relative lack of studies which show the benefits of capsaicin and glucosamine sulfate. The transfer to utility approach for calculating QALY gains has also been questioned in the literature. The study is also from an Australian perspective which may not be transferable to a UK setting.

It is of interest that in the UK 45 g of topical capsaicin costs £15.04. If this size tube was sufficient for one month of treatment the UK yearly cost of treatment with topical capsaicin would be £180.48 (taking into account only drug costs). Some sources suggest this size tube would in fact not be sufficient for one month of treatment (www.pharmac.govt.nz/pdf/0804.pdf). This is significantly more expensive than the $236 cost stated by the Australian study, which equates to £95.57, but does assume that the patient uses the treatment continuously for one year. Using this cost, the incremental cost-effectiveness ratio of topical capsaicin compared with placebo would be (180.48/0.053) £3405 per QALY which is still relatively low.

However, in comparison to other drugs, topical capsaicin appears likely to be closer to the cost of COX-2 inhibitors, and significantly more expensive than some NSAIDs in a UK setting. In the UK celecoxib costs £21.55 per 60-cap 100 mg pack, suggesting a yearly drug cost of approximately £21.55 × 12 = £259 (BNF 51). Diclofenac sodium costs £1.52 for an 84-tab pack of 25 mg, suggesting a yearly drug cost of approximately £1.52 × 12 = £18.24, (BNF 51) although these estimates do not include the adverse event costs of these drugs.

Given this, it is difficult to make reliable recommendations regarding topical capsaicin compared with COX-2 inhibitors and NSAIDs based on this Australian data.

In summary, evidence from an Australian study suggests that topical capsaicin is cost effective compared with placebo, since it brings QALY gains at relatively low cost.

▷ Topical ibuprofen vs oral ibuprofen

The study finds that the effectiveness of the two treatments is not statistically significantly different, but that oral ibuprofen appears slightly better. Oral ibuprofen is generally a more expensive treatment option, due to more gastroprotective drugs and cardiovascular drugs being prescribed alongside it. Overall, oral ibuprofen is generally found to be cost effective compared with topical ibuprofen. However, the authors note that the study considered a population at low risk of adverse events and the prevalence of adverse events in the study was lower than expected. Given the risks known to be associated with taking oral NSAIDs, it may be that in a higher risk population oral NSAIDs would not be cost effective.

In summary:
- in a population at low risk of adverse events, oral ibuprofen is likely to be a cost-effective treatment compared with topical ibuprofen
- treatment with topical ibuprofen is likely to be cheaper than treatment with oral ibuprofen.

7.2.8 From evidence to recommendations

A number of studies, mainly of knee osteoarthritis, have shown short-term (less than four weeks) benefits from topical NSAID gels, creams and ointments when compared with placebo. There are no data on their long-term effectiveness when compared with placebo. There are limited studies comparing other topical gels, creams and ointments with oral NSAIDs. One study with three month follow-up found topical diclofenac in dimethyl sulfoxide to be equivalent to oral diclofenac for knee osteoarthritis over three months.

The data from RCTs have demonstrated a reduction in non-serious adverse effects when compared with oral NSAIDs, although topical preparations may produce local skin irritation. The RCT data do not allow a conclusive judgement on whether using topical NSAIDs reduces the incidence of serious NSAID-related adverse effects. However, it seems logical that there would be a reduced risk given the total dose of NSAIDs from topical application to one joint area is much less than when used orally. Thus, since there are some data supporting the effectiveness of topical NSAIDs, they are likely to be preferred to using oral NSAIDs as early treatment for osteoarthritis, particularly for patients who do not have widespread painful osteoarthritis. However, there are no data comparing topical NSAIDs to paracetamol or on the comparative risk and benefits from the long-term use of oral or topical NSAIDs.

Topical NSAIDs are relatively costly but are cost effective given that they prevent or delay use of oral NSAIDs with their associated serious adverse events. Most of the clinial evidence is for the preparation of diclofenac in DMSO (Pennsaid), but overall there is little evidence and the group did not find sufficient justification to single out this brand in the recommendations. At the time of writing, Pennsaid was not the cheapest alternative in this class.

There are limited data showing some positive effects from topical capsaicin, with short-term follow-up. Although the evidence is limited to knee osteoarthritis, the GDG were aware of widespread use in hand osteoarthritis as part of self-management and felt that the data on efficacy at the knee could reasonably be extrapolated to the hand. No serious toxicity associated with capsaicin use has been reported in the peer-reviewed literature. The evidence base, however, does not support the use of rubefacients.

Topical treatments are used in self-management, which helps change health behaviour positively. Often, people with osteoarthritis will use the topical treatment on top of daily paracetamol and exercise to cope with flare-ups. This is in line with the evidence, which shows short-term benefit. As a safe pharmaceutical option, topical NSAIDs were regarded by the GDG as one of the second-line options for symptom relief after the core treatments. They have therefore been placed on an equal footing with paracetamol.

RECOMMENDATIONS

R23   Healthcare professionals should consider offering topical NSAIDs for pain relief in addition to core treatment (see Fig 3.2) for people with knee or hand osteoarthritis. Topical NSAIDs and/or paracetamol should be considered ahead of oral NSAIDs, COX-2 inhibitors or opioids.

R24   Topical capsaicin should be considered as an adjunct to core treatment for knee or hand osteoarthritis; rubefacients are not recommended for the treatment of osteoarthritis.

7.3   NSAIDs and highly selective COX-2 inhibitors

7.3.1   Clinical introduction

Non-steroidal anti-inflammatory drugs (NSAIDs) have been available for many years and are thought to work by reducing the production of pro-inflammatory and pain-related prostaglandins. The discovery of different cyclooxygenase (COX) enzymes with different physiological actions brought with it the concept that differential blockade of COX-1 (important in normal regulation of the gastro-intestinal (GI) mucosa) and COX-2 (up-regulated at sites of inflammation among other functions and thought responsible for pro-inflammatory mediator production) may provide effective analgesic/anti-inflammatory actions without the common GI complications of traditional NSAIDs. These GI complications are well known to clinicians and include a spectrum of problems from dyspepsia and ulcers to life-threatening perforations, ulcers and bleeds. However the blocking of COX-2 always carried the potential for a pro-thrombotic effect, by changing the balance of pro- and anti-thrombotic mediators.

The first novel agents to be classed COX-2 selective were celecoxib and rofecoxib, although existing agents were also recognised for their high COX-2/COX-1 inhibitory ratios (etodolac, meloxicam). Of these agents, rofecoxib in particular demonstrated the expected outcomes, in that initial studies demonstrated reduced serious GI problems compared with traditional NSAIDs. Importantly, there was no evidence to suggest that any of these agents would differ from traditional NSAIDs with respect to efficacy. However, the initial, pivotal study also demonstrated increased pro-thrombotic cardiovascular problems (an increase in myocardial infarctions). This brought a spotlight to bear on the cardiovascular safety of all such agents, but also on traditional NSAIDs which had varying degrees of COX-2 selectivity. This remains a complex field because of issues including that:

- long-term toxicity must be assessed from longitudinal, observational databases with their inherent problems, including lack of thorough assessment of an individual's cardiovascular risk factors
- more detailed trial data are only available on newer agents
- drug dose in studies do not reflect usual prescribed doses or patient use.

As a result of further scrutiny, there seems less reason to use the terms 'traditional NSAIDs' and 'COX-2' selective agents. It would appear that it may be more useful to return to the generic term NSAIDs with a concomitant awareness of the differing degrees of COX-2 selectivity and different (though not always consequent) side-effect profiles.

7.3.2 Methodological introduction

Three questions were posed in the literature searches for this section of the guideline.

- In adults with osteoarthritis, what are the benefits and harms of COX-2 inhibitors compared with i) non-selective NSAIDs or ii) placebo in respect to symptoms, function and quality of life?
- In adults with osteoarthritis, what are the relative benefits and harms of i) selective COX-2 inhibitors versus nonselective NSAIDs plus GI protective agents and ii) selective COX-2 inhibitors plus GI protective agents versus nonselective NSAIDs plus GI protective agents?
- In adults with osteoarthritis taking aspirin, what are the relative benefits and harms of selective COX-2 inhibitors versus nonselective NSAIDs versus each of these combined with GI protective agents?

We looked firstly at studies that focused on investigating the effects of COX-2 inhibitors compared with non-selective NSAIDs or placebo for the outcomes of symptoms, function, quality of life, and adverse events (AEs) where the latter where reported. Due to the high number of studies in this area only randomised double-blinded controlled trials were considered for inclusion as evidence for all osteoarthritis sites. *However, for knee osteoarthritis studies, only double-blinded RCTs with N≥400 participants and with a duration of longer than 4 weeks were considered for inclusion.*

For the second question, we found two studies (Chan et al. 2007; Scheiman et al. 2006) that investigated the effects of esomeprazole versus placebo in adults with osteoarthritis or RA receiving concomitant COX-2 inhibitors or non-selective NSAIDs. Although these studies included a mixed osteoarthritis/RA population, it was decided to include them, since they were the only studies reporting on the results of well-designed RCTs on this topic. One other RCT (Lai 2005) was found but excluded from the evidence since it was an open-label study and thus did not fulfil the inclusion criteria.

Finally, two studies (Schnitzer et al. 2004; Singh et al. 2006) selected for the first question also included data on adverse gastro-intestinal events in adults with osteoarthritis taking low-dose aspirin. They were therefore relevant to the third question, which focuses on the relative benefits and harms of COX-2 inhibitors and non-selective NSAIDs in adults with osteoarthritis receiving concomitant low-dose aspirin.

The relevant data are reported under the adverse events section of the evidence statements. No other studies were identified that addressed the third question.

7.3.3 Evidence statements: COX-2 inhibitors vs placebo and NSAIDs

▷ Summary

Symptoms: pain

Overall, the studies found that both COX-2 inhibitors were superior to placebo in terms of reducing pain over treatment periods ranging from six weeks to six months. The majority of the data reported here are for outcomes on the VAS and the WOMAC. The limited data on direct comparisons of COX-2 inhibitors and non-selective NSAIDs for this outcome suggested these two drug classes were equivalent. Only a small number of studies reported significant differences when comparing COX-2 inhibitors with NSAIDs:

- knee: two studies reported in favour of celecoxib compared with naproxen (N=1061) (Kivitz 2001); (N=1608) (Zhao et al. 1999)
- knee and hip: one study reported in favour of naproxen compared with etodolac (N=76) (Chikanza and Clarke 1994)
- mixed sites: one study reported in favour of diclofenac compared with meloxicam (N=10,051) (Hawkey 1998).

Knee osteoarthritis

Fifteen RCTs (Bensen et al. 1999; Fleischmann et al. 2006; Gottesdiener et al. 2002; Kivitz et al. 2001; Lehmann 2005; Lund 1998; McKenna 2001; Sheldon 2005; Smugar et al. 2006; Tannenbaum et al. 2004; Williams et al. 2000, 2001; Zhao et al. 1999) focusing on knee osteoarthritis were identified. Two studies (Suarez-Otero 2002; Williams and Osie 1989) were excluded due to multiple methodological limitations, including absence of reported washout period prior to baseline assessment. All other studies were included as evidence.

The studies below reported significant reductions in pain for the following COX-2 inhibitors compared with placebo for treatment periods ranging from 3 to 13 weeks:

- celecoxib 100 to 400 mg (N=1003) (Bensen et al. 1999); (N=1608) (Fleischmann et al. 2006); (N=1061) (Kivitz et al. 2001); (N=1684) (Lehmann 2005); (N=1551) (Sheldon 2005); (N=1702) (Tannenbaum et al. 2004); (N=600) (McKenna 2001); (N=718) (Williams et al. 2001); (N=686) (Williams et al. 2000); (N=1521) (Smugar et al. 2006); (N=1082) (Smugar et al. 2006); (N=599) (Bingham et al. 2007); (N=608) (Bingham et al. 2007)
- lumiracoxib 100 to 400 mg (Fleischmann et al. 2006); (Lehmann 2005); (Sheldon 2005); (Tannenbaum et al. 2004)

- etoricoxib 20 to 360 mg (N=617) (Gottesdiener et al. 2002); (N=599) (Bingham et al. 2007); (N=608) (Bingham et al. 2007)
- meloxicam 7.5 or 15 mg. For the outcome pain at rest meloxicam 7.5 mg (NS) (N=513) (Lund 1998).

The studies below reported on outcomes for the following drug interventions for treatment periods ranging from 12 to 14 weeks:

- celecoxib 100 mg resulted in significant reductions in pain compared with naproxen 2000 mg in WOMAC pain (p<0.001). Celecoxib 200 and 400 mg and naproxen 1000 mg (NS) (N=1061) (Kivitz et al. 2001)
- celecoxib 100 mg and 200 mg had significant reductions in pain scores (WOMAC) compared with naproxen 1000 mg (% change from baseline celecoxib 100 mg –29.5, celecoxib 200 mg –25.2 versus naproxen –21.8) (N=1003) (Zhao et al. 1999)
- celecoxib 100 mg and diclofenac 50 mg (NS) (N=600) (McKenna 2001)
- etoricoxib 20 to 360 mg and diclofenac 150 mg (NS) (N=617) (Gottesdiener et al. 2002)
- etoricoxib 30 mg and celecoxib 200 mg (NS) (N=599 and 608) (Bingham et al. 2007).

Hip osteoarthritis

- etodolac 100 to 400 mg versus placebo joint tenderness on pressure, all measures of weight bearing pain (standing, walking, retiring/arising, standing from chair), and night pain for participants receiving (all p≤0.05) at 12 weeks (N=36) (Sanda et al. 1983)
- melixocam 15 mg and piroxicam 20 mg (NS) (N=285) (Linden et al. 1996)
- celecoxib 100 mg and dexibuprofen 400 mg (NS) (N=148) (Hawel 2003).

Hand osteoarthritis

In favour of lumiracoxib 200 and 400 mg compared with placebo (VAS and AUSCAN) at 4 weeks (N=594) (Grifka 2004).

Foot osteoarthritis

Etodolac 800 mg and naproxen 1000 mg at 5 weeks (NS) (N=60) (Jennings and Alfieri 1997).

Knee and hip osteoarthritis

Eleven RCTs (Chikanza and Clarke 1994; Hosie et al. 1996; Hosie 1997; Leung and Malmstrom 2002; Perpignano 1994; Pincus 2004; Rogind 1997; Sowers and White 2005; Wiesenhutter and Boice 2005; Yocum 2000; Zacher 2003) focusing on knee and hip osteoarthritis were identified.

The studies below compared the following COX-2 inhibitors with placebo, all reporting significant reductions in pain in favour of the active drug treatment(s) for treatment period's ranging from 6 to 12 weeks:

- etoricoxib 30 to 60 mg (N=501) (Leung and Malmstrom 2002); (N=528) (Wiesenhutter and Boice 2005)
- celecoxib 200 mg (N=356) (Pincus 2004)
- meloxicam 7.5 or 15 mg (N=774) (Yocum 2000).

The studies below reported on outcomes for the active drug comparisons for treatment periods ranging from 6 weeks to 6 months:

- naproxen 1000 mg (18/72) was preferred to etodolac 600 mg (7/72) for reducing pain intensity (p=0.044). For the outcome of night pain (NS) (N=76) (Chikanza and Clarke 1994)
- etoricoxib 30 mg and ibuprofen 2400 mg (NS) (N=528) (Wiesenhutter and Boice 2005); etoricoxib 60 mg and diclofenac sodium 150 mg (NS) (N=516) (Zacher 2003)
- meloxicam 7.5 and 15 mg and diclofenac 50 mg (NS) (N=774) (Yocum 2000); meloxicam 15 mg and piroxicam 20 mg (NS) (N=455) (Hosie 1997); meloxicam 7.5 mg and diclofenac sodium 100 mg (NS) (N=336) (Hosie et al. 1996)
- etodolac 600 mg and tenoxicam 20 mg (NS) (N=120) (Perpignano 1994); etodolac 600 mg and piroxicam 20 mg (NS) (N=271) (Rogind 1997)
- celecoxib 200 mg and naproxen 500 mg (NS) (N=404) (Sowers and White 2005) (N=404).

Mixed sites of osteoarthritis

Three RCTs (Dequeker 1998; Hawkey 1998; Hawkey and Svoboda 2004) included populations of adults with knee, hip, hand or spinal osteoarthritis, while two other RCTs (Schnitzer 2004; Singh 2006) included populations of adults with knee, hip or hand osteoarthritis.

The studies below reported on outcomes for the following active drug comparisons over treatment periods ranging from 28 days to 52 weeks:

- diclofenac 100 mg showed a statistically significant reduction in pain on active movement (VAS) compared with meloxicam 7.5 mg at 28 days (mean difference 2.29, 95%CI 1.38 to 3.20). For the outcome of pain at rest (VAS) (NS) (N=10051) (Hawkey 1998)
- lumiracoxib 400 mg, naproxen 1000 mg and ibuprofen 2400 mg (NS) (N=18,325) (Schnitzer et al. 2004)
- celecoxib 200 or 400 mg compared with naproxen 1000 mg and diclofenac 100 mg (NS) (N=13274) (Singh et al. 2006)
- lumiracoxib 200 or 400 mg, celecoxib 200 mg and ibuprofen 2400 mg (NS) (N=1042) (Hawkey and Svoboda 2004)
- meloxicam 7.5 mg and piroxicam 20 mg (NS) (N= 9286) (Dequeker 1998).

▷ Summary

Symptoms: stiffness

Overall, the studies found that both COX-2 inhibitors were superior to placebo in terms of reducing pain over treatment periods ranging from 15 days to six months. The majority of data reported here are for outcomes on the WOMAC and VAS. The limited data available indicated that COX-2 inhibitors and non-selective NSAIDs were comparable with regard to the outcome of stiffness reduction. Only a small number of studies reported a significant difference when comparing COX-2 inhibitors with NSAIDs:

- knee: two studies reported in favour of celecoxib compared with naproxen (Zhao et al. 1999); (N=1061) (Kivitz et al. 2001)
- knee and hip: one study reported in favour of celecoxib compared with naproxen (N=404) (Sowers and White 2005).

Knee osteoarthritis

Twelve RCTs (Bensen et al. 1999; Fleischmann et al. 2006; Gottesdiener et al. 2002; Kivitz et al. 2001; Lehmann 2005; McKenna 2001; Sheldon 2005; Smugar et al. 2006; Tannenbaum et al. 2004; Williams et al. 2000, 2001; Zhao et al. 1999) focusing on knee osteoarthritis were identified.

The studies below all reported significant improvements in stiffness for the COX-2 inhibitors compared with placebo for treatment periods ranging from 6 to 13 weeks:

- celecoxib 100 to 400 mg (N=1003) (Bensen et al. 1999); (N=1608) (Fleischmann et al. 2006); (N=1061) (Kivitz et al. 2001); (N=1551) (Sheldon 2005); (N=1702) (Tannenbaum et al. 2004); (N=600) (McKenna 2001); (N=718) (Williams et al. 2001); (N=686) (Williams et al. 2000); (N=1521) (Smugar et al. 2006); (N=1082) (Smugar et al. 2006)
- lumiracoxib 100 to 400 mg (Fleischmann et al. 2006); (N=1684) (Lehmann 2005); (Sheldon 2005); (Tannenbaum et al. 2004)
- etoricoxib 20 to 360 mg (N=617) (Gottesdiener et al. 2002)
- celecoxib 200 mg and placebo (NS) (Lehmann 2005).

The studies below reported outcomes for the following active drug comparisons in WOMAC stiffness for treatment periods ranging from 6 to 14 weeks:

- celecoxib 100 mg had statistically significant reductions in stiffness scores (WOMAC) compared with naproxen 1000 mg (% change from baseline celecoxib 100 mg –25.5 versus naproxen –22.0) (Zhao et al. 1999)
- celecoxib 100 mg showed significantly reductions in stiffness scores (WOMAC) compared with naproxen (p<0.001). Celecoxib 200 and 400 mg and naproxen 1000 mg on this outcome (NS) (N=1061) (Kivitz et al. 2001)
- etoricoxib 20 to 360 mg and diclofenac 150 mg (NS) (N=617) (Gottesdiener et al. 2002)
- celecoxib 100 mg and diclofenac 50 mg (N=600) (NS) (McKenna 2001).

Hip osteoarthritis

One RCT found that use of etodolac 100 to 400 mg resulted in significant reductions in morning stiffness compared with placebo at 12 weeks (N=36) (Sanda et al. 1983).

Celecoxib 100 mg and dexibuprofen 400 mg (NS) (N=148) (Hawel 2003).

Hand osteoarthritis

One RCT found that at 4 weeks lumiracoxib 200 mg and lumiracoxib 400 mg groups both had statistically significant improvements in pain scores (VAS, AUSCAN) compared with placebo (N=594) (Grifka 2004).

Knee and hip osteoarthritis

Nine RCTs (Chikanza and Clarke 1994; Hosie et al. 1996; Hosie 1997; Leung and Malmstrom 2002; Rogind 1997; Sowers and White 2005; Wiesenhutter and Boice 2005; Yocum 2000; Zacher 2003) focusing on knee and hip osteoarthritis were identified.

The studies below reported a significant difference in favour of the following COX-2 inhibitors compared with placebo for treatment period of 12 weeks:

- etoricoxib 30 to 60 mg (N=501) (Leung and Malmstrom 2002) (N=528); (N=528) (Wiesenhutter and Boice 2005)
- meloxicam 3.75 to 15 mg (N=774) (Yocum 2000).

Out of the studies comparing two active drug comparisons, only one reported a significant reduction in stiffness (WOMAC p=0.02), favouring celecoxib 200 mg versus naproxen 500 mg in participants with hypertension and diabetes after 12 weeks (N=404) (Sowers and White 2005).

The remaining studies reported no statistical differences for the active drug comparisons for treatment period's ranging from 6 weeks to 6 months:

- etoricoxib 30 mg and ibuprofen 2400 mg (NS) (N=528) (Wiesenhutter and Boice 2005); etoricoxib 60 mg and diclofenac sodium 150 mg (N=516) (Zacher 2003)
- meloxicam 3.75 to 15 mg and diclofenac 50 to 100 mg (NS) (N=774) (Yocum 2000); (N=336) (Hosie et al. 1996); meloxicam 15 mg and piroxicam 20 mg (NS) (N=455) (Hosie 1997)
- naproxen 1000 mg and etodolac 600 mg (NS) (N=76) (Chikanza and Clarke 1994)
- etodolac 600 mg and piroxicam 20 mg (NS) (N=271) (Rogind 1997).

▷ Summary: general function/global efficacy measures

Overall, it was found that both COX-2 were superior to placebo in terms of improving patient's and physician's assessments of disease and overall function scores. The data on direct comparisons of COX-2 inhibitors and non-selective NSAIDs indicate these two drug classes had similar effects for these outcomes. Outcomes were assessed using a number of measures including the Patients' and Physicians' Global Assessments and WOMAC. The treatment period's ranged from 15 days to 52 weeks. Only a small number of studies reported a significant difference on comparisons between two active drug interventions:

Knee: one RCT found in favour of celecoxib compared with naproxen (N=1003) (Bensen et al. 1999) and one found in favour of naproxen compared with celecoxib (N=1061) (Kivitz et al. 2001).

Knee osteoarthritis

Fourteen RCTs (Bensen et al. 1999; Bingham et al. 2007; Fleischmann et al. 2006; Gottesdiener et al. 2002; Kivitz et al. 2001; Lehmann 2005; Lund 1998; McKenna 2001; Sheldon 2005; Smugar et al. 2006; Tannenbaum et al. 2004; Williams et al. 2000, 2001) focusing on knee osteoarthritis were identified.

The studies below reported in favour of the COX-2 inhibitors in comparison with placebo for treatment periods ranging from 3 to 13 weeks:

- celecoxib 100 to 400 mg (N=1003) (Bensen et al. 1999); (N=599) (Bingham et al. 2007); (N=608) (Bingham et al. 2007); (N=1608) (Fleischmann et al. 2006) (N=1061); (N=1061) (Kivitz et al. 2001); (N=1684) (Lehmann 2005); (N=600) (McKenna 2001); (N=1551) (Sheldon 2005); (N=1082) (Smugar et al. 2006); (N=1521) (Smugar et al. 2006); (N=1702) (Tannenbaum et al. 2004); (N=718) (Williams et al. 2001); (N=686) (Williams et al. 2000).
- lumiracoxib 100 to 400 mg (Fleischmann et al. 2006); (Lehmann 2005); (Sheldon 2005); (Tannenbaum et al. 2004)

- etoricoxib 20 to 360 mg (N=617) (Gottesdiener et al. 2002); (Bingham et al. 2007);
- meloxicam 7.5 mg and 15 mg. Outcomes of osteoarthritis Index of Severity, and Global Tolerance of study drugs (NS) (N=513) (Lund 1998).

The studies below reported on outcomes for comparisons between two or more drug interventions for treatment period's ranging from 12 to 14 weeks:

- celecoxib 100 mg had a significant improvement in osteoarthritis Severity Index compared with naproxen (p≤0.05) (N=1003) (Bensen et al. 1999)
- naproxen 1000 mg had significantly greater improvements compared with celecoxib 100 mg and 400 mg (p≤0.05) on the outcome of Patient's Global Assessment, with NS differences between naproxen and doses of celecoxib for all other measures (NS) (N=1061) (Kivitz et al. 2001)
- lumiracoxib 100 to 400 mg and celecoxib 200 mg (NS) (N=1608) (Fleischmann et al. 2006); (N=1684) (Lehmann 2005); (N=1551) (Sheldon 2005)
- etoricoxib 20 to 360 mg and diclofenac 150 mg (NS) (N=617) (Gottesdiener 2002); etoricoxib 30 mg and celecoxib 200 mg (NS) (N=599) (Bingham et al. 2007); (N=608) (Bingham et al. 2007)
- celecoxib 100 mg and diclofenac 50 mg (NS) (N=600) (McKenna 2001).

Hip osteoarthritis

Etodolac 100 to 400 mg resulted in significant improvements on global efficacy measures compared with a placebo group in adults with hip osteoarthritis at 12 weeks (N=36) (Sanda et al. 1983). Two other RCTs found non-significant differences between COX-2 inhibitors and non-selective NSAIDs on global efficacy measures, namely meloxicam and piroxicam (N=285) (Linden et al. 1996) and celecoxib 100 mg and dexibuprofen 400 mg (N=148) (Hawel 2003).

Hand osteoarthritis

One RCT found that at 4 weeks lumiracoxib 200 mg and lumiracocib 400 mg groups both had statistically significant improvements in Patient's and Physician's Global Assessments of Disease and patient's functional status (AUSCAN total score) compared with placebo (N=594) (Grifka 2004).

Knee and hip osteoarthritis

Nine RCTs (Hosie et al. 1996; Hosie 1997; Leung and Malmstrom 2002; Perpignano 1994; Rogind 1997; Sowers and White 2005; Wiesenhutter and Boice 2005; Yocum 2000; Zacher 2003) were identified that focused on knee and hip osteoarthritis.

The studies below reported significant improvements on measures of global efficacy and function scores in favour of the following COX-2 inhibitors compared with placebo for a treatment period of 12 weeks:

- etoricoxib 30 and 60 mg (N=501) (Leung and Malmstrom 2002); (N=528) (Wiesenhutter and Boice 2005)
- meloxicam 3.75 to 15 mg (N=774) (Yocum 2000).

The following studies reported on outcomes for comparisons between the active drug comparisons over treatment period's ranging from 6 weeks to 6 months:

- etoricoxib 30 mg and ibuprofen 2400 mg (NS) (N=528) (Wiesenhutter and Boice 2005)
- meloxicam 3.75 to 15 mg and diclofenac 50 mg (NS) (N=774) (Yocum 2000); Meloxicam 15 mg and piroxicam 20 mg (NS) (N=455) (Hosie 1997); meloxicam 7.5 mg and diclofenac sodium 100 mg (NS) (N=336) (Hosie et al. 1996)
- celecoxib 200 mg and naproxen 500 mg (NS) assessed by participants with hypertension and diabetes (N=404) (Sowers and White 2005)
- etodolac 600 mg and tenoxicam 20 mg (NS) (N=120) (Perpignano 1994); etodolac 600 mg and piroxicam 20 mg (NS) (N=271) (Rogind 1997); etoricoxib 60 mg and diclofenac sodium 150 mg (NS) (N=516) (Zacher 2003).

Mixed sites of osteoarthritis

Three RCTs (Dequeker 1998; Hawkey et al. 1998; Hawkey and Svoboda 2004) included populations of adults with knee, hip, hand or spinal osteoarthritis, while two other RCTs (Schnitzer et al. 2004; Singh et al. 2006) included populations of adults with knee, hip or hand osteoarthritis. The treatment period's ranged from 28 days to 52 weeks:

- diclofenac 100 mg showed statistically significant improvements in measures of global efficacy and function outcomes compared with meloxicam 7.5 mg at 28 days. However, these differences did not appear to be clinically significant (NS) (N=10,051) (Hawkey 1998)
- lumiracoxib 400 mg, naproxen 1000 mg and ibuprofen 2400 mg (NS) (N=18325) (Schnitzer et al. 2004)
- lumiracoxib 200 and 400 mg, celecoxib 200 mg and ibuprofen 2400 mg (NS) (N=1042) (Hawkey et al. 2004)
- celecoxib 200 and 400 mg and naproxen 1000 mg and diclofenac 100 mg (NS) (N=13274) (Singh et al. 2006)
- meloxicam 7.5 mg and piroxicam 20 mg (NS) (N= 9286) (Dequeker 1998).

▷ Summary: physical function

Overall, both COX-2 inhibitors were superior to placebo in terms of improving physical function. In general, data are presented for outcomes on the WOMAC. The treatment period's ranged from 6 to 14 weeks. The limited data on direct comparisons of COX-2 inhibitors and non-selective NSAIDs for this outcome suggested these two drug classes may be comparable for this outcome. Only two studies reported a significant difference between active drug interventions in the knee, in favour of celecoxib compared with naproxen (N=1003) (Zhao et al. 1999); (N=1061) (Kivitz et al. 2001).

Knee osteoarthritis

Eleven RCTs (Bensen et al. 1999; Bingham et al. 2007; Fleischmann et al. 2006; Gottesdiener et al. 2002; Kivitz et al. 2001; Lehmann 2005; McKenna 2001; Smugar et al. 2006; Williams et al. 2000, 2001; Zhao 1999) focussed on knee osteoarthritis The studies below reported in favour of the following COX-2 inhibitors in comparison to placebo for treatment period's ranging from 6 to 12 weeks:

- celecoxib 50 to 400 mg (N=1003) (Bensen et al. 1999); (N=599) (Bingham et al. 2007); (N=1061) (Kivitz et al. 2001); (N=600) (McKenna 2001) (N=600); (N=718) (Smugar et al. 2006); (Williams et al. 2001); (N=686) (Williams et al. 2000); (N=1521)
- etoricoxib 20 to 360 mg (N=617) (Gottesdiener 2002); (N=599) (Bingham 2007).

The studies below reported on outcomes for comparisons between for the following active drug comparisons for treatment period's ranging from 12 to 14 weeks:

- celecoxib 100 mg had statistically significant improvements in physical function scores (WOMAC) compared with naproxen (% change from baseline celecoxib 100 mg –26.8 versus naproxen –21.3) (N=1003) (Zhao et al. 1999)
- celecoxib 100 mg showed significantly greater improvement in WOMAC physical function compared with naproxen (p<0.001). There was NS difference between other celecoxib dose groups and naproxen on this outcome (N=1061) (Kivitz et al. 2001)
- etoricoxib 20 to 360 mg and diclofenac 150 mg (NS) (N=617) (Gottesdiener et al. 2002); etoricoxib 30 mg and celecoxib 200 mg (NS) (N=599) (Bingham et al. 2007); (N=608) (Bingham 2007)
- celecoxib 100 mg and diclofenac 50 mg (NS) ((N=600) McKenna 2001).

Hip osteoarthritis

Celecoxib 100 mg and dexibuprofen 400 mg (NS) (N=148) (Hawel 2003)

Knee and hip osteoarthritis

Five RCTs (Leung and Malmstrom 2002; Sowers and White 2005; Wiesenhutter and Boice 2005; Yocum 2000; Zacher 2003) were identified focusing on hip and knee osteoarthritis.

The studies below reported in favour of the following COX-2 inhibitors compared with placebo on WOMAC for a treatment period of 12 weeks:

- etoricoxib 30 to 60 mg (N=501) (Leung and Malmstrom 2002); (N=528) (Wiesenhutter and Boice 2005)
- meloxicam 7.5 to 15 mg (N=774) (Yocum 2000).

The following studies reported outcomes for comparisons between the drug interventions for treatments period's of 6 to 12 weeks:

- etoricoxib 30 mg and ibuprofen 2400 mg (NS) (N=528) (Wiesenhutter and Boice 2005); and etoricoxib 60 mg and diclofenac sodium 150 mg (NS) (N=516) (Zacher 2003)
- meloxicam 7.5 to 15 mg and diclofenac 50 mg (NS) (Yocum 2000 130)
- celecoxib 200 mg and naproxen 500 mg in patients also with hypertension and diabetes (NS) (N=404) (Sowers and White 2005).

▷ Physical examination findings

Hip osteoarthritis

In favour of etodolac 100 to 400 mg compared with placebo on the outcomes of ROM hip adduction, ROM external rotation, and ROM internal rotation (all p≤0.05) at 12 weeks. Outcomes of ROM hip abduction, walking time, and climbing stairs (NS) (N=36) (Sanda et al. 1983).

Celecoxib 100 mg and dexibuprofen 400 mg (NS) (N=148) (Hawel 2003).

Foot osteoarthritis

In favour of etodolac 800 mg compared with naproxen 1000 mg at 5 weeks on walking up steps (p=0.03). Outcomes of walking down stairs, chores, running errands, and walking on a flat surface (NS) (N=60) (Jennings and Alfieri 1997).

Hip osteoarthritis

Celecoxib 100 mg and dexibuprofen 400 mg (NS) (Hawel 2003) (N=148).

Knee and hip osteoarthritis

Two RCTs found NS differences between COX-2 inhibitors and non-selective NSAIDs, meloxicam 15 mg and piroxicam 20 mg (N=455) (Hosie 1997) and meloxicam 7.5 mg and diclofenac sodium 100 mg (N=336) (Hosie et al. 1996) in terms of quality of life outcomes at six month follow-up in adults with hip or knee osteoarthritis.

▷ Gastro-intestinal adverse events

Knee osteoarthritis

Fourteen RCTs (Bensen et al. 1999; Curtis et al. 2005; Fleischmann et al. 2006; Gottesdiener et al. 2002; Kivitz et al. 2001; Lehmann 2005; Lund 1998; McKenna 2001; Sheldon 2005; Smugar et al. 2006; Tannenbaum et al. 2004; Williams et al. 2000, 2001; Zhao et al. 1999) focussed on knee osteoarthritis. Statistical significance testing of differences between treatment groups was not done. COX-2 inhibitors generally had higher percentages of GI AEs compared with placebo, but lower percentages compared with non-selective NSAIDs.

Two RCTs found that celecoxib 200 mg was significantly better than placebo (N=1521) (Smugar et al. 2006); (N=1082) (Smugar et al. 2006) (N=1082) in terms of:

- discontinuation due to lack of efficacy over 6 weeks (end of study)
- use of rescue analgesia over 6 weeks (end of study)
- number of patients with SAEs.

Two RCTs found that there was NS difference between celecoxib 200 mg and placebo (N=1521) (Smugar et al. 2006); (N=1082) in terms of:

- number of patients with drug-related AEs
- number of patients with GI AEs
- number of patients with 1 or more clinical AE.

For the number of withdrawals due to AEs there was no significant difference for etoricoxib 30 mg and placebo (N=599) or celecoxib 200 mg and placebo (N=599) (Bingham et al. 2007); etoricoxib 30 mg and celecoxib 200 mg (NS) (N=599) (Bingham et al. 2007).

One study reported that etoricoxib 30 mg and celecoxib 200 mg were significantly better than placebo for withdrawals due to AEs (N=608) (Bingham et al. 2007) (N=608).

Hip osteoarthritis

Three RCTs focusing on hip osteoarthritis (Hawel 2003, Linden et al. 1996, Sanda et al. 1983) reported on the percentages of GI AEs for COX-2 inhibitors versus non-selective NSAIDs and placebo. Statistical significance testing of differences between treatment groups was not done.

COX-2 inhibitors had higher percentages of GI AEs compared with placebo, but lower percentages compared with non-selective NSAIDs.

Hand osteoarthritis

One RCT (Grifka JK 2004) (N=594) reported percentages of GI AEs for COX-2 inhibitors versus placebo. Statistical significance testing of differences between treatment groups was not done. COX-2 inhibitors had higher percentages of GI AEs compared with placebo.

Knee and hip osteoarthritis

Nine RCTs (Hosie et al. 1996; Hosie 1997; Leung and Malmstrom 2002; Perpignano 1994; Pincus 2004; Rogind 1997; Wiesenhutter and Boice 2005; Yocum 2000; Zacher 2003) reported on the percentages of GI AEs for COX-2 inhibitors versus non-selective NSAIDs and placebo. Statistical significance testing of differences between treatment groups was not done for most studies. COX-2 inhibitors generally had higher percentages of GI AEs compared with placebo, but lower percentages compared with non-selective NSAIDs.

Mixed

Three RCTs (Dequeker 1998; Hawkey 1998; Hawkey and Svoboda 2004) included populations of adults with knee, hip, hand or spinal osteoarthritis, while two other RCTs (Schnitzer et al. 2004, Singh et al. 2006) included populations of adults with knee, hip or hand osteoarthritis. These studies found that generally COX-2 inhibitors were associated with fewer GI AEs than non-selective NSAIDs. In people not taking low-dose aspirin, COX-2 inhibitors were associated with fewer GI AEs than non-selective NSAIDs in one study, but not in another. However, there was no difference between the two drug classes in terms of the incidence of GI AEs for people taking low-dose aspirin.

▷ Cardiovascular adverse events

Knee osteoarthritis

Four RCTs (Curtis et al. 2005; Fleischmann et al. 2006; Lund 1998; Sheldon 2005) focusing on knee osteoarthritis reported percentages of different cardiovascular AEs in the table below. Statistical significance testing of differences between treatment groups was not done. There was no visible trend in the direction of the results across the studies:

Hip osteoarthritis

One RCT focusing on hip osteoarthritis (Hawel 2003) reported on the percentages of cardiovascular complaints for COX-2 inhibitors versus non-selective NSAIDs. Statistical significance testing of differences between treatment groups was not done. COX-2 inhibitors had higher percentages of CV AEs in this study compared with non-selective NSAIDs:

Hand osteoarthritis

One RCT (Grifka 2004) (N=594) reported percentages of cardiovascular AEs for COX-2 inhibitors versus placebo. Statistical significance testing of differences between treatment groups was not done. COX-2 inhibitors had lower percentages of CV AEs in this study compared with placebo:

Knee and hip osteoarthritis

Four RCTs (Leung and Malmstrom 2002, Rogind 1997, Wiesenhutter and Boice 2005, Zacher 2003) reported percentages for CV AEs for COX-2 inhibitors versus non-selective NSAIDs and placebo. Statistical significance testing of differences between treatment groups was not done. COX-2 inhibitors had lower percentages of CV AEs in most of these studies compared with non-selective NSAIDs:

Mixed sites of osteoarthritis

One RCT (Hawkey 1998) included populations of adults with knee, hip, hand or spinal osteoarthritis and reported percentages of cardiac failure events without statistical significance testing. Two other RCTs (Schnitzer et al. 2004, Singh et al. 2006) included populations of adults with knee, hip or hand osteoarthritis. One study (Singh et al. 2006) found NS difference between COX-2 inhibitors and non-selective NSAIDs on the rate of myocardial infarction, but found that non-selective NSAIDs had a higher rate of cardiac failure episodes compared with COX-2 inhibitors. A second study (Schnitzer 2004) with a 52-week treatment and follow-up period found that COX-2 inhibitors and non-selective NSAIDs had similar incidences of cardiovascular AEs in adults with osteoarthritis, regardless of concurrent use or non-use of low dose aspirin.

▷ Renal and hepatic adverse events

Knee osteoarthritis

Four knee osteoarthritis studies reported data on renal AEs. One study (Bensen et al. 1999) found that participants receiving celecoxib had a slightly higher percentage of peripheral edema and hypertension than participants on naproxen or placebo, and had similar percentages of participants with abnormal liver function for each study drug. A second study (McKenna 2001) found that participants receiving diclofenac had significant changes in renal values in comparison with placebo, with celecoxib having lower percentage increases in these values than diclofenac, with most being equivalent to placebo. A third study (Tannenbaum et al. 2004) found that participants receiving celecoxib had slightly higher percentage increases in liver function values than lumiracoxib. The fourth study (Williams et al. 2000) found NS difference between celecoxib and placebo in terms of abnormal renal values.

Knee and hip osteoarthritis

Three studies including participants with knee and/or hip osteoarthritis reported data on renal AEs. One study (Perpignano 1994) reported a significant increase in urea values from baseline in the tenoxicam group, whereas there was NS increase in these levels in the etodolac group. There were NS differences between etodolac and tenoxicam in terms of abnormal changes in any of the other renal values reported. A second study (Rogind 1997) found NS differences between etodolac and piroxicam for renal values reported. The third study (Zacher 2003) found that participants receiving etoricoxib had slightly lower percentages of peripheral edema and hypertension compared with those receiving diclofenac. A lower percentage of participants in the etoricoxib group had abnormal increases in liver values compare to the diclofenac group.

Mixed sites of osteoarthritis

Three studies (Dequeker 1998; Hawkey 1998; Schnitzer et al. 2004) included adults with osteoarthritis in different sites (knee, hip, hand, spine). Two studies (Dequeker 1998; Hawkey 1998) found a significantly lower percentage of abnormalities in a number of renal values for COX-2 inhibitors versus non-selective NSAIDs. The other study (Schnitzer 2004) reported no significant difference between the two drug classes in terms of the percentages of major renal events and serious liver abnormalities found. However, this same study found that significantly more participants taking lumiracoxib had abnormal increases in transaminase levels compared with participants taking NSAIDs.

7.3.4 Evidence statements: co-prescription of a proton pump inhibitor

All evidence statements in section 7.3.4 are level 1++.

▷ Adverse events

One study (Scheiman et al. 2006) reported on two identically designed RCTs (VENUS N=844; PLUTO N=585) that investigated the effect of esomeprazole 20 mg or 40 mg versus placebo in adults with osteoarthritis or RA currently using either COX-2 inhibitors or non-selective NSAIDs over a period of 26 weeks. Outcomes reported included the occurrence of gastric and duodenal ulcers and upper GI AEs. Esomeprazole reduced the occurrence of both types of ulcer and upper GI AEs over a 6-month period in participants receiving either COX-2 inhibitors or non-selective NSAIDs in comparison to users of these anti-inflammatory drugs who received placebo instead of a PPI.

Table 7.56 Incidence of adverse events with PPI				
Study	Ulcer type	Placebo	Esomeprazole 20 mg	Esomeprazole 40 mg
VENUS	Gastric	34/267 (12.7%)	12/267 (4.5%)	10/271 (3.7%)
	Duodenal	10/267 (3.7%)	0/267 (0.0%)	0/271 (0.0%)
	GU + DU	2/267 (0.7%)	0/267 (0.0%)	1/271 (0.4%)
PLUTO	Gastric	19/185 (10.3%)	7/192 (3.6%)	6/196 (3.1%)
	Duodenal	1/185 (0.5%)	1/192 (0.5%)	2/196 (1.0%)
	GU + DU	0/185 (0%)	1/192 (0.5%)	0/196 (0.0%)

▷ Occurrence of GI ulcers in participants receiving NSAIDs or COX-2 inhibitors

In a stratified pooled analysis of the two studies, significantly fewer participants on esomeprazole compared with placebo developed ulcers when taking a non-selective NSAID or a COX-2 inhibitor after 6 months of treatment.

For participants receiving non-selective NSAIDs, 17.1% (95% CI 12.6 to 21.6) of those on placebo developed ulcers compared with 6.8% (95% CI 3.9 to 9.7, p<0.001) of those who received esomeprazole 20 mg and 4.8% (95% CI 2.3 to 7.2, p<0.001) who received esomeprazole 40 mg.

For participants receiving COX-2 inhibitors, 16.5% (95% CI 9.7 to 23.4) of those on placebo developed ulcers over 6 months compared with 0.9% (95% CI 0 to 2.6, p<0.001) of those who received esomeprazole 20 mg and 4.1% (95% CI 0.6 to 7.6, p=0.002) of those who received esomeprazole 40 mg.

Significant reductions in ulcers occurred for COX-2 inhibitor users taking either dose of esomeprazole in each study versus COX-2 inhibitor users taking placebo (p<0.05). For non-selective NSAID users, esomeprazole significantly reduced ulcer occurrence in the VENUS study (p<0.001) but not in the PLUTO study versus NSAIDs users taking placebo.

▷ GI ulcer incidence in low-dose aspirin users

In participants taking concomitant low-dose aspirin, the ulcer incidence at 6 months was similar to that of the whole study population for all treatment groups (placebo: 12.2%, esomeprazole 20 mg: 4.7%, esomeprazole 40 mg: 4.2%).

▷ Serious GI AEs

Overall, there were more serious GI AEs in participants on placebo (12/452 2.7%) than in participants receiving esomeprazole (9/926 1.0%) across the two studies.

7.3.5 Health economic evidence

We looked at studies that focused on economically evaluating nonsteroidal anti-inflammatory drugs (NSAIDs) and COX-2 treatments, GI protective agents, or placebo for the treatment of adults with osteoarthritis. Sixty-one studies (16 through cross-referencing) were identified through the literature search as possible cost-effectiveness analyses in this area. On closer inspection 56 of these studies were excluded for:

- not directly answering the question
- not including sufficient cost data to be considered a true economic analyses
- involving a study population of less than 30 people
- not including cardiovascular adverse events in the analysis.

Five papers were found to be methodologically sound and were included as health economics evidence. However, none of the papers were UK-based and of an acceptable standard to satisfy the GDG as suitable evidence from which to make recommendations. For this reason this area was outlined as important for additional economic modelling. Due to this what follows is simply a brief review of the included studies.

One Canadian study (Maetzel et al. 2003) conducts a detailed cost–utility analysis assessing rofecoxib and celecoxib compared with non-selective NSAIDs. The model involved a Markov model with a decision tree within each health state. Myocardial infarction (MI) was included as a cardiovascular (CV) adverse event, but no other CV adverse events were included. The model had a 5-year duration, but was limited in that once one MI had occurred a patient could not suffer any further CV events. Direct health care costs (in 1999 Canadian $) were calculated and QALYs were estimated using utility values obtained by a standard gamble technique from a survey of 60 randomly selected individuals. The patient population was people with OA or rheumatoid arthritis (RA) who were not prescribed aspirin. The study assumed equal effectiveness of the drugs and only considered differences in adverse events.

The study results were as follows:

- for average-risk patients, the cost per additional QALY of treating patients with rofecoxib rather than naproxen was $455,071
- for average-risk patients, the cost per additional QALY of treating patients with diclofenac rather than ibuprofen was $248,160, and celecoxib was dominated by diclofenac
- for high-risk patients, treatment with rofecoxib dominated treatment with naproxen + PPI; the cost per additional QALY of treating patients with rofecoxib + PPI compared with rofecoxib on its own was $567,820
- for high-risk patients, treatment with celecoxib dominated treatment with ibuprofen + PPI. The cost per additional QALY of treating patients with diclofenac + PPI compared with celecoxib was $518,339. Treating patients with celecoxib + PPI was dominated by treating patients with diclofenac + PPI.

Hence the study concluded that treatment with COX-2 inhibitors is cost effective in high risk patient groups with OA and RA, but not in average risk groups.

A US study considered the cost effectiveness of COX-2 inhibitors compared with non-selective NSAIDs for people with arthritis from the Veterans Health Administration perspective (Schaefer 2005). Two patient groups were considered – those of any age who had a history of perforation, ulcer or bleed (PUB); and those aged 65 years or older, regardless of their PUB history. Both of these groups are regarded as being at 'high risk' of a gastrointestinal (GI) event. CV events included were MI and chronic heart failure (CHF). Costs are in 2001 US$ and QALY weights were obtained from the literature. The time period modelled was one year, but a scenario was also included where the costs for MI were calculated for a 10-year period. The study assumed equal effectiveness of the drugs and only considered differences in adverse events.

The results of the study were as follows:

- the cost per additional QALY for celecoxib compared with non-selective NSAIDs was $28,214 for the PUB history analysis, rofecoxib was dominated by celecoxib and non-selective NSAIDs
- the cost per additional QALY for celecoxib compared with non-selective NSAIDs was $42,036 in the elderly patient analysis, again rofecoxib was dominated by both celecoxib and non-selective NSAIDs
- sensitivity analysis showed that with a threshold cost per QALY value of $50,000, there was an 88% probability that celecoxib would be cost effective in the elderly population, and a 94% probability that it would be cost effective in the PUB history population.

Another US study (Spiegel et al. 2003) conducted a cost-utility analysis comparing COX-2 inhibitors to nonselective NSAIDs. The patient population was 60-year-old patients with OA or RA who were not taking aspirin and who required long-term NSAID therapy for moderate to severe arthritis pain. A lifetime duration was adopted. CV events were included in sensitivity analysis. Patients with a history of ulcer complications were included in sensitivity analysis. A third party payer perspective was adopted for costs (estimated in 2002 US$) and utility values validated by previous investigators were used to allow QALYs to be calculated. The study assumed equal effectiveness of the drugs and only considered differences in adverse events.

The results of the study were as follows:

- the cost per additional QALY of treating patients with a COX-2 inhibitor (celecoxib or rofecoxib) rather than naproxen was $395,324

- the cost per additional QALY of treating patients with a COX-2 inhibitor rather than naproxen assuming a high-risk cohort was $55,803.

A UK study conducted a cost-minimisation analysis based on patients aged 18 or over with acute osteoarthritis of the hip, knee, hand or vertebral spine, taking an NHS perspective (Tavakoli 2003). The treatments considered were meloxicam, diclofenac, and piroxicam, and all resource use associated with GI and non-GI adverse events were included as costs, calculated in 1998 £s. However, the duration of the model was only 4 weeks, giving little time for costs to be accrued.

The results of the study were as follows:

- cost per patient was least for meloxicam (£30), followed by piroxicam (£35) and diclofenac (£51).

An Australian study conducted a cost-utility analysis on a number of different interventions for OA (Segal et al. 2004). One of these analyses involved comparing diclofenac and naproxen with celecoxib. Efficacy was included in the analysis by allocating QALY gains due to pain relief. PUBs and CHF were included as adverse events. Health service costs were considered and are calculated in 2000–2001 Aus$, and QALYs were calculated using the transfer to utility (TTU) technique. The drugs were compared with placebo. The analysis is based on 12 months of treatment. A significant problem with the study is that QALY scores for non-fatal AEs are not incorporated into the modelling, meaning that only fatal AEs are reflected in the results.

The results of the study were as follows:

- the best estimate of cost per additional QALY of treating patients with naproxen rather than placebo (paracetamol) was $7,900 per additional QALY, incorporating a 5% discount rate
- the best estimate of cost per additional QALY of treating patients with diclofenac rather than placebo (paracetamol) was $40,800 per additional QALY, incorporating a 5% discount rate
- the best estimate of cost per additional QALY of treating patients with celecoxib rather than placebo (paracetamol) was $32,930 per additional QALY, incorporating a 5% discount rate
- the study does not directly compare non-selective NSAIDs to COX-2 inhibitors, but the results suggest that net utility gains are similar for the two types of drugs, while non-selective NSAIDs result in lower costs.

7.3.6 Health economic modelling

We conducted a cost-effectiveness analysis, comparing paracetamol, standard NSAIDs and COX-2 inhibitors at doses relevant to clinical practice for which there were robust clinical trial data sufficient to draw reliable conclusions: paracetamol 3000 mg, diclofenac 100 mg, naproxen 750 mg, ibuprofen 1200 mg, celecoxib 200 mg, and etoricoxib 60 mg. We also tested the cost effectiveness of adding omeprazole, a proton pump inhibitor, to each of these NSAIDs/COX-2 inhibitors. It should be noted that we did not consider the cost-effectiveness of other NSAIDs, meloxicam or etodolac, due to a lack of suitable data.

The analysis was based on an assumption that the NSAIDs and COX-2 inhibitors are equally effective at controlling OA symptoms, but that they differ in terms of GI and CV risks. The adverse event risks were taken from three key studies: MEDAL, CLASS and TARGET. As the doses of both standard NSAIDs and COX-2 inhibitors were very high in these trials, we adjusted the observed rates to estimate the impact of more commonly-used and licensed doses. The effectiveness of NSAIDs/COX-2 inhibitors and paracetamol at controlling OA symptoms was estimated from a meta-analysis of RCTs. Given these assumptions, lower doses of a drug will always be more cost effective than a higher dose of the same drug. In practice, though, some individuals may require higher doses than we have assumed in order to achieve an adequate therapeutic response.

One clear result of our analysis is that it is cost effective to add a generic PPI to standard NSAIDs and COX-2 inhibitors. We did not test the relative cost effectiveness of other gastroprotective agents, because of the superior effectiveness evidence for PPIs, and the currently very low cost of omeprazole at this dose.

Given our assumptions and current drug costs, celecoxib 200 mg is the most cost effective of the included NSAIDs/COX-2 inhibitors. This result was not sensitive to the assumed duration of treatment (from 3 months to 2 years), or to the baseline risk of GI events in the population (55 years vs 65 years). It was also relatively insensitive to the baseline risk of CV events. In patients who cannot tolerate celecoxib, etoricoxib 30 mg would be a cost-effective alternative. The relative cost effectiveness of these two options in this context depends primarily on their cost.

However, it is important to note substantial uncertainties over the relative rates of adverse events associated with the COX-2 inhibitors estimated from the MEDAL, TARGET and CLASS studies. In particular, the estimated risk of stroke for celecoxib from CLASS was surprisingly low. If this is an underestimate, then etoricoxib 30 mg could be more cost effective than celecoxib 200 mg. The full data submitted to the American Food and Drug Administration were used for the economic model.

Observational data imply a less attractive cost–effectiveness ratio for celecoxib (around £30,000 per QALY), though this estimate may be biased by its use in selected higher-risk patients in clinical practice. There were no observational data for the other COX-2 inhibitors.

For patients who cannot, or do not wish to, take a COX-2 inhibitor, the relative cost effectiveness of paracetamol and standard NSAIDs depends on their individual risk profile, as well as the dose required to achieve an adequate therapeutic response:

- with low GI and CV risk (patients aged under 65 with no risk factors), standard NSAIDs with a PPI do appear to be relatively cost effective in comparison with paracetamol or no intervention
- for patients with raised GI or CV risk (aged over 65 or with risk factors), standard NSAIDs are not a cost-effective alternative to paracetamol; in our model, the risks of these treatments outweighed the benefits of improved control of OA symptoms, as well as incurring additional costs for the health service.

The model provides cost-effectiveness estimates at a population level, including for NSAIDs in people with increased GI risk. Clearly, for many of these people NSAIDs will be contra-indicated and thus the average cost effectiveness in those who remain eligible will be better than the estimate given here. The relative cost effectiveness of particular NSAIDs and COX-2 inhibitors will vary depending on individual patients' GI and CV risk factors.

The model assesses which of the drugs is most suitable as the first choice for treatment. In instances where the drug is not tolerated or gives inadequate relief, and a different drug from this class is sought as the second choice, treatment needs to be carefully tailored to the individual and it is not possible to provide useful recommendations in a national clinical guideline for this.

The relative costs of the standard NSAIDs employed in this model (diclofenac 100 mg, naproxen 750 mg and ibuprofen 1200 mg) prescribed concurrently with a PPI are similar, and uncertainties over the relative incidence of adverse events with these drugs make it difficult to draw clear conclusions about their comparative cost effectiveness.

The doses and costs considered in the model are shown in Appendix D, available online at www.rcplondon.ac.uk/pubs/brochure.aspx?e=242. Because the incremental cost effectiveness ratios are affected by dose and individual risk factors, the Guideline Development Group felt it would be unwise to single out specific drugs and doses within these classes, except for etoricoxib 60 mg, which was consistently dominated (more expensive and has overall lower gain in QALYs than comparator drugs) in the model results. Readers should be alert to changes in available drug doses and costs after this guideline is published.

7.3.7 From evidence to recommendations

A large amount of clinical trial evidence supports the efficacy of both traditional NSAIDs and COX-2 selective agents in reducing the pain and stiffness of osteoarthritis with the majority of studies reflecting short-term usage and involving knee or hip joint osteoarthritis. There is no strong evidence to suggest a consistent benefit over paracetamol, although some patients may obtain greater symptom relief from NSAIDs. There are again no data to suggest benefits above opioids, but there is a lack of well-designed comparator studies.

All NSAIDs, irrespective of COX-1 and COX-2 selectivity are associated with significant morbidity and mortality due to adverse effects on the GI, renal and cardiovascular system. It should be noted again that clinical trials recruit patients without the serious comorbidities that would be present in routine clinical practice and that supra-normal doses of newer agents are commonly used in clinical trials in order to demonstrate safety.

▷ GI toxicity

There are some data to support that certain COX-2 selective agents reduce the incidence of serious GI adverse events (such as perforations, ulcers and bleeds) when compared with less selective agents, while the evidence for other agents has been more controversial. Dyspepsia, one of the most common reasons for discontinuation, remains a problem with all NSAIDs irrespective of COX-2 selectivity.

▷ Liver toxicity

At the time of writing, lumiracoxib has been withdrawn from the UK market, following concerns about liver toxicity associated with high doses. The model therefore represents the current situation regarding liver toxicity. The GDG were mindful that further safety data will emerge in the lifetime of this guideline; prescribers should be aware of the Summaries of Product Characteristics.

▷ Cardiovascular toxicity

All NSAIDs have the propensity to cause fluid retention and to aggravate hypertension, although for certain agents this effect appears to be larger (etoricoxib). Increasingly a pro-thrombotic risk (including myocardial infarction and stroke) has been identified with COX-2 selective agents in long-term studies, and there does seem to be some evidence for a dose effect. These observational studies also demonstrate an increased cardiovascular risk from older agents such as diclofenac, which has high COX-2 selectivity. It is possible that naproxen does not increase pro-thrombotic risk. All NSAIDs may antagonise the cardio-protective effects of aspirin.

▷ Summary

All potential adverse effects must be put in perspective of patient need and individual risk, including the influence of the patient's age on their GI risk. Best estimates of toxicity data, along with the uncertainty in these values, are detailed in Appendix D, available online at www.rcplondon.ac.uk/pubs/brochure.aspx?e=242. The recommendations mention assessment and monitoring of risk factors, but are unable to specify these because of the rapidly emerging evidence base in this area. Prescribers will be informed by the regularly updated Summaries of Product Characteristics.

There is likely to be a continuing role for NSAIDs/COX-2 inhibitors in the management of some patients with OA. Allowing for the inevitable differences in individual patient response, in general the choice between NSAIDs and COX-2 inhibitors is influenced by their separate side-effect profiles, which tend to favour COX-2 inhibitors, and cost, which tends to favour NSAIDs. Extensive sensitivity analyses showed that these are the two factors which most strongly influence the results of the economic model.

Given that costs are constantly changing and that new data on adverse events will become available, the GDG deemed it unwise to suggest a particular ranking of individual drugs. Indeed, there is no clear distinction between the two sub-classes. Meloxicam and etodolac were not included in the model because of a lack of comparable trial data, and other NSAIDs were excluded because of the rarity of use in the UK, according to the Prescription Pricing Authority (see Appendix D for details, available online at www.rcplondon.ac.uk/pubs/brochure. aspx?e=242). It is beyond the role of a clinical guideline to attempt to categorise meloxicam or etodolac into one of the two sub-classes. However, it is worth noting that each of the drugs in this section varies in its COX-1/COX-2 selectivity.

There was a consistent difference between etoricoxib 60 mg and the other drugs in the model, and therefore in line with the original aim of the economic model, advice is given against the use of etoricoxib 60 mg as the first choice for treatment.

The GDG also noted that the incidence of potentially serious upper GI problems can be reduced by the use of PPIs, and the potential benefit of coprescription of PPIs was an important element of the cost-effectiveness analysis. In fact, the analysis found that it was always more cost effective to coprescribe a PPI than not to do so. The primary paper discussed was the Scheiman paper (Scheiman 2006). The Lai paper was excluded as it was an open-label trial and the Chan paper (Chan 2007) had several limitations: i) a population following hospitalisation for upper GI bleeding (which was not what we were looking at for the model); and ii) it had a zero event rate in the PPI arm of the trial. This meant that we were unable to calculate a relative risk, which is required for the model. Hence the Chan paper corroborates the effectiveness of adding a PPI to a COX-2, but has not been used for the sensitivity analysis. The GDG have attempted to balance all these factors in the following recommendations.

Although NSAIDs and COX-2 inhibitors may be regarded as a single drug class of NSAIDs, these recommendations continue to use the two terms for clarity, and because of the differences in side-effect profile. The recommendations in this section are derived from extensive health economic modelling, which included December 2007 NHS drug tariff costs. This guideline replaces the osteoarthritis aspects only of NICE technology appraisal guidance 27 (National Institute for Health and Clinical Excellence 2001). The guideline recommendations are based on up-to-date evidence on efficacy and adverse events, current costs and an expanded health-economic analysis of cost effectiveness. This has led to an increased role for COX-2 inhibitors, an increased awareness of all potential adverse events (gastrointestinal, liver and cardio-renal) and a recommendation to coprescribe a proton pump inhibitor (PPI).

RECOMMENDATIONS

R25   Where paracetamol or topical NSAIDs are ineffective for pain relief for people with osteoarthritis, then substitution with an oral NSAID/COX-2 inhibitor should be considered.

R26   Where paracetamol or topical NSAIDs provide insufficient pain relief for people with osteoarthritis, then the addition of an oral NSAID/COX-2 inhibitor to paracetamol should be considered.

R27   Oral NSAIDs/COX-2 inhibitors should be used at the lowest effective dose for the shortest possible period of time.

R28   When offering treatment with an oral NSAID/COX-2 inhibitor, the first choice should be either a standard NSAID or a COX-2 inhibitor (other than etoricoxib 60 mg). In either case, these should be coprescribed with a proton pump inhibitor (PPI), choosing the one with the lowest acquisition cost.

R29   All oral NSAIDs/COX-2 inhibitors have analgesic effects of a similar magnitude but vary in their potential GI, liver and cardio-renal toxicity and therefore when choosing the agent and dose, healthcare professionals should take into account individual patient risk factors, including age. When prescribing these drugs, consideration should be given to appropriate assessment and/or ongoing monitoring of these risk factors.

R30   If a person with osteoarthritis needs to take low dose aspirin, healthcare professionals should consider other analgesics before substituting or adding an NSAID or COX-2 inhibitor (with a PPI) if pain relief is ineffective or insufficient.

7.4 Intra-articular injections

7.4.1 Clinical introduction

This section of the guideline is concerned with those therapies that require use of an intra-articular injection, including corticosteroid and hyaluronan injections. It should be noted that all such therapies should be delivered by appropriately trained individuals, and that even experienced clinicians can miss intra-articular placement of such injections, especially in small joints.

▷ Corticosteroids

Corticosteroid injections are used to deliver high doses of synthetic corticosteroids to a specific joint, while minimising systemic side effects. Corticosteroids have marked anti-inflammatory effects, and it is assumed that their analgesic action in osteoarthritis is in some way related to their anti-inflammatory properties. Certainly intra-articular corticosteroids can reduce the volume of synovitis of osteoarthritis (Ostergaard et al. 1996). However, the relationship between osteoarthritis synovitis and pain is less clear. It is recognised that clinical examination is not sensitive in detecting inflammation (synovial hypertrophy or effusions) when compared with imaging methods such as ultrasonography or MRI (D'Agostino et al. 2005), so clinical prediction of response to a corticosteroid injection is unreliable. The presence of an effusion is not in itself an indication for corticosteroid injection, unless there is significant restriction of function associated with the swelling. Rather, the indication should be based on severity of pain and disability.

▷ Hyaluronans

Endogenous hyaluronan (HA, previously known as hyaluronic acid) is a large, linear glycosamino-glycan and is a major non-structural component of both the synovial and cartilage extracellular matrix. It is also found in synovial fluid and is produced by the lining layer cells of the joint. Hyaluronan is removed from the joint via the lymphatic circulation and degraded by hepatic endothelial cells. Its key functions in the joint are to confer viscoelasticity, lubrication and help maintain tissue hydration and protein homeostasis by preventing large fluid movements and by acting as an osmotic buffer.

Synthetic HA was isolated from roosters' comb and umbilical cord tissue and developed for clinical use in ophthalmic surgery and arthritis in the 1960s. The beneficial effects in ophthalmic surgery were followed by the use of HA in osteoarthritis: the rationale was to replace the properties lost by reduced HA production and quality as occurs in osteoarthritis joints, a concept known as viscosupplementation. Commercial preparations of HA have the same structure as endogenous HA although cross-linked HA molecules (known as hylans) were later engineered by linking HA molecules in order to obtain greater elasto-viscosity and intra-articular dwell-time.

However, the mechanism by which HA exerts its therapeutic effect, if any, is not certain, and evidence for restoration of rheological properties is lacking. Given the relatively short intra-articular residency (hours), any hypothesis for its mechanism of action must account for the sometime reported long-duration of clinical efficacy (months).

7.4.2 Methodological introduction: corticosteroids

We looked for studies that investigated the efficacy and safety of intra-articular injection of corticosteroid compared with placebo with respect to symptoms, function and quality of life in adults with osteoarthritis. One Cochrane systematic review and meta-analysis on knee osteoarthritis patients (Bellamy et al. 2006) and three additional RCTs on osteoarthritis of the hip (Flanagan et al. 1988; Qvistgaard et al. 2006) or thumb (Meenagh et al. 2004) were found. No relevant cohort or case-control studies were found.

The meta-analysis assessed the RCTs for quality and pooled together all data for the outcomes of symptoms, function and AEs. However, the outcome of quality of life was not reported. The results for quality of life have therefore been taken from the individual RCTs included in the systematic review.

The meta-analysis included 12 RCTs (with N=653 participants) with comparisons between intra-articular corticosteroids and intra-articular placebo injections in patients with knee osteoarthritis. Studies included in the analysis differed with respect to:

- type of corticosteroid used (one RCT prednisolone acetate; four RCTs triamcinolone hexacetonide; one RCT methylprednisolone; three RCTs hydrocortisone solution; two RCTs triamcinolone acetonide; one RCT cortivazol; one RCT methylprednisolone acetate)
- treatment regimens
- trial design, size and length.

Tests for heterogeneity were performed for any pooled results, but no evidence of heterogeneity was found between studies that were combined. Unless otherwise stated, all evidence statements are derived from data presented in the systematic review and meta-analysis.

The three additional RCTs focused on the outcomes of symptoms, function and quality of life. The three included RCTs were similar in terms of osteoarthritis diagnosis (radiologically). However, they differed with respect to osteoarthritis site, corticosteroid agent, and sample size.

7.4.3 Methodological introduction: hyaluronans

We looked for studies that investigated the efficacy and safety of intra-articular injection of hyaluronic acid/hyaluronans compared with placebo or steroid injection with respect to symptoms, function and quality of life in adults with osteoarthritis. One Cochrane systematic review and meta-analysis on knee osteoarthritis patients (Bellamy et al. 2006) and four additional RCTs on hip/knee/other osteoarthritis sites (Fuchs et al. 2006; Petrella et al. 2006; Qvistgaard et al. 2006; Stahl 2005) were found. No relevant cohort or case-control studies were found.

The meta-analysis assessed the RCTs for quality and pooled all data for the outcomes of symptoms, function and AEs. However, the outcome of quality of life was not reported. The results for quality of life have therefore been taken from the individual RCTs included in the systematic review.

The meta-analysis included 40 RCTs (with N=5257 participants) on comparisons between intra-articular hyaluronic acid/hyaluronans and intra-articular placebo injections in patients with knee osteoarthritis. Studies included in the analysis differed with respect to:

- type of HA used (seven RCTs Artz; one RCT BioHy; one RCT Durolane; 14 RCTs Hyalgan; nine RCTs Synvisc; one RCT Suvenyl; five RCTs Orthovisc; one RCT Replasyn; one RCT Suplasyn)
- treatment regimens
- trial design, size and length
- mode of HA production (includes bacterial and animal sources).

Additionally, the meta-analysis included nine RCTs (with N=755 participants) on comparisons between intra-articular hyaluronic acid/hyaluronans and intra-articular corticosteroid injections. Studies included in the analysis differed with respect to:

- type of HA used (five RCTs Hyalgan; two RCTs Synvisc; two RCTs Orthovisc)
- type of corticosteroid used (five RCTs methylprednisolone acetate; two RCTs triamcinolone hexacetonide; one RCT betamethasone; one RCT betamethasone sodium phosphate-betamethasone acetate)
- treatment regimens
- trial size and length
- mode of HA production (includes bacterial and animal sources).

Results in the Cochrane meta-analysis were presented by product and also pooled by drug-class. This was because products differed in their molecular weight, concentration, treatment schedule and mode of production, and therefore the results for the individual products, rather than pooled class data, are presented here. The chi-squared test for heterogeneity was performed on any pooled results, and evidence of significant heterogeneity ($p<0.10$) was found between pooled studies for many of the outcomes.

Unless otherwise stated, all evidence statements are derived from data presented in the systematic review and meta-analysis.

- The four additional RCTs focused on the outcomes of symptoms, function and quality of life. However, one of these (Stahl et al. 2005) was excluded as evidence due to multiple methodological limitations. The trials were similar in terms of osteoarthritis diagnosis (radiologically).
- However, they differed with respect to osteoarthritis site, study intervention, sample size and study duration. One RCT (Qvistgaard et al. 2006) had a 3-week treatment phase and a follow-up at 3 months; the second RCT (Petrella and Petrella 2006) had a 2-month treatment phase and a follow-up at 12 weeks, and the third RCT (Fuchs et al. 2006) had a 3-week treatment phase and a follow-up at 26 weeks.

7.4.4 Evidence statements: Intra-articular (IA) corticosteroids vs placebo

▷ Knee

Overall, the evidence appraised by the Cochrane review suggests a short-term benefit (up to 1 week) in terms of pain reduction and patient global assessment after IA injections with corticosteroids in the knee. Beyond this period of time there were non-significant differences between IA corticosteroids and IA placebo as reported by most of the studies identified.

There was evidence of pain reduction between two weeks to three weeks but a lack of evidence for efficacy in functional improvement.

No significant differences between corticosteroids and placebo were reported at any time point by studies evaluating the following outcomes in patients with knee OA:

- functional improvement (eg walking distance, range of motion)
- stiffness
- quality of life
- safety
- study withdrawals.

▷ Hip and thumb

No conclusive results were observed in studies evaluating IA injections of corticosteroids and placebo in other joints affected by OA (that is, hip and thumb).

Table 7.57 Pain in knee OA

Knee

Pain outcome	Reference	Intervention	Assessment time	Outcome/effect size
Number of knees improved (pain)	MA (Bellamy et al. 2006a), 1 RCT (N=71)	Hydrocortisone tertiary-butylacetate vs placebo	2 weeks post-injection	RR 1.81, 95%CI 1.09 to 3.00, p=0.02, NNT=3) Favours CS
30% decrease in VAS pain from baseline	MA (Bellamy et al. 2006a), 1 RCT (N=53)	Cortivazol vs placebo vs placebo	1 week post-injection	RR 2.56, 95%CI 1.26 to 5.18, p=0.009 Favours CS
15% decrease in VAS pain from baseline	MA (Bellamy et al. 2006a), 1 RCT (N=118)	Methylprednisolone vs placebo	3 weeks post-injection	RR 3.11, 95%CI 1.61 to 6.01, p=0.0007 Favours CS
Pain (VAS)	MA (Bellamy et al. 2006a), 3 RCTs (N=161)	Cortivazol vs placebo	1 week post-injection	WMD −21.91, 95%CI −29.93 to −13.89, p<0.00001 Favours CS
Pain (VAS)	MA (Bellamy et al. 2006a), 1 RCT (N=53)	Cortivazol vs placebo	12 weeks post-injection	WMD −14.20, 95%CI −27.44 to −0.96, p=0.04 Favours CS
WOMAC pain	MA (Bellamy et al. 2006a), 1 RCT (N=66)	Triamcinolone acetonide vs placebo	1 year post-injection	WMD −13.80, 95% CI −26.79 to −0.81; p=0.04 Favours CS

Knee

Global assessment	Reference	Intervention	Assessment time	Outcome/effect size
Patients global assessment (number of patients preferring treatment)	MA (Bellamy et al. 2006a), 3 RCTs (N=190)	CS vs placebo	Range: 1 to 104 weeks	RR 2.22, 95%CI 1.57 to 3.15, p<0.00001 Favours CS
Overall improvement	MA (Bellamy et al. 2006a), 3 RCTs (N=156)	CS vs placebo	Range: 1 to 104 weeks	RR 1.44, 95%CI 1.13 to 1.82; p=0.003 Favours CS

Table 7.58 Pain in hip and thumb OA

Hip

Pain outcome	Reference	Intervention	Assessment time	Outcome/effect size
Percentage of patients with improved pain relief	1 RCT (Flanagan et al. 1988) (N=30)	Bupivacaine + triamcinolone vs placebo.	1 month post-injection	Improvement: 75% (CS) and 64% (placebo)
Percentage of patients whose pain relief was unchanged	1 RCT (Flanagan et al. 1988) (N=30)	Bupivacaine + triamcinolone vs placebo.	1 and 3 months post-injection	1 month: 8% (CS) and 27% (placebo) 3 months: 17% (CS) and 36% (placebo)
Percentage of patients whose pain had worsened	1 RCT (Flanagan et al. 1988) (N=30)	Bupivacaine + triamcinolone vs placebo.	1 and 3 months post-injection	1 month: 17% (CS) and 9% (placebo) 3 months: 50% (CS) and 8.5% (placebo)
Percentage of patients with improved pain relief at follow-up	1 RCT (Flanagan et al. 1988) (N=30)	Bupivacaine + triamcinolone vs placebo.	3 months and 12 months post-injection	3 months: 33% (CS) and 55% (placebo) 12 months: 8% (CS) and 18% (placebo)
Pain on walking	1 RCT (Qvistgaard et al. 2006) (N=104)	Methylprednisolone vs placebo	14 and 28 days and over the 3-month treatment period	Over 3 months: SMD steroid = 0.6, 95% CI 0.1 to 1.1, p=0.021 14 and 28 days: both p=0.006 Favours CS

Table 7.59 Pain in thumb OA

Thumb (CMC)

Pain outcome	Reference	Intervention	Assessment time	Outcome/effect size
Pain (VAS, mm) change from baseline	1 RCT (Meenagh et al. 2004) (N=40)	Triamcinolone vs placebo	12 weeks and 24 weeks post-injection	12 weeks: 3.5 (CS) and 23.3 (placebo) 24 weeks: 0.0 (CS) and 14.0 (placebo)
Joint tenderness (scale 0–3) change from baseline	1 RCT (Meenagh et al. 2004) (N=40)	Triamcinolone vs placebo	12 weeks and 24 weeks post-injection	12 weeks: 0.5 (CS) and 2.0 (placebo) 24 weeks: 0.5 (CS) 2.5 (placebo)

Table 7.60 Function in hip OA

Hip

Function outcome	Reference	Intervention	Assessment time	Outcome/effect size
OARSI outcome measures	1 RCT (Qvistgaard et al. 2006) (N=104)	Methylprednisolone vs placebo	Day 14 and day 28 (end of treatment)	Day 14: 56% (CS) and 33% (placebo) Day 28: 66% (CS) and 44% (placebo)

Table 7.61 Global assessment in hip OA

Hip

Global assessment outcome	Reference	Intervention	Assessment time	Outcome/effect size
Patient's global assessment	1 RCT (Qvistgaard et al. 2006) (N=104)	Methylprednisolone vs placebo	14 days 28 days and 3 months (end of study)	NS

Table 7.62 Global assessment in thumb OA

Thumb (CMC)

Global assessment outcome	Reference	Intervention	Assessment time	Outcome/effect size
Physician's global assessment	1 RCT (Meenagh et al. 2004) (N=40)	Triamcinolone vs placebo	12 weeks and 24 weeks post-injection	12 weeks: 0.5 (CS) and 2.3 (placebo) 24 weeks: 1.5 (CS) and 5.0 (placebo)
Patient's global assessment	1 RCT (Meenagh et al. 2004) (N=40)	Triamcinolone vs placebo	12 weeks and 24 weeks post-injection	12 weeks: 0.0 (CS) and 2.3 (placebo) 24 weeks: 1.0 (CS) and 5.0 (placebo)

Table 7.63 Adverse events in hip OA

Hip

Adverse events outcome	Reference	Intervention	Assessment time	Outcome/effect size
SAEs or infection	1 RCT (Qvistgaard et al. 2006) (N=104)	Methylprednisolone vs placebo	Over 3 months study	None for either group

Table 7.64 Withdrawals in thumb OA

Thumb (CMC)

Total withdrawals	Reference	Intervention	Assessment time	Outcome/effect size
Number of withdrawals	1 RCT (Meenagh et al. 2004) (N=40)	Triamcinolone vs placebo	Over 24 weeks study	Both N=3

7.4.5 Evidence statements: Intra-articular (IA) hyaluronans vs placebo

▷ Knee

Overall, the evidence suggests that hyaluronans and hylan derivatives seem to be superior to placebo in terms of efficacy* and quality of life outcomes in patients with OA in the knee at different post-injection periods but especially at the 5- to 13-week post injection period.

No major safety issues were identified relating to these agents when compared with placebo but a definitive conclusion is precluded due to sample-size restrictions.

It should be noted that alongside the by drug class (pooled) results, outcomes are presented by therapeutic agent due to the differential efficacy effects for different products on different variables at different timepoints** found by the Cochrane review (Bellamy 2006).

▷ Hip

No significant differences between hyaluronans and placebo were reported at any time point by the RCT (Qvistgaard 2006) evaluating efficacy and function outcomes in patients with hip OA.

Table 7.65 Pain in knee OA

Knee

Pain outcome	Reference	Intervention	Assessment time	Outcome/effect size
HA (general)				
WOMAC knee pain score (mean change from baseline)	One RCT (Petrella and Petrella 2006) (N=106)	HA vs placebo	End of treatment (3 weeks).	8.0 (HA) 2.8 (placebo); p<0.02 Favours HA
WOMAC knee pain score, pain walking (VAS) and pain stepping (VAS) at 6–12 weeks	One RCT (Petrella and Petrella 2006) (N=106)	HA vs placebo	6 and 12-weeks (ie 3 and 9-weeks post-injection)	NS
HA Artz				
Pain (VAS)	1 MA (Bellamy et al. 2006) 1–4 weeks, 5–13 weeks (3 RCTs, N=507) and 14–26 weeks post-injection (2 RCTs, N=312)	HA Artz vs placebo	1–4 weeks, 5–13 weeks and 14–26 weeks post-injection	NS
HA Durolane				
WOMAC pain (change from baseline, 0–20 Likert)	1 MA (Bellamy et al. 2006) 1 RCT, N=346	HA durolane vs placebo	Week 2	WMD 0.74, 95% CI 0.02 to 1.46, p=0.04 Favours placebo

continued

* Efficacy was assessed in terms of pain relief, function improvement and patient global assessment.
** There was a high variability observed across the agents evaluated (different molecular weight, concentration, treatment schedules, and mode of production) and the heterogeneity of the RCTs included.

Table 7.65 Pain in knee OA – *continued*

Knee

Pain outcome	Reference	Intervention	Assessment time	Outcome/effect size
HA Durolane – *continued*				
WOMAC pain (change from baseline, 0–20 Likert)	1 MA (Bellamy et al. 2006b) 1 RCT, N=346	HA durolane vs placebo	Weeks 6, 13 and 26	NS
HA Hyalgan				
Pain on weight bearing during walking (VAS)	1 MA (Bellamy et al. 2006b) 4 RCTs, N=878	Hyalgan vs placebo	14–26 weeks post-injection	WMD –4.57, 95% CI –8.72 to –0.42, p=0.03 Favours HA
Pain spontaneous (VAS)	1 MA (Bellamy et al. 2006b) 1–4 weeks: 2 RCTs, N=73 5–13 weeks: 2 RCTs, N=73	Hyalgan vs placebo	1–4 weeks and 5–13 weeks post-injection	1–4 weeks: WMD –23.88, 95% CI –33.50 to –14.25, p<0.00001 5–13 weeks: WMD –21.03, 95% CI –30.26 to –11.80, p<0.00001 Favours HA
Pain at rest (VAS)	1 MA (Bellamy et al. 2006b) 5 RCTs, N=155	Hyalgan vs placebo	5–13 weeks post-injection	WMD –9.65, 95% CI –14.18 to –5.13, p=0.00003) Favours HA
WOMAC pain (VAS)	1 MA (Bellamy et al. 2006b) 1 RCT, N=177	Hyalgan vs placebo	14–26 weeks post-injection	WMD –5.66, 95% CI –10.06 to –1.26, p=0.01 Favours HA
Number of joints improved for pain under load at end of treatment	1 MA (Bellamy et al. 2006b) end of treatment: 1 RCT, N=37; 1 week post-injection: 1 RCT, N=38; and 5–13 weeks post-injection: 1 RCT, N=37	Hyalgan vs placebo	End of treatment 1 week and 5–13 weeks post-injection	End of treatment: RR 2.68, 95% CI 1.37 to 5.25, p=0.004 1 week post-injection: RR 3.60, 95% CI 1.48 to 8.78, p=0.005 5–13 weeks post-injection: RR 4.03, 95% CI 1.67 to 9.69, p=0.002 Favours HA
Number of joints with improvement in pain on touch	1 MA (Bellamy et al. 2006b) 1 RCT, N=38	Hyalgan vs placebo	Not mentioned	RR 2.25, 95% CI 1.12 to 4.53, p=0.02 Favours HA
Pain (number of patients improved)	1 MA (Bellamy et al. 2006b) 1 RCT, N=408	Hyalgan vs placebo	32 weeks post-injection	RR 1.36, 95% CI 1.06 to 1.75, p=0.02 Favours HA

continued

| Table 7.65 Pain in knee OA – *continued* | | | | |

Knee

Pain outcome	Reference	Intervention	Assessment time	Outcome/effect size
HA Hyalgan – *continued*				
Number of joints improved for walking pain	1 MA (Bellamy et al. 2006b) end of treatment: 1 RCT, N=37, 5–13 weeks post-injection: 1 RCT, N=38, 5–13 weeks post-injection 1 RCT, N=37	Hyalgan vs placebo	At end of treatment 1 week post-injection, 5–13 weeks post-injection	End of treatment: RR 1.68, 95% CI 1.02 to 2.78, p=0.04 5–13 weeks post-injection: RR 3.60, 95% CI 1.48 to 8.78, p=0.005 5–13 weeks post-injection (1 RCT, N=37; RR 2.30, 95% CI 1.26 to 4.19, p=0.006 Favours HA
Pain (VAS)	1 MA (Bellamy et al. 2006b)	Hyalgan vs placebo	45–52 weeks post-injection	NS
WOMAC pain (VAS), number of knee joints without rest pain, number of knee joints without night pain, number of patients with moderate/ marked pain, pain (number of patients improved), number of patients with none/ slight/mild pain	1 MA (Bellamy et al. 2006b), 1 RCT, N=177	Hyalgan vs placebo	1–4 weeks and 5–13 weeks post-injection	NS
HA Hylan G-F20				
Pain on walking (VAS)	1 MA (Bellamy et al. 2006b) 1 RCT, N=30	Hylan G-F20 vs placebo	5–13 weeks post-injection	WMD –13.80, 95% CI –19.74 to –7.86, p<0.00001 Favours HA
WOMAC pain	1 MA (Bellamy et al. 2006b) 1–4 weeks: 2 RCTs, N=60 14–26 weeks: 1 RCT, N=30	Hylan G-F20 vs placebo	1–4 weeks and 14–26 weeks post-injection	1–4 weeks: SMD –1.26, 95% CI –1.86 to –0.66, p=0.00004 14-26 weeks: SMD –1.09, 95% CI –1.92 to –0.25, p=0.01 Favours HA
Pain at night at 1–4 weeks	1 MA (Bellamy et al. 2006b) 1–4 weeks: 6 RCTs, N=391; 14–26 weeks: 3 RCTs, N=182	Hylan G-F20 vs placebo	1–4 weeks and 14–26 weeks post-injection	1–4 weeks: WMD –8.03, 95% CI –11.95 to –4.12, p=0.00006 14–26 weeks: WMD –17.12, 95% CI –23.22 to –11.02, p=0.00001 Favours HA

continued

Table 7.65 Pain in knee OA – *continued*

Knee

Pain outcome	Reference	Intervention	Assessment time	Outcome/effect size
HA Hylan G-F20 – *continued*				
Pain at rest (VAS)	1 MA (Bellamy et al. 2006b) 1–4 weeks: 2 RCTs, N=124, 5–13 weeks: 1 RCT, N=30	Hylan G-F20 vs placebo	1–4 weeks and 5–13 weeks post–injection	1–4 weeks: 2 RCTs, N=124; WMD –9.44, 95% CI –14.07 to –4.82, p=0.00006) 5–13 weeks: 1 RCT, N=30; WMD –18.67, 95% CI –23.32 to –14.02, p<0.00001 Favours HA
Pain overall (VAS) and pain on walking (VAS)	1 MA (Bellamy et al. 2006b)	Hylan G-F20 vs placebo	1–4 weeks post–injection	NS
HA Suvenyl				
Pain (VAS) change from baseline and percentage of painful days (VAS) change from baseline	1 MA (Bellamy et al. 2006b) 1 RCT, N=174	HA Suvenyl vs placebo	45–52 weeks post–injection	NS
HA Orthovisc				
WOMAC pain (5–25 Likert)	1 MA (Bellamy et al. 2006b) 5–13 weeks: 2 RCTs, N=69 45–52 weeks: 1 RCT, N=40	HA Orthovisc vs placebo	5–13 weeks and 45–52 weeks post–injection	5–13 weeks: WMD –5.40, 95% CI –6.92 to –3.89, p<0.00001 45–52 weeks: WMD –5.30, 95% CI –7.02 to –3.58, p<0.00001 Favours HA
Number of patients with a 40% improvement from baseline in WOMAC pain score	1 MA (Bellamy et al. 2006b) 2 RCTs, N=394	HA Orthovisc vs placebo	5–13 weeks post-injection.	RR 1.30, 95% CI 1.08 to 1.57, p=0.006
WOMAC pain (several variables)	1 MA (Bellamy et al. 2006b)	HA Orthovisc vs placebo	5–26 weeks	NS
HA Suplasyn				
Pain at rest (VAS)	1 MA (Bellamy et al. 2006b) 1 RCT, N=53	HA Suplasyn vs placebo	1 week post-injection	WMD 0.83, 95% CI 0.03 to 1.63, p=0.04 Favours placebo
Pain after walking, VAS and WOMAC pain, VAS	1 MA (Bellamy et al. 2006b) 1 RCT, N=53	HA Suplasyn vs placebo	1 week post-injection	NS

Table 7.66 Stiffness in knee OA

Knee

Stiffness	Reference	Intervention	Assessment time	Outcome/effect size
HA (general)				
WOMAC stiffness	1 RCT (Petrella and Petrella 2006) (N=106)	HA vs placebo	End of treatment (3 weeks)	Mean change from baseline −1.9 and −2.0 respectively, p<0.05 Favours HA
WOMAC stiffness	1 RCT (Petrella and Petrella 2006) (N=106)	HA vs placebo	6 and 12 weeks (ie 3 and 9-weeks post-injection)	NS
HA Artz				
WOMAC stiffness (0–8 Likert)	1 MA (Bellamy et al. 2006b) 1 RCT, N=123	HA Artz vs placebo	5–13 weeks post-injection	NS
HA Durolane				
WOMAC stiffness (change from baseline, 0–20 Likert)	1 MA (Bellamy et al. 2006b) 1 RCT, N=346	HA durolane vs placebo	Week 2	WMD 0.51, 95% CI 0.16 to 0.86, p=0.005 Favours placebo
WOMAC stiffness (change from baseline, 0–8 Likert)	1 MA (Bellamy et al. 2006b) 1 RCT, N=346	HA durolane vs placebo	Weeks 6, 13 and 26	NS
HA Hylan G-F20				
WOMAC stiffness (2–10 Likert)	1 MA (Bellamy et al. 2006b) 1–4 weeks: 2 RCTs, N=60 5–13 weeks: 2 RCTs, N=60 4–26 weeks post-injection: 1 RCT, N=39	Hylan G-F20 vs placebo	1–4 weeks, 5–13 weeks and 14–26 weeks post-injection	1–4 weeks: WMD −1.08, 95% CI −1.73 to −0.44, p=0.001 5–13 weeks: WMD −1.34, 95% CI −2.13 to −0.55, p=0.0009 14-26 weeks: WMD −1.00, 95% CI -1.89 to −0.11, p=0.03 Favours HA
HA Orthovisc				
WOMAC stiffness (2–10 Likert)	1 MA (Bellamy et al. 2006b) 5–13 weeks: 1 RCT, N=29 14–26 weeks: 1 RCT, N=29	HA Orthovisc vs placebo	5–13 weeks and 14–26 weeks post-injection	5–13 weeks: WMD −1.50, 95% CI −2.84 to −0.16, p=0.03) 14–26 weeks: WMD −1.50, 95% CI -2.71 to −0.29, p=0.02. Favours HA

Table 7.67 Function in knee OA

Knee

Function	Reference	Intervention	Assessment time	Outcome/effect size
HA (general)				
WOMAC physical function	1 RCT (Petrella and Petrella 2006) (N=106)	HA vs placebo	End of treatment (3 weeks).	p<0.05 Favours HA
WOMAC physical function and range of motion (flexion)	1 RCT (Petrella and Petrella 2006) (N=106)	HA vs placebo	6 and 12-weeks (ie 3 and 9-weeks post-injection)	NS
HA Artz				
WOMAC function (0–68 Likert) Range of motion (1 RCT, N=98) Lequesne Index (0–24, range of motion	1 MA (Bellamy et al. 2006b)	HA Artz vs placebo	5–13 weeks post-injection and 14–26 weeks post-injection	NS
HA Durolane				
WOMAC physical function (change from baseline, 0–68 Likert)	1 MA (Bellamy et al. 2006b) 1 RCT, N=346	HA durolane vs placebo	Week 2, 6, 13 and 26	NS
HA Hyalgan				
Lequesne Index (0–24)	1 MA (Bellamy et al. 2006b) 1–4 weeks: 6 RCTs, N=400 5–13 weeks: 5 RCTs, N=201	Hyalgan vs placebo	1–4 weeks and 5–13 weeks post-injection	1–4 weeks: WMD –1.50, 95% CI –2.36 to –0.65, p=0.0006 5–13 weeks: WMD –2.34, 95% CI –3.41 to –1.27, p=0.00002 Favours HA
Flexion (degrees)	1 MA (Bellamy et al. 2006b) 1 RCT, N=35	Hyalgan vs placebo	5–13 weeks post-injection	WMD 7.60, 95% CI 0.46 to 14.74, p=0.04 Favours HA
WOMAC function (VAS), Lequesne Index (0–24), and Flexion (degrees)	1 MA (Bellamy et al. 2006b)	Hyalgan vs placebo	1–4 weeks and 5–13 weeks and 14–26 weeks post-injection	NS
HA Hylan G-F20				
Lequesne Index (0–24)	1 MA (Bellamy et al. 2006b) 1 RCT, N=110	Hylan G-F20 vs placebo	5–13 weeks post-injection	WMD –1.60, 95% CI –2.98 to –0.22, p=0.02 Favours HA
WOMAC physical function	1 MA (Bellamy et al. 2006b) 5–13 weeks: 3 RCTs, N=170 4–26 weeks: 1 RCT, N=30	Hylan G-F20 vs placebo	5–13 weeks and 4–26 weeks post-injection	5–13 weeks: WMD –11.91, 95% CI –15.06 to –8.76, p<0.00001 4–26 weeks: WMD –17.00, 95% CI –26.90 to –7.10, p=0.0008

continued

Table 7.67 Function in knee OA – *continued*

Knee

Function	Reference	Intervention	Assessment time	Outcome/effect size
HA Hylan G-F20 – *continued*				
Improvement in most painful knee movement (VAS)	1 MA (Bellamy et al. 2006b) 1–4 weeks post-injection: 4 RCTs, N=267	Hylan G-F20 vs placebo	4 weeks post-injection	4 weeks post-injection: WMD 19.29, 95% CI 12.26 to 26.31, p<0.00001.
Lequesne Index (0–24) and 15 metre walking time	1 MA (Bellamy et al. 2006b)	Hylan G-F20 vs placebo	Up to 26 weeks post-injection	NS
HA Suvenyl				
Lequesne Index (the changes from baseline), 0–100 modified scale and joint space width (percentage of progressors: joint space narrowing >0.5 mm)	1 MA (Bellamy et al. 2006b) 1 RCT, N=131	HA Suvenyl vs placebo	45–52 weeks post-injection	NS
HA Orthovisc				
WOMAC total score (VAS, change from baseline)	1 MA (Bellamy et al. 2006b) 2 RCTs, N=336	HA Orthovisc vs placebo	5–13 weeks and 14–26 weeks post-injection	NS
WOMAC physical function	1 MA (Bellamy et al. 2006b) 1–4 weeks: 3 RCTs, N=110 5–13 weeks: 2 RCTs, N=69 14–26 weeks: 2 RCTs, N=69	HA Orthovisc vs placebo	5–13 weeks and 45–52 weeks post-injection	1–4 weeks: WMD –7.20, 95% CI –8.84 to –5.56, p<0.00001 5–13 weeks: WMD –12.87, 95% CI –18.60 to –7.14, p=0.00001 4–26 weeks post-injection: WMD –10.88, 95% CI –16.97 to –4.79, p=0.0005
25-metre walking time (seconds) and knee circumference (mm)	1 MA (Bellamy et al. 2006b) 1 RCT, N=41	HA Orthovisc vs placebo	1–4 weeks post-injection	NS
WOMAC physical function	1 MA (Bellamy et al. 2006b) 1–4 weeks: 3 RCTs, N=110 5–13 weeks and 14–26 weeks: 2 RCTs, N=69	HA Orthovisc vs placebo	1–4 weeks, 5–13 weeks and 14–26	1–4 weeks: WMD –7.20, 95% CI –8.84 to –5.56, weeks post-injection p<0.00001 5–13 weeks: WMD –12.87, 95% CI –18.60 to –7.14, p=0.00001 14–26 weeks post-injection: WMD –10.88, 95% CI –16.97 to –4.79, p=0.0005 Favours HA

continued

Table 7.67 Function in knee OA – *continued*

Knee

Function	Reference	Intervention	Assessment time	Outcome/effect size
HA Orthovisc – *continued*				
Range of motion – flexion (degrees)	1 MA (Bellamy et al. 2006b) 1 RCT, N=41	HA Orthovisc vs placebo	1–4 weeks post-injection	WMD 4.00, 95% CI 2.02 to 5.98, p=0.00007 Favours HA
WOMAC physical function	1 MA (Bellamy et al. 2006b) 2 RCTs, N=60	HA Orthovisc vs placebo	1–4 weeks post-injection	Significant heterogeneity
HA Suplasyn				
WOMAC function at 1 week post-injection; and walk time second at 1 week post-injection	1 MA (Bellamy et al. 2006b) 1 RCT, N=53	HA Suplasyn vs placebo	1 week post-injection	NS

Table 7.68 Global assessment in knee OA

Knee

Global assessment	Reference	Intervention	Assessment time	Outcome/effect size
HA (general)				
Patient global assessment of knee condition.	1 RCT (Petrella and Petrella 2006) (N=106)	HA vs placebo	6 and 12-weeks (ie 3 and 9-weeks post-injection)	NS
HA Artz				
Patient's global assessment (number of patients improved)	1 MA (Bellamy et al. 2006b) 3 RCTs, N=495	HA Artz vs placebo	1–4 weeks post-injection	Favours HA
Patient's global assessment (number of patients improved)	1 MA (Bellamy et al. 2006b) 5–13 weeks: 2 RCTs, N=384 14–26 weeks: 1 RCT, N=189	HA Artz vs placebo	5–13 weeks and 14–26 weeks post-injection	NS
HA Hyalgan				
Patient global assessment (number of patients improved)	1 MA (Bellamy et al. 2006b) 5–13 weeks: 2 RCTs, N=75 14–26 weeks: 3 RCTs, N=363	Hyalgan vs placebo	5–13 weeks and 14–26 weeks post-injection	5–13 weeks: RR 2.44, 95% CI 1.43 to 4.16, p=0.001 14–26 weeks: RR 1.24, 95% CI 1.03 to 1.50, p=0.02 Favours HA

continued

Table 7.68 Global assessment in knee OA – *continued*

Knee

Global assessment	Reference	Intervention	Assessment time	Outcome/effect size
HA Hyalgan – *continued*				
Patient global assessment (number of joints fairly good/ good/very good) at 5–13 weeks	1 MA (Bellamy et al. 2006b) 5–13 weeks: 2 RCTs, N=61	Hyalgan vs placebo	5–13 weeks post-injection	RR 2.12, 95% CI 1.22 to 3.70, p=0.008 Favours HA
Patient global assessment (number of patients improved) and physician global assessment (VAS)	1 MA (Bellamy et al. 2006b)	Hyalgan vs placebo	1–4 weeks and up to 45–52 weeks post-injection	NS
HA Hylan G-F20				
Patient global assessment (VAS)	1 MA (Bellamy et al. 2006b) 1–4 weeks: 1 RCT, N=30 5–13 weeks: 1 RCT, N=30	Hylan G-F20 vs placebo	1–4 weeks and 5–13 weeks post-injection	1–4 weeks: WMD –20.00, 95% CI –33.16 to –6.84, p=0.003 5–13 weeks: WMD –20.00, 95% CI –30.57 to –9.43, p=0.0002 Favours HA
Patient global evaluation of efficacy due to treatment at 1–4 weeks and 5–13 weeks post-injection	1 MA (Bellamy et al. 2006b) 1–4 weeks: 5 RCTs, N=298 5–13 weeks: 5 RCTs, N=298	Hylan G-F20 vs placebo	1–4 weeks and 5–13 weeks post-injection	1–4 weeks: WMD 0.70, 95% CI 0.46 to 0.93, p<0.00001 5–13 weeks: WMD 1.23, 95% CI 0.97 to 1.48, p<0.00001 Favours HA
Physician global assessment (VAS) at 1-4 weeks and 5–13 weeks post-injection	1 MA (Bellamy et al. 2006b) 1–4 weeks: 1 RCT, N=30; 5–13 weeks: 1 RCT, N=30	Hylan G-F20 vs placebo	1–4 weeks and 5–13 weeks post-injection	1-4 weeks: WMD –20.00, 95% CI –37.64 to –2.36, p=0.03 5–13 weeks: WMD –20.00, 95% CI –36.10 to –3.90, p=0.01 Favours HA
Patient global assessment (VAS), patient global assessment (number of patients good or very good), physician global assessment (VAS)	1 MA (Bellamy et al. 2006b) 1 RCT, N=30	Hylan G-F20 vs placebo	Up to 14–26 weeks post-injection	NS

continued

Table 7.68 Global assessment in knee OA – *continued*

Knee

Global assessment	Reference	Intervention	Assessment time	Outcome/effect size
HA Suvenyl				
Patient global assessment (change from baseline)	1 MA (Bellamy et al. 2006b) 1 RCT, N=174	HA Suvenyl vs placebo	45–52 weeks post-injection	NS
HA Orthovisc				
Patient global assessment (VAS)	1 MA (Bellamy et al. 2006b) 1 RCT, N=29	HA Orthovisc vs placebo	1–4 weeks post-injection.	WMD –20.00, 95% CI –33.22 to –6.78, p=0.003 Favours HA
Patient global assessment (VAS), patient global assessment (number of patients rating treatment as effective or very effective), physician global assessment (VAS)	1 MA (Bellamy et al. 2006b)	HA Orthovisc vs placebo	Up to 14–26 weeks post-injection	NS

Table 7.69 Quality of life in knee OA

Knee

Quality of life	Reference	Intervention	Assessment time	Outcome/effect size
HA (general)				
SF-36 dimensions of physical function and vitality	1 RCT (Petrella and Petrella 2006) (N=106)	HA vs placebo	End of treatment (3 weeks)	p<0.05 Favours HA
SF-36 dimensions of physical function and vitality	1 RCT (Petrella and Petrella 2006) (N=106)	HA vs placebo	6 and 12-weeks (ie 3 and 9-weeks post-injection	NS
HA Artzal				
SF-36 dimensions physical functioning, role physical, bodily pain, general health and vitality	1 RCT (Karlsson et al. 2002) (N=210) in the systematic review	HA Artzal vs placebo	Improvement between weeks 0 and 26	Both groups improved
SF-36 dimensions of social functioning, role emotional and of mental health	1 RCT (Karlsson et al. 2002) (N=210) in the systematic review	HA Artzal vs placebo	Improvement between weeks 0 and 26	Placebo improved, HA deteriorated. Favours placebo.

continued

Table 7.69 Quality of life in knee OA – *continued*

Knee

Quality of life	Reference	Intervention	Assessment time	Outcome/effect size
HA Synvisc				
SF-12 physical component score	1 RCT (Kahan et al. 2003 105) (N=445) in the systematic review	HA Synvisc vs placebo	9 months (end of treatment)	+5.5 points (Synvisc) +2.3 points (placebo) p<0.0001 Favours HA
SF-12 mental component	1 RCT (Kahan et al. 2003 105) (N=445) in the systematic review	HA Synvisc vs placebo	9 months (end of treatment)	+2.9 points (Synvisc) +1.6 points (placebo) P values not given Favours Synvisc
SF-36 dimensions physical functioning, role physical, bodily pain, general health, vitality, social functioning, role emotional and mental health	1 RCT (Karlsson et al. 2002) (N=210) in the systematic review	HA Synvisc vs placebo	Improvement between weeks 0 and 26	Both groups improved
HA Hyalgan				
SF-36 dimension of 'vitality'	1 RCT (Jubb et al. 2003) (N=408) in the systematic review	Hyalgan vs placebo	52 weeks post-injection	p=0.03 Favours HA
Any other SF-36 dimensions	1 RCT (Jubb et al. 2003) (N=408) in the systematic review	Hyalgan vs placebo	52 weeks post-injection	NS

Table 7.70 Adverse events in knee OA

Knee

Adverse events	Reference	Intervention	Assessment time	Outcome/effect size
HA Artz				
Number of AEs probably/possibly related to treatment	1 MA (Bellamy et al. 2006b) 2 RCTs, N=432	HA Artz vs placebo	5–13 weeks post-injection	RR 1.59, 95% CI 1.12 to 2.26, p=0.009 Favours placebo
Number of patients reporting AEs	1 MA (Bellamy et al. 2006b) 1 RCT, N=156	HA Artz vs placebo	45–52 weeks post-injection	NS
HA BioHy				
Number of AEs for injection site pain	1 MA (Bellamy et al. 2006b) 1 RCT, N=49	HA BioHy vs placebo	Not mentioned	NS

continued

Table 7.70 Adverse events in knee OA – *continued*

Knee

Adverse events	Reference	Intervention	Assessment time	Outcome/effect size
HA Durolane				
Number of patients affected by device-related AEs; number of patients with AEs related to injection only; number of patients with non-serious treatment-related AEs; number of patients with non-serious AEs	1 MA (Bellamy et al. 2006b) 1 RCT, N=347	HA Durolane vs placebo	Not mentioned	NS
HA Hyalgan				
Number of patients with adverse reaction but study drug continued	1 MA (Bellamy et al. 2006b) 6 RCTs, N=666	Hyalgan vs placebo	Not mentioned	RR 1.42, 95% CI 1.10 to 1.84, p=0.007 Favours placebo
Number of patients with local adverse reaction and study drug discontinued	1 MA (Bellamy et al. 2006b) 4 RCTs, N=941	Hyalgan vs placebo	5–13 weeks post-injection	RR 3.34, 95% CI 1.31 to 8.56, p=0.01 Favours placebo
Number of patients reporting AEs; number of patients with serious or severe AEs and post-injection; number of knee joints with local adverse reaction; number of patients with injection site pain or painful intra-articular injection	1 MA (Bellamy et al. 2006b)	Hyalgan vs placebo	14–26 weeks and 45–52 weeks post-injection	NS
HA Hylan G-F20				
Number of patients not requiring additional treatment for study knee	1 MA (Bellamy et al. 2006b) 1 RCT, N=152	Hylan G-F20 vs placebo	45–52 weeks post-injection	NS
Number of clinical failures	1 MA (Bellamy et al. 2006b) 14–26 weeks: 1 RCT, N=152 45–52 weeks: 1 RCT, N=118	Hylan G-F20 vs placebo	14–26 weeks and 45–52 weeks post-injection	5–13 weeks: WMD –NS

continued

Table 7.70 Adverse events in knee OA – *continued*

Knee

Adverse events	Reference	Intervention	Assessment time	Outcome/effect size
HA Hylan G-F20 – *continued*				
Number of patients with local reaction	1 MA (Bellamy et al. 2006b) 6 RCTs, N=469	Hylan G-F20 vs placebo	Not mentioned	NS
Number of patients with local adverse reactions but study drug continued	1 MA (Bellamy et al. 2006b) 1 RCT, N=30	Hylan G-F20 vs placebo	Not mentioned	NS
HA Suvenyl				
Patient assessment of treatment efficacy (number of patients rating very good or good vs moderate, bad or very bad; number of patients reporting knee pain during or after intra-articular injection	1 MA (Bellamy et al. 2006b)	HA Suvenyl vs placebo	Not mentioned	NS
HA Orthovisc				
Number of patients with treatment-related AEs; number of patients with local skin rash or musculoskeletal AEs	1 MA (Bellamy et al. 2006b)	HA Orthovisc vs placebo	Not mentioned	NS
HA Replasyn				
Number of patients with local adverse reaction but study drug continued	1 MA (Bellamy et al. 2006b) 1 RCT, N=39	HA Replasyn vs placebo	Not mentioned	NS

Table 7.71 Withdrawals in knee OA

Knee

Study withdrawals	Reference	Intervention	Assessment time	Outcome/effect size
HA (general)				
Discontinuation due to AEs	1 RCT (Petrella and Petrella 2006) (N=106)	HA vs placebo	End of treatment (3 weeks)	N=2 (HA) N=1 (placebo) Both groups similar
HA Artz				
Total withdrawals overall; withdrawals due to AEs	1 MA (Bellamy et al. 2006b)	HA Artz vs placebo	1–4 weeks, 5–13 weeks and 14–26 weeks post-injection	NS
HA BioHy				
Total withdrawals overall	1 MA (Bellamy et al. 2006b) 1 RCT, N=49	HA BioHy vs placebo	14–26 weeks post-injection	NS
HA Durolane				
Total withdrawals overall, withdrawals due to inefficacy AEs	1 MA (Bellamy et al. 2006b) 1 RCT, N=347	HA durolane vs placebo	Not mentioned	NS
HA Hyalgan				
Total withdrawals overall Withdrawals due to lack of efficacy/ painful injection/AEs	1 MA (Bellamy et al. 2006b)	Hyalgan vs placebo	During treatment	NS
HA Hylan G-F20				
Total withdrawals overall	1 MA(Bellamy et al. 2006b) 1–4 weeks: 1 RCT, N=94; 5–13 weeks: 4 RCTs, N=329; 14–26 weeks: 1 RCT, N=52	Hylan G-F20 vs placebo	1–4 weeks (1 RCT, N=94), 5–13 weeks (4 RCTs, N=329) and 14–26 weeks post-injection (1 RCT, N=52)	NS
HA Suvenyl				
Total withdrawals overall, withdrawals due to inefficacy and number of withdrawals due to AEs	1 MA (Bellamy et al. 2006b) 1 RCT, N=216	HA Suvenyl vs placebo	Not mentioned	NS
HA Orthovisc				
Total withdrawals overall; withdrawals due to lack of efficacy/local AEs	1 MA (Bellamy et al. 2006b)	HA Orthovisc vs placebo	Not mentioned	NS
HA Suplasyn				
Total withdrawals overall	1 MA (Bellamy et al. 2006b) 1 RCT, N=60	HA Suplasyn vs placebo	Not mentioned	NS

7.4.6 Evidence statements: Intraarticular (IA) therapy: Hyaluronans vs Corticosteroid

▷ Knee

Data from the Cochrane meta-analysis (Bellamy et al. 2006b) suggest that IA therapy with hyaluronans may have a more prolonged effect than IA with corticosteroids.

▷ Hip and hand

No significant differences between hyaluronans and corticosteroids were reported at any time point by the two studies evaluating efficacy and function outcomes in patients with OA in the hip (Qvistgaard 2006) and the hand (Fuchs 2006).

Table 7.72 Pain in knee OA

Knee

Pain	Reference	Intervention	Assessment time	Outcome/effect size
Hyalgan				
Spontaneous pain intensity (VAS)	1 MA (Bellamy et al. 2006b) 3 RCTs, N=170	Hyalgan vs corticosteroid (methylprednisolone acetate)	5–13 weeks post-injection	WMD –7.73, 95% CI –12.81 to –2.64, p=0.003 Favours HA
Number of patients with moderate or severe pain under load	1 MA (Bellamy et al. 2006b) 2 RCTs, N=169	Hyalgan vs corticosteroid (methylprednisolone acetate)	5–13 weeks post-injection	RR 0.61, 95% CI 0.44 to 0.84, p=0.003 Favours HA
Number of patients with moderate or greater rest pain	1 MA (Bellamy et al. 2006b) 2 RCTs, N=169	Hyalgan vs corticosteroid (methylprednisolone acetate)	5–13 weeks post-injection	RR 0.39, 95% CI 0.19 to 0.78, p=0.008 Favours HA
Spontaneous pain intensity (VAS), number of joints with moderate or severe walking pain and number of joints with moderate or severe pain under load, number of patients with at least moderate or greater night pain, number of patients with moderate or greater rest pain	1 MA (Bellamy et al. 2006b)	Hyalgan vs corticosteroid (methylprednisolone acetate)	1–4 weeks, 5–13 weeks and 45–52 weeks post-injection	NS
Pain at night	1 MA (Bellamy et al. 2006b) 1 RCT, N=20	Hyalgan vs corticosteroid (triamcinolone hexacetonide)	14–26 weeks post-injection	WMD –37.74 to –3.66 Favours HA

continued

Table 7.72 Pain in knee OA – *continued*

Knee

Pain	Reference	Intervention	Assessment time	Outcome/effect size
Hyalgan – *continued*				
Pain on nominated activity (VAS), pain at rest (VAS) and pain at night (VAS)	1 MA (Bellamy et al. 2006b)	Hyalgan vs corticosteroid (triamcinolone hexacetonide)	End of treatment (week 4) and 14–26 weeks post-injection	NS
HA Hylan G-F20				
WOMAC pain walking on a flat surface (0–4 Likert)	1 MA (Bellamy et al. 2006b) 5–13 weeks: 1 RCT, N=215 14–26 weeks: 1 RCT, N=215	Hylan G-F20 vs corticosteroid triamcinolone hexacetonide	5–13 weeks and 14–26 weeks post-injection	5–13 weeks: WMD −0.40, 95% CI −0.65 to −0.15, p=0.002 14–26 weeks: WMD −0.40, 95% CI −0.68 to −0.12, p=0.005 Favours HA
HA Orthovisc				
Pain on weight bearing (VAS)	1 MA (Bellamy et al. 2006b) 1 RCT, N=55	Orthovisc vs corticosteroid 6-methylprednisolone acetate	5–13 weeks and 14–26 weeks post-injection	5–13 weeks: WMD −15.64, 95% CI −24.51 to −6.77, p=0.0006 14-26 weeks: WMD −15.40, 95% CI −25.91 to −4.89, p=0.004 Favours HA
Pain on walking (VAS)	1 MA (Bellamy et al. 2006b) 1 RCT, N=55	Orthovisc vs corticosteroid 6-methylprednisolone acetate	5–13 and 14–26 weeks post-injection	5–13 weeks: WMD −18.43, 95% CI −29.19 to −7.67, p=0.0008 14-26 weeks: WMD −14.90, 95% CI −25.91 to −3.89, p=0.008 Favours HA
Pain at rest (VAS)	1 MA (Bellamy et al. 2006b) 1 RCT, N=55	Orthovisc vs corticosteroid 6-methylprednisolone acetate	6–13 weeks post-injection	WMD −7.70, 95% CI −13.50 to −1.00, p=0.009 Favours HA
Pain on weight bearing (VAS) and Pain on walking (VAS)	1 MA (Bellamy et al. 2006b) 1 RCT, N=55	Orthovisc vs corticosteroid 6-methylprednisolone acetate	1–4 weeks post-injection	NS
Pain at rest (VAS)	1 MA (Bellamy et al. 2006b) 1 RCT, N=55	Orthovisc vs corticosteroid 6-methylprednisolone acetate	1–4 weeks and 14–26 weeks post-injection	NS

Table 7.73 Function in knee OA

Knee

Function	Reference	Intervention	Assessment time	Outcome/effect size
Hylan G-F20				
WOMAC total score (0–96 Likert)	1 MA (Bellamy et al. 2006b) 1 RCT, N=215	Hylan G-F20 vs corticosteroid triamcinolone hexacetonide	5–13 weeks and 14–26 weeks post-injection	5–13 weeks: WMD –7.40, 95% CI –12.74 to –2.06, p=0.007 14–26 weeks: WMD –7.30, 95% CI –12.76 to –1.84, p=0.009 Favours HA
WOMAC physical function (0-68 Likert)	1 MA (Bellamy et al. 2006b) 1 RCT, N=215	Hylan G-F20 vs corticosteroid triamcinolone hexacetonide	5–13 weeks and 14–26 weeks post-injection	5–13 weeks: WMD –5.00, 95% CI –8.86 to –1.14, p=0.01 14–26 weeks: WMD –5.20, 95% CI –9.10 to –1.30, p=0.009
HA Orthovisc				
WOMAC function (VAS)	1 MA (Bellamy et al. 2006b) 1 RCT, N=40	Orthovisc vs corticosteroids betamethasone	5–13 weeks post-injection	WMD –9.00, 95% CI –14.15 to –3.85, p=0.0006 Favours HA
WOMAC function (VAS) and flexion (degrees	1 MA (Bellamy et al. 2006b) 1 RCT, N=40	Orthovisc vs corticosteroids betamethasone	1–4 weeks post-injection	NS
Lequesne Index (0–24)	1 MA (Bellamy et al. 2006b) 1 RCT, N=55	Orthovisc vs corticosteroid 6-methylprednisolone acetate	5–13 weeks and 14–26 weeks post-injection	5–13 weeks: WMD –1.40, 95% CI –2.13 to –0.67, p=0.0002 14–26 weeks: WMD –1.14, 95% CI –2.16 to –0.12, p=0.03
Lequesne Index (0–24)	1 MA Bellamy et al. 2006b) 1 RCT, N=55	Orthovisc vs corticosteroid 6-methylprednisolone acetate	1–4 weeks post-injection	NS

Table 7.74 Adverse events in knee OA

Knee

Adverse events	Reference	Intervention	Assessment time	Outcome/effect size
Hyalgan				
Number of patients with local or systemic reactions, number of joints with local reactions but continued in trial	1 MA (Bellamy et al. 2006b)	Hyalgan vs corticosteroid methylprednisolone acetate	Up to 5–13 weeks post-injection	NS
HA Orthovisc				
Number of patients with local AEs	1 MA (Bellamy et al. 2006b) 1 RCT, N=40	Orthovisc vs corticosteroids betamethasone	Not mentioned	NS
Number of patients reporting musculo-skeletal AEs, number of patients reporting skin AEs, number of patients reporting general AEs, number of patients reporting knee pain after injection	1 MA (Bellamy et al. 2006b) 1 RCT, N=55	Orthovisc vs corticosteroid 6-methylprednisolone acetate	Not mentioned	NS

Table 7.75 Withdrawals in knee OA

Knee

Study withdrawals	Reference	Intervention	Assessment time	Outcome/effect size
Hyalgan				
Total withdrawals overall; number of patients withdrawn due to lack of efficacy, number of patients withdrawn due to AEs	1 MA (Bellamy et al. 2006b)	Hyalgan vs corticosteroid (methylprednisolone acetate)	1–4 weeks, 5–13 weeks 14–26 weeks and 45–52 weeks post-injection	NS
Total withdrawals overall, withdrawals due to lack of efficacy and withdrawals due to AEs	1 MA (Bellamy et al. 2006b) 1 RCT, N=63	Hyalgan vs corticosteroid (triamcinolone hexacetonide)	Week 4 (end of treatment) and 14–26 weeks post-injection	NS
HA Hylan G-F20				
Total withdrawals overall and with-drawals due to lack of efficacy/local reaction	1 MA (Bellamy et al. 2006b)	Hylan G-F20 vs corticosteroids betamethasone	Not mentioned	NS

continued

Table 7.75 Withdrawals in knee OA – *continued*

Knee

Study withdrawals	Reference	Intervention	Assessment time	Outcome/effect size
HA Hylan G-F20 – *continued*				
Withdrawals due to lack of efficacy	1 MA (Bellamy et al. 2006b) 1 RCT, N=216	Hylan G-F20 vs corticosteroid triamcinolone hexacetonide	Not mentioned	RR 0.03, 95% CI 0.00 to 0.48, p=0.01 Favours HA
Total withdrawals overall and withdrawals due to AEs	1 MA (Bellamy et al. 2006b) 1 RCT, N=216	Hylan G-F20 vs corticosteroid triamcinolone hexacetonide	Not mentioned	NS
HA Orthovisc				
Total withdrawals overall and number of patients withdrawn due to AEs.	1 MA (Bellamy et al. 2006b) 1 RCT, N=40	Orthovisc vs corticosteroid betamethasone	Not mentioned	NS
Total withdrawals overall and number of patients withdrawn due to increased pain	1 MA (Bellamy et al. 2006b) 1 RCT, N=60	Orthovisc vs corticosteroid 6-methylprednisolone acetate	Not mentioned	NS

7.4.7 Health economic evidence

We looked at studies that conducted economic evaluations involving corticosteroids or hyaluronans versus placebo or compared with each other. Four papers: one French, one Canadian, one Taiwanese and one from the USA, and all evaluating hyaluronans, are included here as a summary of the health economic evidence currently available. However, due to some methodological limitations the use of these papers is limited and evidence statements cannot be made from them.

The French study (Kahan et al. 2003) compared treatment including hyaluronan with 'conventional treatment' for patients with knee OA. The authors carried out a cost-effectiveness analysis using the Lequesne index, WOMAC and the SF-12. The duration of the analysis was 9 months, and the hyaluronan treatment arm involved three intratricular injections spaced one week apart. No information is given on what the conventional treatment arm involved so unfortunately it is difficult to interpret the results precisely.

An additional problem with the study is that the full costs of hyaluronan were not included, since its cost was based on the 65% reimbursement rate instituted in France in September 2000. All other costs were reported in 1998 euros.

Table 7.76 Results of Kohan's economic evaluation			
	Conventional treatment	**Hyaluronan treatment (Synvisc)**	**p value**
Total cost (societal)	€829.40	€829.10	
Total cost (medical only)	€777.90	€785.30	
Total cost (medical only, including total Hyaluronan cost	€777.90	€848.14	
Reduction in:			
Lequesne index	−1.6	−3.6	0.0001
WOMAC (total)	−8.1	−19.8	0.0001
WOMAC (pain)	−12.2	−24.6	0.0001
WOMAC (stiffness)	−7.7	−20.7	0.0001
WOMAC (function)	−7.0	−18.4	0.0001
Pain on walking (VAS)	−24.4	−37.4	0.0001
Improvement in quality of life (SF12):			
Physical	2.3	5.5	0.0001
Mental	1.6	2.9	Not stated

The results taken from the French paper are shown in the table above (Kahan et al. 2003). They appear to show hyaluronan treatment with Synvisc dominating (less expensive and more effective) conventional treatment. If only medical costs are considered, Synvisc does not appear dominant, but given it was found to be significantly more effective than conventional treatment for the outcome measures considered for a small cost increment, then Synvisc would appear to be cost effective.

Including the full hyaluronan costs, the cost difference per patient becomes more substantial and the cost effectiveness of the treatment becomes more uncertain. For example, the cost per one point improvement in the SF12 Physical Quality of Life scale over a 9-month period is €21.95 when comparing hyaluronan treatment to conventional treatment.

The lack of detail included regarding what treatment 'conventional treatment' involves, and the fact that the total cost of the hyaluronan treatment was not included due to the reimbursement regime in France means that this study cannot be used to make evidence statements.

The Canadian study (Torrance et al. 2002) conducted a cost–utility analysis to compare appropriate care with hyaluronan treatment to appropriate care without hyaluronan treatment for patients with knee OA. Appropriate care is described as the preferred management strategy of specialists, rheumatologists or orthopaedic surgeons, encouraged to follow treatment guidelines published by the American College of Rheumatology and instructed to treat conservatively. Appropriate care did include corticosteroid injections for some patients. The clinical data were taken from the clinical trial run alongside the economic analysis, which was a 1-year prospective, randomised, open-label, parallel design trial (Raynauld 2002). The unblinded nature of the trial may bias the results.

The base-case analysis took the societal perspective, but a healthcare payer perspective was considered in sensitivity analysis and this had little effect on costs differences between treatment groups, and so affected results only minimally. All costs were reported in Canadian dollars at 1999 prices.

Table 7.77 Costs from Torrance's economic evaluation

	Appropriate care	Appropriate care + Hyaluronan	Difference
Total societal cost (Canadian $)	$1,414.58	$2,124.71	$710.13
Total healthcare payer cost (Candian $)	Not stated	Not stated	$705

Table 7.78 Results of Torrance's economic evaluation

	Incremental cost	QALY gain	Cost per QALY gain
Base case	$705	0.071	$9,930
SA on outcomes			
High	$705	0.117	$6,026
Low	$705	0.025	$28,200
SA on costs			
High	$1,008	0.071	$14,197
Low	$402	0.071	$5,662

The results of the Canadian study are shown in the tables above. The study provided little information on what appropriate care involves. The cost data provided show that some patients in both treatment arms received corticosteroid injections, with the cost per patient of this treatment being higher for patients in the appropriate care arm. However, the cost per patient ($18.45) is still very low and the difference in 'medication' costs (for example, NSAIDs) per patient between the groups is far larger ($237.32 vs $305.10). Hence it is not clear that this analysis allows a comparison of hyaluronan treatment and corticosteroid treatment as there are no data that suggest that patients substitute one treatment for another depending on which group they are in, particularly as some patients in the hyaluronan arm clearly receive both treatments.

Hyaluronan can also not be compared with placebo using this study as a placebo was not used in the study. The fact that the study was not blinded may also weaken any evidence statements made, and so again, given these problems no evidence statements are made.

The study conducted in Taiwan was well conducted, but is of limited use for the questions being addressed here. This is because the study compared hyaluronan with celecoxib and naproxen in a cost-effectiveness analysis (Yen et al. 2004). Being set in Taiwan makes the study of limited use for a UK guideline, and also CV adverse events were not included, which severely harms the credibility of the naproxen and celecoxib analysis. Given that a placebo arm was not included, this harms the interpretation of the hyaluronan treatment arm as the treatments it is compared with may not be credible. All costs were reported in US dollars at 2002 prices. Table 7.79 shows the results of the study.

Table 7.79 Results of Yen's economic evaluation

Strategy	Expected cost (US$)	Incremental cost (US$)	Effectiveness (QALY)	Incremental effect (QALY)	Incremental cost-effectiveness ratio (ER)
Naproxen	498.98	–	0.4357	–	–
Celecoxib	547.80	48.82	0.4380	0.0023	21,226
Hyaluronan	678.00	130.20	0.4411	0.0031	42,000

These results meant that hyaluronan was not considered cost effective compared with celecoxib and naproxen in Taiwan. If CV effects were included, celecoxib and naproxen would appear slightly worse, making hyaluronan appear better in comparison. However, due to the setting of the study and the comparators used, no useful evidence statements can be made from this study.

The US study (Waddell et al. 2001) builds a pharmacoeconomic model to calculate the cost effects of including hyaluronan treatment in a standard osteoarthritis treatment pathway for patients with mild, moderate, and severe OA. This treatment path does include steroid injections for some patients. The study is not a formal cost-effectiveness or cost–utility analysis as it does not include a measure of health gain attributable to the treatment. Instead, it assumes that hyaluronan treatment reduces the need for other treatments, and delays total knee replacement operations, and analyses the difference this makes to costs from a health-insurer perspective.

The chief problem with this study is that the duration used is not appropriate for the modelling assumptions. It is assumed that hyaluronan treatment delays total knee replacement (a key cost driver) by approximately one year. The authors analyse a 3-year time period and then include no future costs. Given that a certain proportion of the theoretical cohort has a total knee replacement each year, and that it is assumed that the hyaluronan treatment delays such treatment by a year, it is obvious that the hyaluronan treatment group will incur much less costs in a fixed time period. However, these costs would simply be accrued the following year in reality, unless the treatment actually prevents total knee replacement surgery, which is not what the paper assumes. For this reason the results of the paper are very misleading, and so again no evidence statements can be made.

7.4.8   From evidence to recommendations

▷   Corticosteroids

Generally the research evidence demonstrates that intra-articular corticosteroid injections provide short-term (1–4 weeks) reduction in osteoarthritis pain, although effects on function appear less marked. The effects have been best demonstrated for knee osteoarthritis, although there are some data for efficacy in hip and hand osteoarthritis. The GDG noted that these injections are widely used in many osteoarthritis sites. There is no clear message from this evidence on whether any particular corticosteroid preparation is more effective than another, or on which dose of a given preparation is most effective. In clinical practice, the short-term pain relief may settle flares of pain and also allow time for patients to begin other interventions such as joint-related muscle strengthening.

The risks associated with intra-articular corticosteroid injection are generally small. A small percentage of patients may experience a transient increase in pain following injection. Subcutaneous deposition of steroid may lead to local fat atrophy and cosmetic defect. Care should always be taken when injecting small joints (such as finger joints) to avoid traumatising local nerves. There is a very small risk of infection. The question of steroid-arthropathy, that is, whether intra-articular steroids may increase cartilage loss, remains controversial and is currently based on animal model and retrospective human studies. Nevertheless, caution should be applied if injecting an individual joint on multiple occasions and other osteoarthritis therapies should be optimised.

▷ Hyaluronans

The research evidence on the efficacy of HAs is often difficult to interpret because of confounders including:

- different molecular weights of HA
- different injection schedules (ranging from once weekly to a series of five injections)
- poor trial design despite large numbers of studies, for example lack of intention-to-treat analyses, limitations in blinding.

On balance, the evidence seems to suggest a benefit for reducing pain up to 3 months after a series of three to five injections, although the effect size is generally small. Given this, and the cost of the therapies together with increased clinician visits required for injections, hyaluronan injections were assessed in the cost-consequence analysis (see Appendix C for details, available online at www.rcplondon.ac.uk/pubs/brochure.aspx?e=242). The Cochrane review (Bellamy 2006b) regarded pooled estimates across different products as potentially misleading, and also warned about pooled estimates because of different study designs. Also, meta-analysis was only possible for two of the WOMAC sub-scales, ruling out the use of the transfer to utility technique. With this in mind, and given the effect that different injection schedules have on cost estimates, the cost-consequence analysis looked at three products individually, using estimates from individual trials in each case. This allows a more thorough sensitivity analysis across different hyaluronan products. In all cases, the cost-effectiveness estimate is outside the realms of affordability to the NHS, and in one case is dominated by placebo. Sensitivity analyses on the individual estimates give a consistent message: that the efficacy would have to be three to five times higher than the estimates from the trials before reaching the standard threshold for cost effectiveness to the NHS.

Clinical trials do not suggest sub-groups of osteoarthritis patients may have greater benefit from HA therapies thereby improving cost effectiveness. A research recommendation is therefore made in section 10 to this effect.

The toxicity of intra-articular HA appears small. A small percentage of patients may experience a transient increase in pain following injection, and some get a frank flare of arthritis with marked effusion. As with any injection procedure there is a very small risk of infection.

RECOMMENDATIONS

R31   Intra-articular corticosteroid injections should be considered as an adjunct to core treatment for the relief of moderate to severe pain in people with osteoarthritis.

R32   Intra-articular hyaluronan injections are not recommended for the treatent of osteoarthritis.
      See p 297 for the associated recommendation for future research.

8 | Referral for specialist services

8.1 Referral criteria for surgery

8.1.1 Clinical introduction

Prosthetic joint replacement is the removal of articular surfaces from a painful joint and their replacement with synthetic materials, usually metal and plastic (although a variety of surfaces are now in widespread use including ceramic and metal). It has been successfully performed for over 40 years and is now one of the most common planned surgical procedures performed. Over 120,000 are performed annually in the UK accounting for 1% of the total healthcare budget. It is performed in the vast majority of cases for pain which originates from the joint, limits the patient's ability to perform their normal daily activities, disturbs sleep and does not respond to non-surgical measures. Joint replacement is very effective at relieving these symptoms and carries relatively low risk both in terms of systemic complications and suboptimal outcomes for the joint itself. Joint replacement allows a return to normal activity with many patients able to resume moderate levels of sporting activity including golf, tennis and swimming.

Successful outcomes require:
- careful selection of patients most likely to benefit
- thorough preparation in terms of general health and information
- well-performed anaesthesia and surgery
- appropriate rehabilitation and domestic support for the first few weeks.

For most patients the additional risk of mortality as a consequence of surgery, compared with continuing conservative treatment, is small. The recovery from joint replacement is rapid with patients commencing rehabilitation the day following surgery and normal activities within 6–12 weeks. Although knee recovery may be slower than hip; 95% of hip and knee replacements would be expected to continue functioning well into the second decade after surgery, with the majority providing lifelong pain-free function. However, around one in five patients are not satisfied with their joint replacements and a few do not get much improvement in pain following joint replacement.

Joint replacement is one of the most effective surgical procedures available with very few contraindications. As a result the demand from patients for these treatments continues to rise along with the confidence of surgeons to offer them to a wider range of patients in terms of age, disability and comorbidities.

8.1.2 Methodological introduction: indications for joint replacement

We looked for studies that investigated the indications for referring osteoarthritis patients for total/partial joint replacement surgery. Due to the large volume of evidence, studies were excluded if they used a mixed arthritis population of which less than 75% had osteoarthritis or if the population was not relevant to the UK.

Seven expert opinion papers (Anon 1995; Coyte et al. 1995; Dreinhofer et al. 2006; Imamura et al. 1996; Mancuso et al. 1996; Naylor and Williams 1996; Quintana et al. 2000), one cross-sectional study (Juni et al. 2003), one observational study (Dolin et al. 2003) and one observational-correlation study (Hawker et al. 2001) were found.

The seven expert opinion papers consisted of surveys and consensus group findings from rheumatologists, orthopaedic surgeons and other clinicians and their opinions of the indications for referral for joint replacement surgery.

The cross-sectional study (Juni et al. 2003) studied patients suitable for total knee arthroplasty (TKA) and assessed their willingness to undergo TKA surgery. The observational study (Dolin et al. 2003) assessed criteria that surgeons used as indications for total hip arthroplasty (THA) surgery. The observational-correlation study (Hawker 2001) assessed the willingness of patients (from low-rate and high-rate surgery areas) to undergo arthroplasty.

8.3.1 Methodological introduction: predictors of benefit and harm

We looked for studies that investigated the patient-centred factors that predict benefits and harms from osteoarthritis-related surgery. Due to the large volume of evidence, studies were excluded if they used a mixed arthritis population of which less than 75% had osteoarthritis or if the population was not relevant to the UK. Additionally, studies were categorised into groups of predictive factors and for each category the largest trials and those that covered each outcome of interest were included.

Two cohort studies (**level 2+**) (Caracciolo and Giaquinto 2005; Nilsdotter et al. 2001), two case-control studies (**level 2+**) (Amin et al. 2006; Spicer et al. 2001) and 20 case-series' (**level 3**) (Chakrabarti et al. 1997; De Leeuw and Villar 1998; Degreef and De 2006; Elson and Brenkel 2006; Escobar et al. 2007; Gill et al. 2003; Goutallier et al. 2006; Harrysson et al. 2004; Iannotti and Norris 2003; Jain et al. 2003; Johnsen et al. 2006; Jones et al. 2001; Kennedy et al. 2003; Lingard et al. 2004; Meding et al. 2000; Messieh 1999; Roder et al. 2007; Sadr et al. 2006; Schmalzried et al. 2005; Solomon et al. 2006) were found focusing on factors that predict the outcome of joint replacement surgery.

The two cohort studies (Caracciolo and Giaquinto 2005; Nilsdotter et al. 2001) were methodologically sound and differed with respect to osteoarthritis/surgery site, trial size and follow-up time. The first cohort study (Caracciolo and Giaquinto 2005) investigated N=100 patients who had either TKA or THA compared with N=46 controls, with a follow-up time of 6 months. The second cohort study (Nilsdotter et al. 2001) investigated N=184 patients who had THA compared with N=2960 controls, with a follow-up time of 6 and 12 months.

The two case-control studies (Amin et al. 2006; Spicer et al. 2001) were methodologically sound and both assessed the effect of knee replacement surgery on knee society score and survival of the prosthesis in obese and non-obese patients.

8.1.4 Evidence statements: indications for joint replacement

▷ Age

Four studies (Anon 1995; Coyte et al. 1995; Juni et al. 2003; Mancuso et al. 1996) looked at the effect of age on indications for surgery in knee osteoarthritis patients and found that age was associated with the decision to perform surgery.

Three studies (Dolin et al. 2003; Mancuso et al. 1996; Quintana et al. 2000) looked at the effect of age on indications for surgery in hip osteoarthritis patients and found that age was associated with the decision to perform surgery.

One study (Hawker et al. 2001) looked at the effect of age on indications for surgery in hip or knee osteoarthritis patients and found that age was associated with the decision to perform surgery.

Table 8.1 Effect of age on attitudes towards surgery for OA

Age outcome	Reference	Outcome/effect size
Knee osteoarthritis		
Patient's willingness to undergo surgery	1 cross-sectional study (Juni et al. 2003) (N=26,046)	OR per 10-year increase in age: 0.71, 95% CI 0.65 to 0.77 Favours younger persons (more willing)
Indication for surgery	1 study of expert opinions (Mancuso et al. 1996) (N=378 orthopaedic surgeons)	• Age >80 = neutral factor • Age <50 = sway decision against surgery for most surgeons
Referral for surgery	1 study of expert opinions (Coyte et al. 1996) (N=244 family physicians and N=96 rheumatologists)	• Age <55 years: 52% FPs = less likely and 35% = more likely to refer • Age >80 years: >70% of FPs who treated more patients with severe knee osteoarthritis = less likely to refer
Indications for surgery	1 study of expert opinions (Anon 1995) (N=13 experts)	• Age <55 years: alternative surgical procedures considered • Poor outcomes do not appear to be related to age • Data for risk factors is insufficient for age
Hip		
Priority for surgery	1 observational study (Dolin et al. 2003) (N=74 patients, N=8 surgeons)	Aged ≥70 years: RR 1.43, 95% CI 1.02 to 2.01 Favours older age (Higher priority)
Decision to perform arthroplasty	1 study of expert opinions (Quintana et al. 2000) (N=125 orthopaedic surgeons)	Age = significantly associated
Indications for surgery	1 study of expert opinions (Mancuso et al. 1996) (N=378 orthopaedic surgeons)	• Age >80 = neutral factor • Age <50 = sway decision against surgery for most surgeons • Age >80 and < 2years to live as neutral factors • Age <50, cachexia and alcohol abuse = less likely
Hip or knee		
Definite willingness to undergo arthroplasty	1 observational-correlation study (Hawker et al. 2001) (N=1027)	OR 0.57 for 65–74 years of age vs 55–64 years of age, p=0.0008 Favours younger age (more willing)

▷ Gender

Two studies (Coyte et al. 1996; Juni et al. 2003) looked at the effect of gender on indications for surgery in knee osteoarthritis patients and found that gender was not associated with the decision to refer for surgery but was associated wit the patient's willingness to undergo surgery.

One study (Dolin et al. 2003) looked at the effect of gender on indications for surgery in hip osteoarthritis patients and found that gender was associated with priority to undergo surgery.

One study (Hawker et al. 2001) looked at the effect of gender on indications for surgery in hip or knee osteoarthritis patients and found that gender was not associated with willingness to undergo surgery.

Table 8.2 Effect of gender on attitudes towards surgery for OA

Gender outcome	Reference	Outcome/effect size
Knee osteoarthritis		
Patient's willingness to undergo surgery	1 cross-sectional study (Juni et al. 2003) (N=26,046)	OR 0.60, 95% CI 0.49 to 0.74 Favours men (more willing)
Referral for surgery	1 study of expert opinions (Coyte et al. 1996) (N=244 family physicians and N=96 rheumatologists)	• Age <55 years: 52% FP's = less likely and 35% = more likely to refer • Age >80 years: >70% of FPs who treated more patients with severe knee osteoarthritis = less likely to refer
Hip		
Priority for surgery	1 observational study (Dolin et al. 2003) (N=74 patients, N=8 surgeons)	RR 1.41, 95% CI 1.03 to 1.91 Favours women (higher priority)
Hip or knee		
Definite willingness to undergo arthroplasty	1 observational-correlation study (Hawker et al. 2001) (N=1027)	No association

▷ Weight/BMI

Two studies (Mancuso et al. 1995, 1996) looked at the effect of weight on indications for surgery in knee osteoarthritis patients and found that weight was associated with the decision against surgery.

Three studies (Dolin et al. 2003; Imamura et al. 1996; Mancuso et al. 1996) looked at the effect of weight on indications for surgery in hip osteoarthritis patients and found that obesity was associated with the decision against surgery in two studies but was not associated with decision for surgery in one study.

Table 8.3 Effect of weight/BMI on attitudes towards surgery for OA

Weight/BMI outcome	Reference	Outcome/effect size
Knee osteoarthritis		
Indication for surgery	1 study of expert opinions (Mancuso et al. 1996) (N=378 orthopaedic surgeons)	Obesity = sway decision against surgery for most surgeons
Indications for surgery	1 study of expert opinions (1995) (N=13 experts)	• Obesity = possible contraindication (higher mechanical failure rate) • Obese = similar to normal population for reduction in pain and disability • Data for risk factors is insufficient for weight
Hip		
Priority for surgery	1 observational study (Dolin et al. 2003) (N=74 patients, N=8 surgeons)	Not associated with obesity (BMI >30)

continued

Table 8.3 Effect of weight/BMI on attitudes towards surgery for OA – *continued*

Weight/BMI outcome	Reference	Outcome/effect size
Hip – *continued*		
Indications for surgery	1 study of expert opinions (Mancuso et al. 1996) (N=378 orthopaedic surgeons)	• Obesity = sway decision against surgery for most surgeons • Obesity = neutral or sway slightly against surgery
Appropriateness of surgery	1 study of expert opinions (Imamura et al. 1996) (N=8 orthopaedic surgeons, N=8 GPs)	• Severe obesity in Grade 3 osteoarthritis patients = surgery not appropriate (for most surgeons) and sometimes in Grade 1 or 2 osteoarthritis patients • Weight more influential than comorbidities
Hip or knee		
Definite willingness to undergo arthroplasty	1 observational-correlation study (Hawker et al. 2001) (N=1027)	OR 0.57 for 65–74 years of age vs 55–64 years of age, p=0.0008 Favours younger age (more willing)

▷ Smoking/drugs/alcohol

Three studies (Anon 1995; Coyte et al. 1996; Mancuso et al. 1996) looked at the effect of smoking, drugs or alcohol on indications for surgery in knee osteoarthritis patients. Two studies found that drug and/or alcohol use was associated with the decision against surgery. However, one study found that smoking data was insufficient to make a conclusion.

One study (Mancuso et al. 1996) looked at the effect of smoking, drugs or alcohol on indications for surgery in knee osteoarthritis patients. Two studies found that alcohol use was associated with the decision against surgery.

Table 8.4 Effect of smoking/drugs/alcohol on attitudes towards surgery for OA

Smoking/drugs/ alcohol outcome	Reference	Outcome/effect size
Knee osteoarthritis		
Indication for surgery	1 study of expert opinions (Mancuso et al. 1996) (N=378 orthopaedic surgeons)	Alcohol use = sway decision against surgery for most surgeons
Referral for surgery	1 study of expert opinions (Coyte et al. 1996) (N=244 family physicians and N=96 rheumatologists)	History of drug/alcohol abuse: >70% of FPs and rheumatologists who treated more patients with severe knee osteoarthritis = less likely to refer
Indications for surgery	1 study of expert opinions (Anon 1995) (N=13 experts)	Data for risk factors is insufficient for smoking
Hip		
Indications for surgery	1 study of expert opinions (Mancuso et al. 1996) (N=378 orthopaedic surgeons)	Alcohol use = sway decision against surgery for most surgeons

▷ Comorbidities

Three studies (Anon 1995; Coyte et al. 1996; Mancuso et al. 1996) looked at the effect of comorbidities on indications for surgery in knee osteoarthritis patients. Overall, all 3 studies found that comorbidities were associated with the decision against surgery.

Two studies (Imamura et al. 1996; Mancuso et al. 1996) looked at the effect of comorbidities on indications for surgery in hip osteoarthritis patients. One study found that comorbidities were associated with the decision against surgery, in the second study experts were not sure about the role of comorbidities.

Table 8.5 Effect of comorbidities on attitudes towards surgery in OA

Comorbidities outcome	Reference	Outcome/effect size
Knee osteoarthritis		
Indication for surgery	1 study of expert opinions (Mancuso et al. 1996) (N=378 orthopaedic surgeons)	Comorbidities = sway decision against surgery for most surgeons
Referral for surgery	1 study of expert opinions (Coyte et al. 1996) (N=244 family physicians and N=96 rheumatologists)	Patello-femoral arthritis, peripheral vascular disease and sometimes local active skin infection = less likely to refer
Indications for surgery	1 study of expert opinions (1995) (N=13 experts)	Comorbidities associated with poor outcomes. Comorbidities = local or systemic infection and other medical conditions that substantially increase the risk of serious perioperative complications or death
Hip		
Indications for surgery	1 study of expert opinions (Mancuso et al. 1996) (N=378 orthopaedic surgeons)	Comorbidities = sway decision against surgery for most surgeons. Comorbidities = neutral or sway slightly against surgery
Appropriateness of surgery	1 study of expert opinions (Imamura et al. 1996 2827) (N=8 orthopaedic surgeons, N=8 GPs)	Disagreement about role of comorbidities; comorbidities not useful in resolving uncertain indications for surgery

▷ Structural features

One study (Mancuso et al. 1996) looked at structural features as indications for surgery in knee osteoarthritis patients and found that destruction of joint space was an indication for surgery.

Four studies (Dolin et al. 2003; Dreinhofer et al. 2006; Mancuso et al. 1996; Quintana et al. 2000) looked at structural features as indications for surgery in hip osteoarthritis patients. Overall, all three studies found that joint space damage/high X-ray scores were required as an indicator for surgery. One study found bone quality was not an indication for surgery.

Table 8.6 Effect of structural features on attitudes to surgery for OA

Structural features outcome	Reference	Outcome/effect size
Knee osteoarthritis		
Indication for surgery	1 study of expert opinions (Mancuso et al. 1996) (N=378 orthopaedic surgeons)	Majority of joint space destroyed = indication
Hip		
Priority for surgery	1 observational study (Dolin et al. 2003) (N=74 patients, N=8 surgeons)	Higher X-ray ratings (score of >9/15: RR 1.98, 95% CI 1.23 to 3.19) Higher priority
Decision to perform arthroplasty	1 study of expert opinions (Quintana et al. 2000) (N=125 orthopaedic surgeons)	Quality of the bone = no association
Indications for surgery	1 study of expert opinions (Mancuso et al. 1996) (N=378 orthopaedic surgeons)	Majority of joint space destroyed = indication for surgery
Indications for surgery	1 study of expert opinions (Dreinhofer et al. 2006) (N=304 orthopaedic surgeons, N=314 referring physicians)	X-ray changes = not very important 50% JSN or total loss of joint space = indicator

▷ Symptoms, function, global assessment, QoL

Five studies (Dolin et al. 2003; Dreinhofer et al. 2006; Imamura et al. 1996; Mancuso et al. 1996; Quintana et al. 2000) looked at osteoarthritis symptoms and function as indications for surgery in hip osteoarthritis patients and found mixed results. However, pain was found by most studies to be an important requirement for surgery.

▷ Hip or knee

One study (Hawker et al. 2001) looked at osteoarthritis symptoms as indications for surgery in hip or knee osteoarthritis patients and found no association between WOMAC disease severity and willingness to undergo surgery.

Table 8.7 Effect of symptoms, function and quality of life on attitudes to surgery for OA

Symptoms, function and QoL outcome	Reference	Outcome/effect size
Knee osteoarthritis		
Indication for surgery	1 study of expert opinions (Mancuso et al. 1996) (N=378 orthopaedic surgeons)	Indications: • at least have severe daily pain and rest pain several days/week and transfer pain (eg standing up from a sitting position) several days/week • unable to walk more than 3 blocks • difficulty climbing stairs • not require marked abnormalities on physical examination – nearly normal or somewhat decreased flexion and a stable knee joint can be consistent with TKA

continued

Table 8.7 Effect of symptoms, function and quality of life on attitudes to surgery for OA – *continued*

Symptoms, function and QoL outcome	Reference	Outcome/effect size
Knee osteoarthritis – *continued*		
Referral for surgery	1 study of expert opinions (Coyte et al. 1996) (N=244 family physicians and N=96 rheumatologists)	• Pain not responsive to drug therapy = more likely to refer • Walking limited to <1 block without pain = more likely to refer • Persistent non-weight-bearing knee pain, night pain and limitations of active flexion or extension = more likely to refer
Indications for surgery	1 study of expert opinions (Anon 1995) (N=13 experts)	Indications = radiographic evidence of joint damage, moderate to severe persistent pain or disability or both (not substantially relieved by an extended nonsurgical management) usually includes trials of analgesic and NSAIDs, physical therapy, use of walking aids, reduction in physical activities that provoke discomfort)
Hip		
Priority for surgery	1 observational study (Dolin et al. 2003) (N=74 patients, N=8 surgeons)	• Higher priority = pain distress (RR 1.91, 95% CI 1.43 to 2.56); Pain intensity (RR 1.91, 95% CI 1.43 to 2.56); higher patient ratings of average pain distress (RR 1.57, 95% CI 1.13 to 2.19); higher patient ratings of average pain disruption (RR 1.41, 95% CI 1.04 to 1.92); AIMS total >50 (RR: 1.75, 95% CI 1.324 to 2.48) • Not associated with priority = patient pain intensity rating, health anxiety and walk performance
Decision to perform arthroplasty	1 study of expert opinions (Quintana et al. 2000) (N=125 orthopaedic surgeons)	• Uncertain indicators: pain and functional limitations described as 'moderate' • Significant indicators: pain and functional limitation • Panel scoring of appropriateness was more related to level of pain and to functional limitation than the other variables (age, surgical risk, previous nonsurgical treatment) for the decision to perform arthroplasty
Indications for surgery	1 study of expert opinions (Mancuso et al. 1996) (N=378 orthopaedic surgeons)	Indications: • at least have severe daily pain rest pain and transfer pain (eg standing up from a sitting position) several days/week • unable to walk more than 3 blocks or up to 10 blocks • difficulty climbing stairs and any difficulty putting on shoes and socks • reduced ROM of the hip need not be marked – flexion >45° • unable to walk up to 10 blocks

continued

Table 8.7 Effect of symptoms, function and quality of life on attitudes to surgery for OA – *continued*

Symptoms, function and QoL outcome	Reference	Outcome/effect size
Hip – *continued*		
Indications for surgery	1 study of expert opinions (Dreinhofer et al. 2006) (N=304 orthopaedic surgeons, N=314 referring physicians)	• Rest pain and pain with activity = highly important indicators • Range of motion = much less important indicator • Pain severity = important: severe pain, rest pain or night pain and need for analgesics should be present on several days/week before this is considered • Functional items such as difficulty climbing stairs and putting on shoes and socks: more referring physicians than surgeons indicated that these were very important criteria • Heterogeneity within each group on appropriate levels of pain and functional impairment • Reduced walking distance = important indicator (degree of restriction ranged from <1 km and <0.5 km) • Other impairments (including climbing stairs, putting on shoes and socks and the need for a crutch): referring physicians required more advanced disease as prerequisite than surgeons. • Quality of life issues, activities of daily living, sports and sex = most important additional items • Overall ranking of importance for pain symptoms: rest pain, night pain and pain with activities
Appropriateness of surgery	1 study of expert opinions (Imamura et al. 1996) (N=8 orthopaedic surgeons, N=8 GPs)	• Presence or absence of disability = not influential factor
Hip or knee		
Definite willingness to undergo arthroplasty	1 observational-correlation study (Hawker et al. 2001) (N=1027)	Willingness not associated with WOMAC disease severity score

▷ Osteoarthritis grade

Two studies (Coyte et al. 1996; Juni et al. 2003) looked at osteoarthritis grade as indications for surgery in knee osteoarthritis patients. Both studies found that patients with more severe disease were more willing to undergo surgery and were more likely to be referred for surgery.

Two studies (Imamura et al. 1996; Naylor and Williams 1996) looked at osteoarthritis grade as indications for surgery in hip osteoarthritis patients. Both studies found that more severe disease was a more important indicator for surgery.

Table 8.8 Effect of grade of OA on attitudes towards surgery for OA

Osteoarthritis grade outcome	Reference	Outcome/effect size
Knee osteoarthritis		
Patient's willingness to undergo surgery	1 cross-sectional study (Juni et al. 2003) (N=26,046)	OR per 10-point increase of NZ score 1.57, 95% CI 1.47 to 1.66 Favours more severe disease (more willing)
Referral for surgery	1 study of expert opinions (Coyte et al. 1996) (N=244 family physicians and N=96 rheumatologists)	Moderate-severe knee osteoarthritis by radiography = more likely to refer
Hip		
Indications for surgery	1 study of expert opinions (Naylor and Williams 1996) (N=11 experts)	• Functional class I: pain is mild or osteotomy an option = inappropriate; moderate pain osteotomy no option = case-specific judgement • Functional class III: patients <60 years old = osteotomy preferable and mild pain = cautious for surgery unless good chance of prosthesis survival Patients >60 years old = moderate and severe pain + impaired ADLs are strong indicators • Functional class IV: patients usually bedbound/wheelchair so pain on activity not a factor; severe rest pain = potentially appropriate regardless of other factors, as surgery may be only way to relieve pain; some expectation of improvement in function = surgery appropriate; mild to moderate pain + little expectation of functional improvement = need careful weighing of risks and benefits.
Urgency for surgery	1 study of expert opinions (Naylor and Williams 1996) (N=11 experts)	• Functional class I: mild pain on activity and no rest pain = low priority; moderate pain during activity = higher priority; rest pain and/or work or caregiving impeded = high priority • Functional class III: severe pain on activity (unless rest pain absent or mild) = higher priority Severe pain on activity and at rest = surgery must be provided as soon as possible • Functional class IV: most patients have severe and longstanding arthritis affecting most joints thus surgery = limited benefits for function; moderate to severe rest pain = surgery should be provided quickly; high priority = those few patients with moderate rest pain who may only recently have become confined to a wheelchair or bed and have good prospects of walking again Delay may reduce their chances of rehabilitation
Indications for surgery	1 study of expert opinions (Imamura et al. 1996) (N=8 orthopaedic surgeons, N=8 GPs)	• Severity of hip = most important indicator • Least severe grades (Charnley class 4 and 5) = inappropriate • Charnley grades 1 or 2 = appropriate for those with low comorbidity or medium comorbidity if not severely overweight

▷ Willingness

One study (Juni et al. 2003) looked at willingness of knee osteoarthritis patients to undergo surgery and found that approximately one third of patients would not accept surgery if offered and they were concerned with the risks and benefits of surgery.

One study (Hawker et al. 2001) looked at willingness of hip or knee osteoarthritis patients in high and low-rate surgery areas to undergo surgery and found that patients in high rate arthroplasty areas were more willing to undergo surgery.

Table 8.9 Willingness to undergo surgery for OA

Willingness outcome	Reference	Outcome/effect size
Knee osteoarthritis		
Patient's willingness to undergo surgery	1 cross-sectional study (Juni et al. 2003) (N=26,046)	• Approximately one third of participants considered for TKA indicated that they would not accept surgery if offered • Majority concerned about risks and benefits of TKA
Hip or knee		
Willingness to undergo arthroplasty	1 observational-correlation study (Hawker et al. 2001) (N=1027)	For patients with severe arthritis: • definitely willing: 8.5% and 14.9% (in low-rate and high-rate arthroplasty areas) • probably willing: 17.5% and 21.5% (in low-rate and high-rate arthroplasty areas) • unsure: 18.5% and 19.4% (in low-rate and high-rate arthroplasty areas) • definitely or probably unwilling: 55.5% and 44.2% (in low-rate and high-rate arthroplasty areas) • needs for arthroplasty, adjusted for willingness (expressed per 1000 phase in respondents): 2.4% and 5.4% (in low-rate and high-rate arthroplasty areas) • patients in the high-rate area were significantly more likely to know someone who had undergone joint arthroplasty, compared with those in the low-rate area (94.3% and 72.7% respectively, $p<0.001$)

▷ Use of assistive devices

One study (Mancuso et al. 1996) looked at the effect of usage of assistive devices by knee osteoarthritis patients on the decision to undergo surgery and found that assistive device use did not affect the decision to perform surgery.

One study (Mancuso et al. 1996) looked at the effect of usage of assistive devices by hip osteoarthritis patients on the decision to undergo surgery and found that overall, assistive device use did not affect the decision to perform surgery.

Osteoarthritis

Table 8.10 Effect of assistive device use on attitude towards surgery for OA

Assistive devices outcome	Reference	Outcome/effect size
Knee osteoarthritis		
Indication for surgery	1 study of expert opinions (Mancuso et al. 1996) (N=378 orthopaedic surgeons)	Assistive device was not a uniform requirement – use of a cane or crutch several days/week or less often to be consistent with TKA
Hip		
Indication for surgery	1 study of expert opinions (Mancuso et al. 1996) (N=378 orthopaedic surgeons)	• Assistive device was not a uniform requirement – use of a cane or crutch several days/week or less often to be consistent with TKA • More Canadian than US surgeons required an assistive device to be used every day and the use of a cane with stairs

▷ Patient psychological factors (including expectations)

Three studies (Anon 1995; Coyte et al. 1996; Mancuso et al. 1996) (N=13 experts) looked at the effect of psychological factors on indications for surgery in knee osteoarthritis patients and all studies found that psychological factors were important indicators affecting the decision to perform surgery.

One study (Mancuso et al. 1996) looked at the effect of psychological factors on indications for surgery in hip osteoarthritis patients and all studies found that psychological factors were important indicators affecting the decision to perform surgery.

Table 8.11 Effect of psychological factors in attitudes towards surgery for OA

Patient psychological factors outcome	Reference	Outcome/effect size
Knee osteoarthritis		
Indication for surgery	1 study of expert opinions (Mancuso et al. 1996) (N=378 orthopaedic surgeons)	• Desire to derive psychological benefit from surgery, desire to return to sports, unrealistic expectations, poor motivation, limited cooperation, hostile personality, depression and dementia = sway decision against surgery • Wanting to be independent and return to work = sway decision for surgery and was the most favourable factor • US surgeons had a greater tendency to rate borderline mental status and other psychiatric diagnoses more unfavourably than Canadian surgeons
Referral for surgery	1 study of expert opinions (Coyte et al. 1996) (N=244 family physicians and N=96 rheumatologists)	• Patient demands TKA and sensation of instability by patient = more likely to refer • Major psychiatric disorders = less likely to refer

continued

Table 8.11 Effect of psychological factors in attitudes towards surgery for OA – *continued*

Patient psychological factors outcome	Reference	Outcome/effect size
Knee osteoarthritis – *continued*		
Indications for surgery	1 study of expert opinions (Anon 1995) (N=13 experts)	The patient's goals and expectations should be ascertained prior to THA to determine whether they are realistic and attainable by the recommended therapeutic approach. Any discrepancies between the patient's expectations and the likely outcome should be discussed in detail with the patient and family members before surgery.
Hip		
Indications for surgery	1 study of expert opinions (Mancuso et al. 1996) (N=378 orthopaedic surgeons)	• Desire to derive psychological benefit from surgery, desire to return to sports, unrealistic expectations, poor motivation, limited cooperation, hostile personality, depression and dementia = sway decision against surgery • Wanting to be independent and return to work = sway decision for surgery

▷ Postoperative care and physician advice

One study (Mancuso et al. 1996) looked at the effect of home care on the decision to perform surgery in knee osteoarthritis patients and found that limited home care did not affect the decision to perform surgery.

Two studies (Mancuso et al. 1996; Quintana et al. 2000) looked at the effect of limited home care and previous nonsurgical treatment and surgical risk on indications for surgery in hip osteoarthritis patients and found that limited home care did not affect the decision to perform surgery but previous nonsurgical treatment and surgical risk significantly affected the decision.

One study (Hawker et al. 2001) looked at the effect of interaction with their physician on willingness to undergo surgery in patients with hip or knee osteoarthritis and found mixed results.

Table 8.12 Effect of postoperative care and physician advice on attitudes to surgery for OA

Postoperative care and physician advice outcome	Reference	Outcome/effect size
Knee osteoarthritis		
Indication for surgery	1 study of expert opinions (Mancuso et al. 1996) (N=378 orthopaedic surgeons)	• Limited home care = no effect on decision for surgery • Limited home care and inadequate available rehabilitation = mostly rated neutral
Hip		
Decision to perform arthroplasty	1 study of expert opinions (Quintana et al. 2000) (N=125 orthopaedic surgeons)	Surgical risk and previous nonsurgical treatment = significantly associated with decision

continued

Table 8.12 Effect of postoperative care and physician advice on attitudes to surgery for OA – *continued*

Postoperative care and physician advice outcome	Reference	Outcome/effect size
Hip – *continued*		
Indications for surgery	1 study of expert opinions (Mancuso et al. 1996) (N=378 orthopaedic surgeons)	Limited home care = no effect on decision for surgery
Hip or knee		
Definite willingness to undergo arthroplasty	1 observational-correlation study (Hawker et al. 2001) (N=1027)	• There was NS difference between patients suitable for arthroplasty in the low-and high-rate arthroplasty areas for: number of patients under the care of a physician for their arthritis and number of patients having discussed arthroplasty with their physician • Patients suitable for arthroplasty in the low-rate arthroplasty area had a significantly higher number of patients who were recommended by their physician for arthroplasty (20% and 28% of potential candidates respectively, p<0.001) • Definite willingness to undergo arthroplasty was significantly associated with having ever spoken with a physician (OR 2.93, p=0.0001)

8.1.5 Evidence statements: predictors of benefit and harm

▷ Age

Knee osteoarthritis

Peri-operative complications/hospital stay

One case-series (Jones et al. 2001) (N=454) found that for TKA patients:

• there was non-significant difference between younger and older patients for length of stay in the acute care setting or rehabilitation facilities and in-hospital complications

• older age groups were more likely to be transferred to rehabilitation facilities regardless of joint type replaced (older patients with TKA = 83%, younger patients 40%).

One case-series (Solomon et al. 2006) (N=124) found that:

• older age (71–80 years or ≥81 years versus 65–70 years) was a significant predictor of AEs

• patients at low risk of AEs included those with fewer than two of the following risk factors: age more than 70 years, male gender, one or more comorbid illnesses:
  – age 71–80 years: OR 1.3 (95% CI 1.0 to 1.6)
  – age 81–95 years: OR 1.6 (95% CI 1.1 to 2.4).

One case-series (Gill et al. 2003) (N=3048) found that older patients had a much higher mortality rate post TKA:

• patients aged <65 years: mortality rate 0.13% (N=1 out of N=755 patients)

• patients aged ≥85 years: mortality rate 4.65% (N=4 out of N=86 patients)

• risk ratio was 14 times higher in patients aged ≥85 years than the rest of the patients (OR 13.7, 95% CI 3.0 to 44.8).

Long-term survival of prosthesis

One case-series (Harrysson et al. 2004) (N=35, 857) found that for TKA:

- the cumulative revision rate for TKA due to:
  - any cause was higher in younger patients (<60 years old) than the older group (≥60 years old) at 8.5 years post-surgery (13% and 6% respectively)
  - loosening of components was higher in younger patients (<60 years old) than the older group (≥60 years old) at 8.5 years post-surgery (6% and 2.5% respectively).

While for TKA patients, regression analysis showed that risk for revision due to:
  - any cause was significantly lower (risk ratio 0.49, 95% CI 0.38 to 0.62, p<0.0001) in the older patients (≥60 years) compared with younger patients (<60 years)
  - loosening of components was significantly lower (risk ratio 0.41, 95% CI 0.27 to 0.62, p<0.0001) in the older patients (≥60 years) compared with younger patients (<60 years)
  - any cause attributable to year of surgery decreased each year (risk ratio 0.92, 95% CI 0.89 to 0.96, p<0.0001) in the older patients (≥60 years) compared with younger patients (<60 years)
  - loosening of components attributable to year of surgery decreased each year (risk ratio 0.87, 95% CI 0.82 to 0.94, p=0.0001) in the older patients (≥60 years) compared with younger patients (<60 years)
  - infection attributable to year of surgery decreased each year (risk ratio 0.91, 95% CI 0.85 to 0.96, p=0.0015) in the older patients (≥60 years) compared with younger patients (<60 years)
  - and that there was no significant difference between the older (≥60 years) and younger patients (<60 years), for risk of revision due to infection.

The same case-series (Harrysson et al. 2004) (N=35, 857) found that for unicompartmental KA cumulative revision rate due to:

- any cause was higher in younger patients (<60 years old) than the older group (≥60 years old) at 9.2 years post-surgery (22% and 14% respectively)
- loosening of components was higher in younger patients (<60 years old) than the older group (≥60 years old) at 9.5 years post-surgery (8% and 6.5% respectively).

While regression analysis showed that for unicompartmental KA patients:
  - risk for revision due to any cause was significantly lower (risk ratio 0.55, 95% CI 0.45 to 0.65, p<0.0001) in the older patients (≥60 years) compared with younger patients (<60 years)
  - risk for revision due to loosening of components was significantly lower (risk ratio 0.63, 95% CI 0.48 to 0.83, p=0.0012) in the older patients (≥60 years) compared with younger patients (<60 years)
  - there was no significant difference between the older (≥60 years) and younger patients (<60 years), for risk of revision due to infection
  - risk for revision (due to any cause) attributable to year of surgery decreased each year (risk ratio 0.94, 95% CI 0.91 to 0.97, p=0.0001) in the older patients (≥60 years) compared with younger patients (<60 years)
  - risk for revision (due to loosening of components) attributable to year of surgery decreased each year (risk ratio 0.91, 95% CI 0.87 to 0.96, p=0.0002) in the older patients (≥60 years) compared with younger patients (<60 years)

- there was no significant difference between the older (≥60 years) and younger patients (<60 years), for risk of revision due to infection attributable to year of surgery.

Symptoms (pain, stiffness), function, QoL

One case-series (Elson and Breknel 2006) (N=512) found that:
- younger age was a predictor of poor outcome (high pain score)
- age was a significant predictor of TKA outcome:
  - younger patients were significantly associated with poor outcome (high pain score), pain at 5 years post-surgery (17% aged <60 years vs 7% aged 60–64, p<0.05; 13% aged 60–70; 7% aged >70)
  - patients aged less than 60 years are more than twice as likely to report poor outcome scores (high pain at 5 years post-surgery) than those older than 60 years
  - patients who had unilateral TKA (first knee) and those who had staged unilateral TKA (second knee) were significantly more likely to have poor outcome scores (high pain at 5 years post surgery) than those who had bilateral TKA at the same time (13%, 6% and 2% respectively, p<0.01).

One case-series (Jones et al. 2001) (N=454) found that for TKA patients, age was not a strong predictor of postoperative WOMAC pain or function.

One case-series (Lingard et al. 2004) (N=860) found that older age was a strong predictor of SF-36 physical functioning at 2 years post-surgery.

One case-series (Escobar et al. 2007) (N=855) found that age was:
- associated with postoperative SF-36 scores and WOMAC scores
- not a predictor of postoperative SF-36 physical function, bodily pain, vitality, social functioning, role emotional, mental health, role physical
- a predictor of postoperative SF-36 general health
- a predictor of postoperative WOMAC pain, and stiffness
- not a predictor of postoperative WOMAC function.

Hip osteoarthritis

Peri-operative complications/hospital stay

One case-series (Jones et al. 2001) (N=454) found that for THA patients there was a NS difference between younger and older patients for:
- length of stay in the i) acute care setting; ii) rehabilitation facilities
- in-hospital complications.

While the older age group were more likely to be transferred to rehabilitation facilities regardless of joint type replaced.

Long-term survival of prosthesis

One case-series (Johnsen et al. 2006) (N=36, 984) found that:

- older age was associated with increased RR of failure in patients aged ≥80 years (RR 1.6, 95% CI 1.0 to 2.6) compared with patients aged 60–69 years at 0–30 days after primary THA
- younger age was associated with increased RR of failure in patients aged 10 to 49 years (RR 1.7, 95% CI 1.3 to 2.3) and patients aged 50 to 59 years (RR 1.3, 95% CI 1.0 to 1.6) compared with patients aged 60–69 years. Patients aged 70–79 years and ≥80 years were associated with a lower RR for failure (RR 0.9, 95% CI 0.7 to 1.0) and (RR 0.6, 95% CI 0.5 to 0.8) respectively at 6 months to 8.6 years after primary THA.

Symptoms (pain, stiffness), function, QoL

One case-series (Jones et al. 2001) (N=454) found that for THA patients, age was not a strong predictor of postoperative WOMAC pain or function.

One case-series (Roder et al. 2007) (N=12,925) found by linear regression that patients were an average of 1.6 years older per category of reduced preoperative walking capacity (p<0.01; effect size 0.4), indicating that age had a moderate effect on deterioration of preoperative walking capacity.

Thumb osteoarthritis

Symptoms (pain, stiffness), function, QoL

One case-series (Degreef and De 2006) (N=36) found that age at operation was not a significant predictor of surgical outcome (DASH score – disabilities of the arm, shoulder and hand).

▷ Gender

Knee osteoarthritis

Peri-operative complications/hospital stay

One case-series (Solomon et al. 2006) (N=124) found that:

- male gender was a significant predictor of AEs.

Patients at low risk of AEs included those with fewer than two of the following risk factors; age >70 years, male gender, one or more comorbid illnesses.

Long-term survival of prosthesis

- One case-series (Harrysson et al. 2004) (N=35, 857) found that for TKA there was no significant risk of TKA revision due to any cause or component loosening associated with gender.
- Men were significantly more likely than women to have TKA revision due to infection (risk ratio 1.64, 95% CI 1.23 to 2.18, p=0.0007).
- The same case-series (Harrysson et al. 2004) (N=35, 857) found that for unicompartmental KA there was no significant risk of revision due to any cause or component loosening associated with gender.

- Men were significantly more likely than women to have unicompartmental KA revision due to infection (risk ratio 1.88, 95% CI 1.13 to 3.14, p=0.0156).

Symptoms (pain, stiffness), function, QoL

One case-series (Elson and Breknel 2006) (N=512) found that gender was not associated with outcome of TKA (pain at 5 years post-surgery).

One case-series (Escobar et al. 2007) (N=855) found that gender was:
- associated with postoperative SF-36 scores and WOMAC scores
- a predictor of postoperative WOMAC stiffness
- not a predictor of postoperative:
    - SF-36 physical function, bodily pain, role physical, vitality, role emotional, mental health
    - WOMAC pain.

While male gender was:
- not a predictor of postoperative SF-36 general health
- a predictor of postoperative SF-36 social functioning and WOMAC function.

And female gender was:
- not a predictor of postoperative SF-36 social functioning
- a predictor of postoperative SF-36 general health.

▷ Hip osteoarthritis

Long-term survival of prosthesis/hospital stay

One case-series (Johnsen et al. 2006) (N=36, 984) found that:
- male gender was associated with an increased RR of THA failure of any cause (RR 1.5, 95% CI 1.1 to 2.0) at 0–30 days (RR 1.2, 95% CI 1.0 to 1.4) at 6 months to 8.6 years after primary THA
- there was no association between THA failure and gender or age at 31 days to 6 months after primary THA.

Symptoms (pain, stiffness), function, QoL

One cohort study (Nilsdotter et al. 2001) (N=3144) found that:
- there was no difference between men and women for postoperative outcome (WOMAC and SF-36) at 6 months and 12 months post-THA surgery
- gender was not associated with postoperative WOMAC pain or physical function at 12 months post-THA surgery.

▷ Thumb osteoarthritis

Long-term survival of prosthesis

One case-series (Chakrabarti et al. 1997) (N=71) found that women had a higher prosthesis survival rate than men (N=7, 85% and N=4, 36% respectively).

▷ Weight/BMI

Knee osteoarthritis

One case-series (Messieh 1999) (N=124) found that body weight of 180 lbs or more was not significantly associated with symptomatic pulmonary embolism.

One case-control study (Amin et al. 2006) (N=79) found that overall rate of complications following TKA was significantly higher in the morbidly obese group compared with the non-obese group (32% and 0% respectively, p=0.001).

Long-term survival of prosthesis

One case-control study (Spicer et al. 2001) (N=656) found that:
- there was NS difference between obese and non-obese patients for percentage of revisions (4.9% and 3.1% respectively)
- revision due to osteolysis was significantly higher in the obese group compared with the non-obese group (p=0.016)
- higher BMI was associated with an increase in incidence of focal osteolysis
- survival analysis showed NS difference for revision of any component between obese and non-obese patients (98.1% and 99.9% survival rates respectively). This similarity was maintained until the 10th year post-operatively (97.2% and 95.5% respectively).

One case-control study (Amin et al. 2006) (N=79) found that overall rate of TKA revisions and revisions plus pain (5-year survivorship) was significantly higher in the morbidly obese group compared with the non-obese group (p=0.01 and p=0.02 respectively).

Symptoms (pain, stiffness), function, QoL

- One case-series (De Leeuw and Villar 1998) (N=101) found that improvement in postoperative QoL was significantly greater in the obese groups compared with the non-obese group.
- Two case-control studies (Amin et al. 2006; Spicer et al. 2001) found that there was NS difference between obese and non-obese patients for KSS score at the most recent follow-up for function, absolute improvement and knee scores.

One case-series (Escobar et al. 2007) (N=855) found that BMI was not associated with postoperative SF-36 scores and WOMAC scores.

▷ Hip osteoarthritis

Peri-operative complications/hospital stay

One case-series (Sadr et al. 2006) (N=3309) found that:
- increasing BMI was significantly associated with length of stay in hospital (p<0.001)
- compared with the normal weight group, mean length of hospital stay increased by 4.7% in the overweight group and 7.0% in the obese group (multivariate logistic regression)
- there was NS association between increasing BMI and risk of systemic postoperative complications
- in the obese group, there was a 58% risk (OR 1.58, 95% CI 1.06 to 2.35) of systemic postoperative complications compared with those of normal weight.

Symptoms (pain, stiffness), function, QoL

One case-series (Jain et al. 2003) (N=78) found that:
- there was no correlation between pre-operative BMI and post-operative mobility, WOMAC pain, function or other complications.

▷ Smoking

Hip osteoarthritis

Peri-operative complications/hospital stay

One case-series (Sadr et al. 2006) (N=3309) found that:
- there was NS association between smoking status or tobacco preference and the mean length of stay (after adjusting for covariates of age, BMI and so on)
- smoking status significantly increased the risk of systemic postoperative complications (p=0.013)
- previous and current smokers had increased risks of suffering from postoperative complications compared with non-smokers (multivariate logistic regression analysis): 43% (OR 1.32, 95% CI 1.04 to 1.97) and 56% (OR 1.56, 95% CI 1.14 to 2.14) respectively
- there was NS association between postoperative complications and preference for different tobacco products
- number of pack years of tobacco smoking was significantly associated with increased risk of systemic postoperative complications (p=0.004)
- the heaviest tobacco smoking group was associated with a 121% (OR 2.21, 95% CI 1.28 to 3.82) increased risk of systemic complications compared with non-smokers (multivariate logistic regression analysis)
- there was NS difference between smoking for:
  - 0–19.9 pack years and non-smokers for risk of systemic complications
  - status, preference of tobacco product or pack years and local complications.

▷ Comorbidities

Knee

Peri-operative complications/hospital stay

One case-series (Gill et al. 2003) (N=3048) found that cardiovascular comorbidities significantly influenced mortality rate after TKA (p<0.0001). Risk of mortality associated with comorbidities was 16 times higher than when comorbidities were absent (OR 15.9, 95% CI 3.4 to 143.5).

Symptoms (pain, stiffness), function, QoL

One case-series (Lingard et al. 2004) (N=860) found that a greater number of comorbid conditions was a strong predictor of SF-36 physical functioning at 2 years post-surgery.

One case-series (Escobar et al. 2007) (N=855) found that:
- low back pain and comorbidities were associated with postoperative SF-36 scores and WOMAC scores

- low back pain and Charlson Index were not predictors of postoperative SF-36 physical function
- low back pain and Charlson Index were predictors of postoperative SF-36 bodily pain
- Charlson index 1 and low back pain were not predictors of postoperative SF-36 general health
- Charlson Index ≥2 was a predictor of postoperative SF-36 general health
- low back pain and Charlson Index were not predictors of postoperative SF-36 role physical
- low back pain and Charlson Index were predictors of postoperative SF-36 vitality
- low back pain was not a predictor of postoperative SF-36 social functioning
- Charlson Index was a predictor of postoperative SF-36 social functioning
- low back pain and Charlson Index ≥2 were not predictors of postoperative SF-36 role emotional
- Charlson Index 1 was a predictor of postoperative SF-36 role emotional
- gender, age and Charlson Index were not predictors of postoperative SF-36 mental health
- low back pain was a predictor of postoperative SF-36 mental health
- Charlson Index 1 was not a predictor of postoperative WOMAC pain
- low back pain and Charlson Index ≥2 were predictors of postoperative WOMAC pain
- Charlson Index 1 was not a predictor of postoperative WOMAC Function
- low back pain and Charlson Index ≥2 were predictors of postoperative WOMAC function
- Charlson Index was not a predictor of postoperative WOMAC stiffness
- low back pain and Charlson Index were predictors of postoperative WOMAC stiffness.

Hip osteoarthritis

Peri-operative complications/hospital stay

One case-series (Solomon et al. 2006) (N=124) found that:

- comorbid illnesses (1 or 2+ versus none) was a significant predictor of AEs
- patients at low risk of AEs included those with fewer than two of the following risk factors: age >70 years, male gender 1 or more comorbid illnesses.

Long-term survival of prosthesis

One case-series (Johnsen et al. 2006) (N=36, 984) found that:

- a high comorbidity index score was a strong predictor of THA failure compared with a low comorbidity index score (RR 2.3, 95% CI 1.6 to 3.5) at 0–30 days and (RR 3.0, 95% CI 2.1 to 4.5) at 31 days to 6 months after primary THA
- a medium comorbidity index score was associated with reduced RR of failure (RR 0.7, 95% CI 0.6 to 0.8) compared with a low comorbidity score whereas a high comorbidity index score was a strong predictor of THA failure compared with a low comorbidity index score (RR 2.8, 95% CI 2.3 to 3.3) at 6 months to 8.6 years after primary THA.

Symptoms (pain, stiffness), function, QoL

One case-series (Roder et al. 2007) (N=12,925) found that comorbidities influenced the post-operative walking capacity: there was a consistent increase in the percentage of Charnley class-C patients with each decrease in category of pre-operative walking capacity at each of the follow-up years.

▷ Structural features

Knee osteoarthritis

Symptoms (pain, stiffness), function, QoL

One cohort study (Caracciolo and Giaquinto 2005) (N=146) found that in TKA patients preoperative Charnley or modified Charnley Class C was not a predictor of postoperative WOMAC function.

One case-series (Goutallier et al. 2006) (N=68) found that preoperative medial femorotibial narrowing did not influence postoperative (valgus tibial osteotomy) functional outcome at the time of last follow-up or radiographic outcome at one year post-surgery.

Hip osteoarthritis

Symptoms (pain, stiffness), function, QoL

One cohort study (Caracciolo and Giaquinto 2005) (N=146) found that in THA patients, pre-operative Charnley or modified Charnley Class C was not a predictor of postoperative WOMAC function.

One case-series (Meding et al. 2000) (N=1015) found that:
- patients with a greater degree of pre-surgery cartilage space loss had significantly less hip pain at 6 months (p=0.0016) and 1 year (p=0.0028) post-THA surgery
- there was non-significant association between degree of cartilage space loss and hip pain at 3, 5 and 7 years post-THA surgery
- patients with pre-surgery superior cartilage space loss (femoral head migration) had significantly less pain at 6 months post-THA surgery (p<0.05) compared with those with mainly global or medial hip cartilage space
- there was non-significant association between pre-surgery osteophyte formation and post-THA pain
- there was non-significant association between the pre-surgery degree of cartilage space loss, direction of cartilage space loss or osteophyte formation and post-operative Harris hip score at 1 month, 3 months, 5 years and 7 years post-THA surgery.

Shoulder osteoarthritis

Symptoms (pain, stiffness), function, QoL

One case-series (Iannotti and Norris 2003) (N=154) found that:
- patients with rotator cuff tear that were treated with total shoulder arthroplasty had better postoperative active external rotation that those treated with hemiarthroplasty
- preoperative glenoid erosion significantly affected postoperative ROM for patients with hemiarthroplasty
- patients with moderate-severe glenoid erosion treated with total arthroplasty had significantly greater increase in postoperative active external rotation compared with hemiarthroplasty (p=0.0013)

- there was NS difference between total and hemi-arthroplasty patients with glenoid erosion for postoperative active forward flexion
- there was NS difference between total and hemi-arthroplasty patients with or without glenoid erosion for postoperative American shoulder and elbow surgeons' scores
- degree of glenoid erosion did not affect the outcome of shoulder arthroplasty in any of the patients
- for patients treated with total or hemi-arthroplasty, there was NS difference between shoulders with or without preoperative posterior subluxation of the humeral head for:
  - postoperative American shoulder and elbow surgeons' scores
  - postoperative pain
  - postoperative active external rotation
- there was non-significant difference between total or hemi-arthroplasty patients who were without preoperative glenoid erosion or humeral head subluxation, for postoperative American shoulder and elbow surgeons' scores.

Thumb osteoarthritis

Symptoms (pain, stiffness), function, QoL

One case-series (Degreef and De 2006) (N=36) found that preoperative web angle, hyperextension of the MCP and flexion of the MCP were all significant predictors (p<0.05) of surgical outcome (DASH score – disabilities of the arm, shoulder and hand).

▷ Symptoms, function, QoL

Knee osteoarthritis

Symptoms (pain, stiffness), function, QoL

One case-series (Elson and Breknel 2006) (N=512) found that preoperative pain scores as well as mobility on stairs was a predictors of poor outcome (high pain score).

One cohort study (Caracciolo and Giaquinto 2005) (N=146) found that in TKA patients, preoperative WOMAC function was:
- significantly associated with postoperative function (p<0.001)
- a significant predictor of higher postoperative WOMAC function (OR 1.15, 95% CI 1.04 to 1.28).

One case-series (Lingard et al. 2004) (N=860) found that:
- preoperative WOMAC pain score was a strong determinant of postoperative WOMAC pain at 1 and 2 years post surgery
- preoperative SF-36 score was a strong determinant of postoperative WOMAC pain at 1 and 2 years post surgery
- preoperative WOMAC function score was a strong determinant of postoperative WOMAC function at 1 and 2 years post surgery
- there was NS difference between men and women with respect to WOMAC function at 1 year and 2 years post surgery

- patients with preoperative WOMAC function in the lowest quartile (<34) had considerable functional disability after TKA (mean scores 62.1 and 59.8 for 1 year and 2 years post surgery)
- patients with preoperative WOMAC function in the lowest quartile (<34) had considerable functional disability after TKA (mean scores 62.1 and 59.8 for 1 year and 2 years post surgery)
- patients with preoperative WOMAC function in the lowest quartile (<34) had the greatest improvement in WOMAC function after TKA compared with other groups: they were over four times more likely (OR 4.12, 95% CI 2.86 to 6.25) to have a score of ≤60 at 2 years post surgery than patients with preoperative WOMAC function score of >35
- preoperative SF-36 physical functioning score was a strong predictor of SF-36 physical functioning at 1 year and 2 years post surgery
- older age and greater number of comorbid conditions were also strong predictors of SF-36 physical functioning at 2 years post surgery.

One case-series (Kennedy et al. 2003) (N=812) found that:
- there was NS difference between men and women for postoperative improvement in AKS score at 5 years post-TKR
- increased age (up to 70–73 age-group) was associated with an increase in postoperative improvement in AKS score at 5 years post-TKR
- older age (>73 years) was associated with a significant decrease (p<0.05) in postoperative improvement in AKS score at 5 years post-TKR – the 79–86 year age-group showed the least improvement
- patients with the worst preoperative AKS scores had significantly greater improvement (p<0.001) in AKS score at 5 years post-TKR compared with those with higher preoperative AKS scores.

One case-series (Escobar et al. 2007) (N=855) found that preoperative SF-36 domains for mental health and:
- physical function were predictors of postoperative SF-36 physical function
- bodily pain were predictors of postoperative SF-36 bodily pain
- general health were predictors of postoperative SF-36 general health
- role physical were predictors of postoperative SF-36 role physical
- vitality were predictors of postoperative SF-36 vitality
- social functioning were predictors of postoperative SF-36 social functioning
- role emotional were predictors of postoperative SF-36 role emotional
- preoperative WOMAC pain were predictors of postoperative WOMAC pain
- preoperative WOMAC function were predictors of postoperative WOMAC function
- preoperative WOMAC stiffness were predictors of postoperative WOMAC stiffness.

Hip osteoarthritis

Symptoms (pain, stiffness), function, QoL

One cohort study (Caracciolo and Giaquinto 2005) (N=146) found that in THA patients, preoperative WOMAC function was:
- significantly associated with postoperative function (p<0.005)
- a significant predictor of higher postoperative WOMAC function (OR 1.44, 95% CI 1.07 to 1.92).

One cohort study (Nilsdotter et al. 2001) (N=3144) found that preoperative:
- pain was significantly associated with postoperative pain at 12 months (p=0.011)
- physical function was significantly associated with postoperative physical function at 12 months (p<0.006).

One case-series (Roder et al. 2007) (N=12,925) found that:
- there was NS difference between the proportion of pain-free patients in any of the preoperative pain categories
- there were significant differences (p<0.01) between the preoperative walking capacity groups with respect to postoperative walking capacity >60 minutes.
  - patients with the worst preoperative walking capacity had the worst postoperative recovery of walking capacity
  - patients with the highest preoperative walking capacity had the best postoperative walking capacity.
- there were significant differences (p<0.01) between the preoperative hip flexion groups with respect to postoperative hip flexion.
  - patients with preoperative flexion ≤70 had the worst postoperative recovery of motion (flexion)
  - patients with excellent range of preoperative flexion sustained a slight loss of flexion range post surgery.
- patients with excellent preoperative hip ROM (flexion) were an average of 3 years older (p<0.01) than those with the poorest preoperative ROM.

▷ Shoulder

Symptoms (pain, stiffness), function, QoL

One case-series (Iannotti and Norris 2003) (N=154) found that:
- severity of preoperative loss of passive external rotation was found to significantly affect the postoperative range of external motion (p=0.006):
  - hemiarthroplasty: patients with preoperative external rotation of <10° had mean postoperative external rotation of 25°, compared with those with preoperative ≥10° had mean 47° postoperatively
  - total arthroplasty: patients with preoperative external rotation of <10° had mean postoperative external rotation of 43°, compared with those with preoperative ≥10° had mean 50° postoperatively
- preoperative internal rotation contracture did not have an adverse effect on results of total shoulder arthroplasties

- the severity of preoperative loss of forward flexion had no effect on postoperative forward flexion after either hemi- or total-arthroplasty
- presence of full thickness repairable rotator cuff tear (isolated to the supraspinatus tendon) did not affect post-operative American shoulder and elbow surgeons' scores for pain or function, decrease in pain or patient satisfaction.

Thumb osteoarthritis

Symptoms (pain, stiffness), function, QoL

One case-series (Degreef and De 2006) (N=36) found that range of motion was not a significant predictors of surgical outcome (DASH score).

▷ Osteoarthritis grade

Hip osteoarthritis

Symptoms (pain, stiffness), function, QoL

One cohort study (Nilsdotter et al. 2001) (N=3144) found that:
- patients with severe preoperative radiographic osteoarthritis did not differ from the moderate osteoarthritis group with respect to postoperative SF-36 and WOMAC scores at 6 months and 12 months post-THA surgery
- preoperative radiographic grade of osteoarthritis was not associated with postoperative WOMAC pain or physical function at 12 months post-THA surgery.

One case-series (Schmalzried et al. 2005) (N=147) found that:
- preoperative hip grade was not associated with postoperative Harris Hip score
- postoperative UCLA activity scores were similar for all preoperative hip grades
- preoperative hip grade influenced the amount of postoperative pain
- mild-moderate pain was significantly less frequent at latest follow-up in Grade A hips compared with Grade B and C combined (3% and 18% respectively, p=0.03)
- preoperative lower grade hips showed greater postoperative improvement in ROM
- improvement in flexion, extension, abduction and external rotation were significantly greater in Grade B and C hips combined compared with Grade A (all: p<0.04).

Thumb osteoarthritis

Symptoms (pain, stiffness), function, QoL

One case-series (Degreef and De 2006) (N=36) found that radiographic stage was not a significant predictor of surgical outcome (DASH score).

▷ Other outcomes

Knee osteoarthritis

Symptoms (pain, stiffness), function, QoL

One case-series (Escobar et al. 2007) (N=855) found that social support was:
- associated with postoperative SF-36 scores and WOMAC scores
- not a predictor of postoperative SF-36 physical function, bodily pain, vitality, social functioning, WOMAC stiffness
- a predictor of postoperative SF-36 general health, role physical, role emotional, mental health, WOMAC pain, WOMAC function, hospital was not associated with postoperative SF-36 scores and WOMAC scores.

Peri-operative complications/hospital stay

One case-series (Messieh 1999) (N=124) found that:
- preoperative Hb level ≥14 g/L was significantly associated with the development of symptomatic pulmonary embolism (p=0.011)
- bilateral TKA was significantly associated with the development of symptomatic pulmonary embolism (p≤0.05)
- preoperative Hb level ≥14 g/L was a predictor of pulmonary embolism (OR 2.4, 95% CI 1.2 to 4.6)
- bilateral TKA was a predictor of pulmonary embolism (OR 7.2, 95% CI 1.3 to 39.6).

Thumb osteoarthritis

Symptoms (pain, stiffness), function, QoL

One case-series (Degreef and De 2006) (N=36) found that surgical procedure and hand dominance were not significant predictors of surgical outcome (DASH score).

8.1.6 Health economic evidence

We looked at studies that conducted economic evaluations involving referral to joint surgery for patients with osteoarthritis. One paper from New Zealand investigating 153 patients on orthopaedic waiting lists was found (Fielden et al. 2005). The paper investigates the waiting times for patients, and the cost incurred by the patients, as well as considering the health status of patients at different time points before and after surgery. The paper concludes that the cost is significantly higher for patients who wait longer than 6 months for surgery compared with patients who wait less than 6 months. However, it is interesting to note that this is from a societal perspective. Costs are significantly higher for personal and societal costs for the group that waits over 6 months, but for medical costs alone the cost is higher but not statistically significantly so. The paper also finds that the health of patients generally worsens over time up until their operation, after which health improves, suggesting that the longer a patient waits the more health losses they accrue as opposed to someone who is treated more quickly.

8.1.7 From evidence to recommendations

Although demand and frequency of joint replacement continues to rise there is very little evidence on which to base decisions about who to refer. The most effective techniques for defining criteria to guide appropriate referral have been the development of expert guided consensus. The purpose of these criteria is to quantify the benefit/risk ratio in order to inform patients and referrers of the appropriateness of treatment. However, each decision remains individual and ultimately it is the patient who must decide on their own risk/benefit calculation based upon the severity of their symptoms, their general health, their expectations of lifestyle and activity and the effectiveness of any non-surgical treatments. Referral for consideration of surgery should allow all patients who may benefit to have access to a health worker, usually the surgeon, who can inform that decision.

The use of orthopaedic scores and questionnaire-based assessments has become widespread. These usually assess pain, functional impairment and sometimes radiographic damage. The most common are the New Zealand score and the Oxford hip or knee score. Many (such as the Oxford tools) were designed to measure population-based changes following surgery, and none have been validated for the assessment of appropriateness of referral.

Similarly the use of radiographic reports as a basis for referral decisions is unreliable. This is because radiographs appearances do not correlate well with symptoms, significant painful lesions may not be detectable on plain radiographs and the radiographs are often inadequately performed, for example, non-weight bearing radiographs of the knee.

The restriction of referral for consideration of surgery based on other health issues such as BMI age or comorbidities has no basis in evidence. There are some groups of patients for whom the risks of postoperative complication may be slightly higher or the long-term outcomes of joint replacement worse but there is no evidence supporting these as reasons to deny treatment. Indeed there is evidence to suggest these patients can have greater benefit than other groups.

RECOMMENDATIONS

R33   Clinicians with responsibility for referring a person with osteoarthritis for consideration of joint surgery should ensure that the person has been offered at least the core (non-surgical) treatment options (see Fig 3.2).

R34   Referral for joint replacement surgery should be considered for people with osteoarthritis who experience joint symptoms (pain, stiffness, reduced function) that have a substantial impact on their quality of life and are refractory to non-surgical treatment. Referral should be made before there is prolonged and established functional limitation and severe pain.

R35   Patient-specific factors (including age, gender, smoking, obesity and comorbidities) should not be barriers to referral for joint replacement therapy.

R36   Decisions on referral thresholds should be based on discussions between patient representatives, referring clinicians and surgeons, rather than using current scoring tools for prioritisation.

9 | Areas for future research

What are the factors influencing, and methods of improving, adherence to osteoarthritis therapies?

Many therapies for osteoarthritis, for example, paracetamol or muscle strengthening, will have benefits but are often only used by people for a limited duration. For example, when using muscle strengthening there is little information on how optimal contact with a physiotherapist can be achieved, and how this can be sustained over the long term for a chronic condition like osteoarthritis.

What are the short- and long-term benefits of non-pharmacological and pharmacological osteoarthritis therapies in the very elderly?

There is very little data on the use of all osteoarthritis therapies (non-pharmacological and pharmacological) in the very elderly. This is of increasing concern with our ageing population. For example, exercise therapies may need to be tailored, and use of opioids requires more careful titration.

What are the benefits of combination (non-pharmacological and pharmacological) osteoarthritis therapies and how can they be included in clinically useful, cost-effective algorithms for long term use?

Most people with osteoarthritis get a combination of non-pharmacological and pharmacological therapies, but most of the trial evidence only evaluates single therapies. Often trials are of short duration (for example, 6 weeks) when people may live with osteoarthritis for more than 30 years! The optimal content and frequency of review by front-line clinicians is not known.

What are the predictors of good outcome following total and partial joint replacement?

Although joint replacement provides very good pain relief for many people with osteoarthritis, it does not provide a good outcome in a substantial number of people. It would be very useful to have preoperative tools to help choose people who would derive most benefit.

What are the benefits of individual and combination osteoarthritis therapies in people with multiple joint region pain?

Most people over 55 have more than one painful joint, for example, it is common to have osteoarthritis in both knees, and there may be excess strain put on the upper limbs if painful knee osteoarthritis is present. Most trials of osteoarthritis therapies have examined efficacy of therapies on a single joint.

Is it possible to identify subsets of people with osteoarthritis in whom existing treatments are more beneficial and cost effective (for example, acupuncture or hyaluronans)?

Osteoarthritis is complex in terms of pain and range of structural pathology. It may be that certain treatments have increased efficacy if targeted to subsets of the general osteoarthritis population. At present, there are few useful subclassifications of osteoarthritis.

Who are the people with osteoarthritis who would benefit from devices (including footwear, insoles, braces and splints)?

There are a range of devices available to help people with osteoarthritis, but there are very few trials to demonstrate their efficacy, and in particular little data to guide health professionals on which people would benefit most from these aids.

What are effective strategies for weight loss in people with painful knee or hip osteoarthritis, and how much weight should they lose?

Weight loss appears effective for reducing pain in overweight people with osteoarthritis, but losing weight is very difficult and probably requires multiple strategies to be effective. Taking exercise when joints are already very painful may be extremely difficult.

What are the benefits of treatment of comorbidities (for example, depression) in people with osteoarthritis?

Pain is a complex problem and many of the effect sizes for treatments listed in this guideline are small to moderate. As well as obesity, there are many other comorbid conditions in people with osteoarthritis, many of which may influence pain and quality of life. How treatment of these conditions influences outcomes has not been explored.

What social and psychological outcome measures are the most effective indicators to identify patient-perceived benefits of effective self-management strategies for osteoarthritis?

For individuals with knee and hip osteoarthritis, what benefits can be achieved using a patient-centred approach to information giving and pain management compared with group self-management programmes (as measured by pain, changes in prescriptions for symptom control, positive health-seeking behaviours and participation in activities of daily living, quality of life)?

References

Anon (1995) NIH consensus conference: Total hip replacement. NIH Consensus Development Panel on Total Hip Replacement. *Journal of the American Medical Association* 273 (24): 1950–6.

Ajzen I, Fishbein M (1980) *Understanding attitudes and predicting social behaviour.* USA: Prentice Hall.

Algozzine GJ, Stein GH, Doering PL (1982) Trolamine salicylate cream in osteoarthritis of the knee. *Journal of the American Medical Association* 247 (9): 1311–3.

Altman RD, Asch E, Bloch D et al. (1986) Development of criteria for the classification and reporting of osteoarthritis. Classification of osteoarthritis of the knee. Diagnostic and Therapeutic Criteria Committee of the American Rheumatism Association. *Arthritis & Rheumatism* 29 (8): 1039–49.

Altman RD, Aven A, Holmburg CE et al. (1994) Capsaicin cream 0.025% as monotherapy for osteoarthritis: a double-blind study. *Seminars in Arthritis & Rheumatism* 23 (suppl 3): 25–33.

Altman RD, Zinsenheim JR, Temple AR et al. (2007) Three-month efficacy and safety of acetaminophen extended-release for osteoarthritis pain of the hip or knee: a randomized, double-blind, placebo-controlled study. *Osteoarthritis & Cartilage* 15 (4): 454–61.

Amadio P, Cummings D (1983) Evaluation of acetaminophen in the management of osteoarthritis of the knee. *Current Therapeutic Research, Clinical & Experimental* 34 (1): 59–66.

Amin AK, Clayton RA, Patton JT et al. (2006) Total knee replacement in morbidly obese patients. Results of a prospective, matched study. *Journal of Bone & Joint Surgery – British Volume* 88 (10): 1321–6.

Andrews CJ, Cohen L, Crail RB et al. (1976) A trial of Fortagesic and Paramol 118 in osteoarthritis. *Journal of International Medical Research* 4 (6): 432–4.

Arcury TA, Gesler WM, Cook HL (1999) Meaning in the use of unconventional arthritis therapies. *American Journal of Health Promotion* 14 (1): 7–15.

Arthritis and Musculoskeletal Alliance (2004) *Standards of care for people with osteoarthritis.* London: ARMA.

Arthritis Care (2004) *OA nation.* London: Arthritis Care.

Arthritis Research Campaign (2002) *Arthritis: the big picture.* London: Arthritis Research campaign.

Baker K, Goggins J, Xie H et al. (2007) A randomized crossover trial of a wedged insole for treatment of knee osteoarthritis. *Arthritis & Rheumatism* 56 (4): 1198–203.

Baker K, Robertson V, Duck F (2001) A review of therapeutic ultrasound: biophysical effects. *Physical Therapy* 81: 1351–8.

Ballantyne PJ, Gignac MA, Hawker GA (2007) A patient-centered perspective on surgery avoidance for hip or knee arthritis: lessons for the future. *Arthritis & Rheumatism* 57 (1): 27–34.

Battisti E, Piazza E, Rigato M et al. (2004) Efficacy and safety of a musically modulated electromagnetic field (TAMMEF) in patients affected by knee osteoarthritis. *Clinical & Experimental Rheumatology* 22 (5): 568–72.

Baxter D (1996) Low intensity laser therapy. In: Kitchen S, Bazin S, editors. *Clayton's electrotherapy 10E.* London: WB Saunders, p197–217.

Bellamy N, Bourne R, Campbell J et al. (2006a) Intra-articular corticosteroids for osteoarthritis of the knee. *Cochrane Database of Systematic Reviews*

Bellamy N, Campbell J, Robinson V et al. (2006b) Viscosupplementation for the treatment of osteoarthritis of the knee. *Cochrane Database of Systematic Reviews* (2): CD005321.

Belza B, Topolski T, Kinne S et al. (2002) Does adherence make a difference? Results from a community-based aquatic exercise program. *Nursing Research* 51 (5): 285–91.

Bennell KL, Hinman RS, Metcalf BR (2005) Efficacy of physiotherapy management of knee joint osteoarthritis: a randomised, double blind, placebo controlled trial. *Annals of the Rheumatic Diseases* 64 (6): 906–12.

Bensen WG, Fiechtner JJ, McMillen JI (1999) Treatment of osteoarthritis with celecoxib, a cyclooxygenase-2 inhibitor: a randomized controlled trial. *Mayo Clinic Proceedings* 74 (11): 1095–105.

Berry H (1992) Controlled trial of a knee support ('Genutrain') in patients with osteoarthritis of the knee. *European Journal of Rheumatology and Inflammation* 12 (3): 30–4.

Bianchi M, Broggini M, Balzarini P et al. (2003) Effects of tramadol on synovial fluid concentrations of substance P and interleukin-6 in patients with knee osteoarthritis: comparison with paracetamol. *International Immunopharmacology* 3 (13–14): 1901–8.

Bingham CO, Sebba AI, Rubin BR et al. (2007) Efficacy and safety of etoricoxib 30 mg and celecoxib 200 mg in the treatment of osteoarthritis in two identically designed, randomized, placebo-controlled, non-inferiority studies. *Rheumatology* 46 (3): 496–507.

Bird HA, Hill J, Stratford ME et al. (1995) A double-blind cross-over study comparing the analgesic efficacy of tramadol with pentazocine in patients with osteoarthritis. *Journal of Drug Development & Clinical Practice* 7 (3): 181–8.

Bjordal JM, Klovning A, Ljunggren AE et al. (2007) Short-term efficacy of pharmacotherapeutic interventions in osteoarthritic knee pain: A meta-analysis of randomised placebo-controlled trials. *European Journal of Pain* 11 (2): 125–38.

Borjesson M, Robertson E, Weidenhielm L et al. (1996) Physiotherapy in knee osteoarthrosis: effect on pain and walking. *Physiotherapy Research International* 1 (2): 89–97.

Boureau F, Delecoeuillerie G, Orvain J (1990) Comparative study of the efficacy and tolerance of 2 dosages of the paracetamol 400 mg codeine 25 mg association versus paracetamol 1000 mg in non-inflammatory rheumatic pain. *Rhumatologie - Revue International de Rhumatologie* 20 (1): 41–7.

Bradley JD, Heilman DK, Katz.B.P (2002) Tidal irrigation as treatment for knee osteoarthritis: a sham-controlled, randomized, double-blinded evaluation. *Arthritis & Rheumatism* 46 (1): 100–8.

Brenes GA, Rapp SR, Rejeski WJ et al. (2002) Do optimism and pessimism predict physical functioning? *Journal of Behavioral Medicine* 25 (3): 219–31.

Brismee JM, Paige RL, Chyu MC et al. (2007) Group and home-based tai chi in elderly subjects with knee osteoarthritis: a randomized controlled trial. *Clinical Rehabilitation* 21 (2): 99–111.

Brosseau L, Gam A, Harman K et al. (2006) Low level laser therapy (Classes I, II and III) for treating osteoarthritis. *Cochrane Database of Systematic Reviews* (1): CD002046.

Brosseau L, Welch V, Wells G et al. (2000) Low level laser therapy for osteoarthritis and rheumatoid arthritis: a meta-analysis. *Journal of Rheumatology* 27 (8): 1961–9.

Brosseau L, Yonge KA, Robinson V et al. (2003) Thermotherapy for treatment of osteoarthritis. *Cochrane Database of Systematic Reviews* (4): CD004522.

Brouwer RW, Jakma TS, Verhagen AP et al. (2005) Braces and orthoses for treating osteoarthritis of the knee. *Cochrane Database of Systematic Reviews* (1): CD004020.

Brouwer RW, van Raaij TM, Verhaar JA et al. (2006) Brace treatment for osteoarthritis of the knee: a prospective randomized multi-centre trial. *Osteoarthritis & Cartilage* 14 (8): 777–83.

Buszewicz M, Rait G, Griffin M et al. (2006) Self management of arthritis in primary care: randomised controlled trial. *British Medical Journal* 333 (7574): 879.

Calfas KJ, Kaplan RM, Ingram RE (1992) One-year evaluation of cognitive-behavioral intervention in osteoarthritis. *Arthritis Care & Research* 5 (4): 202–9.

Callaghan MJ, Oldham JA, Hunt J (1995) An evaluation of exercise regimes for patients with osteoarthritis of the knee: a single-blind randomized controlled trial. *Clinical Rehabilitation* 9 (3): 213–8.

Callaghan MJ, Whittaker PE, Grimes S et al. (2005) An evaluation of pulsed shortwave on knee osteoarthritis using radioleucoscintigraphy: a randomised, double blind, controlled trial. *Joint, Bone, Spine: Revue du Rhumatisme* 72 (2): 150–5.

Caracciolo B, Giaquinto S (2005) Determinants of the subjective functional outcome of total joint arthroplasty. *Archives of Gerontology & Geriatrics* 41 (2): 169–76.

Carr AJ, Donovan JL (1998) Why doctors and patients disagree. *British Journal of Rheumatology* 37 (1): 1–4.

Cepeda MS, Camargo F, Zea C et al. (2006) Tramadol for osteoarthritis. *Cochrane Database of Systematic Reviews*

Chakrabarti AJ, Robinson AHN, Gallagher P (1997) De la Caffiniere thumb carpometacarpal replacements. 93 cases at 6 to 16 years follow-up. *Journal of Hand Surgery – British Volume* 22 B (6): 695–8.

Chamberlain MA, Care G (1982) Physiotherapy in osteoarthrosis of the knees. A controlled trial of hospital versus home exercises. *International Rehabilitation Medicine* 4 (2): 101–6.

Chan FK, Wong VW, Suen BY et al. (2007) Combination of a cyclo-oxygenase-2 inhibitor and a proton-pump inhibitor for prevention of recurrent ulcer bleeding in patients at very high risk: a double-blind, randomised trial. *Lancet* 369 (9573): 1621–6.

Chan GN, Smith AW (2005) Changes in knee moments with contralateral versus ipsilateral cane usage in females with knee osteoarthritis. *Clinical Biomechanics* 20 (4): 396–404.

Chang RW, Falconer J (1993) A randomized, controlled trial of arthroscopic surgery versus closed-needle joint lavage for patients with osteoarthritis of the knee. *Arthritis & Rheumatism* 36 (3): 289–96.

Cheing GL, Hui-Chan CWY (2004) Would the addition of TENS to exercise training produce better physical performance outcomes in people with knee osteoarthritis than either intervention alone? *Clinical Rehabilitation* 18 (5): 487–97.

Cheing GL, Huichan CWY, Chan KM (2002) Does four weeks of TENS and/or isometric exercise produce cumulative reduction of osteoarthritic knee pain? *Clinical Rehabilitation* 16 (7): 749–60.

Cheing G, Hui-Chan C (2003a) Analgesic effects of transcutaneous electrical nerve stimulation and interferential currents on heat pain in healthy subjects. *Journal of Rehabilitation Medicine* 35: 62–8.

Cheing G, Tsui A, Lo S et al. (2003b) Optimal stimulation duration of TENS in the management of osteo-arthritic knee pain. *Journal of Rehabilitation Medicine* 35: 62–8.

Chikanza IC, Clarke B (1994) A comparative study of the efficacy and toxicity of etodolac and naproxen in the treatment of osteoarthritis. *British Journal of Clinical Practice* 48 (2): 67–9.

Chodosh J, Morton SC, Mojica W et al. (2005) Meta-analysis: chronic disease self-management programs for older adults. *Annals of Internal Medicine* 143 (6): 427–38.

Christensen R, Bartels EM, Astrup A et al. (2007) Effect of weight reduction in obese patients diagnosed with knee osteoarthritis: a systematic review and meta-analysis. *Annals of the Rheumatic Diseases* 66 (4): 433–9.

Cibere J, Kopec JA, Thorne A et al. (2004) Randomized, double-blind, placebo-controlled glucosamine discontinuation trial in knee osteoarthritis. *Arthritis Care & Research* 51 (5): 738–45.

Clegg DO, Reda DJ, Harris CL et al. (2006) Glucosamine, chondroitin sulfate, and the two in combination for painful knee osteoarthritis. *New England Journal of Medicine* 354 (8): 795–808.

Cliborne AV, Wainner RS, Rhon DI et al. (2004) Clinical hip tests and a functional squat test in patients with knee osteoarthritis: reliability, prevalence of positive test findings, and short-term response to hip mobilization. *Journal of Orthopaedic & Sports Physical Therapy* 34 (11): 676–85.

Cochrane T, Davey RC, Edwards SMM (2005) Randomised controlled trial of the cost-effectiveness of water-based therapy for lower limb osteoarthritis. *Health Technology Assessment* 9 (31): iii–xi, 1.

Cohen M, Wolfe R, Mai T et al. (2003) A randomized, double blind, placebo controlled trial of a topical cream containing glucosamine sulfate, chondroitin sulfate, and camphor for osteoarthritis of the knee. *Journal of Rheumatology* 30 (3): 523–8.

Cook C, Pietrobon R, Hegedus E (2007) Osteoarthritis and the impact on quality of life health indicators. *Rheumatology International* 27 (4): 315–21.

Corben S and Rosen R (2005) *Self management for long term conditions: patients' perspectives on the way ahead.* London: King's Fund.

Coulter A and Ellins J (2006) *Patient-focused interventions: a review of the evidence.* London: The Health Foundation.

Coupe VM, Veenhof C, van Tulder MW et al. (2007) The cost effectiveness of behavioural graded activity in patients with osteoarthritis of hip and/or knee. *Annals of the Rheumatic Diseases* 66 (2): 215–21.

Cox F, Stevenson F, Britten N (2004) *A systematic review of communication between patients and healthcare professionals about medicine taking and prescribing.* London: Medicines Partnership.

Coyte PC, Hawker Croxford GR, Croxford R et al. (1996) Variation in rheumatologists' and family physicians' perceptions of the indications for and outcomes of knee replacement surgery. *Journal of Rheumatology* 23 (4): 730–8.

Cross MJ, March LM, Lapsley HM et al. (2006) Patient self-efficacy and health locus of control: relationships with health status and arthritis-related expenditure. *Rheumatology* 45 (1): 92–6.

Curtis, L and Netten, A (2006) *Unit costs of health & health social care.* Kent: PSSRU, University of Kent.

Curtis SP, Bockow B, Fisher C et al. (2005) Etoricoxib in the treatment of osteoarthritis over 52-weeks: A double-blind, active-comparator controlled trial. *BMC Musculoskeletal Disorders* 6: 58.

Cushnaghan J, McCarthy C, Dieppe P (1994) Taping the patella medially: a new treatment for osteoarthritis of the knee joint? *British Medical Journal* 308 (6931): 753–5.

D'Agostino MA, Conaghan PG, Le Bars M et al. (2005) EULAR report on the use of ultrasonography in painful knee osteoarthritis. Part 1: prevalence of inflammation in osteoarthritis. *Annals of the Rheumatic Diseases* 64: 1703–9.

Das A, Jr., Hammad TA (2000) Efficacy of a combination of FCHG49(TM) glucosamine hydrochloride, TRH122(TM) low molecular weight sodium chondroitin sulfate and manganese ascorbate in the management of knee osteoarthritis. *Osteoarthritis & Cartilage* 8 (5): 343–50.

Dawes PT, Kirlew C, Haslock I (1987) Saline washout for knee osteoarthritis: results of a controlled study. *Clinical Rheumatology* 6 (1): 61–3.

Day R, Brooks P, Conaghan PG et al. (2004) A double blind, randomized, multicenter, parallel group study of the effectiveness and tolerance of intraarticular hyaluronan in osteoarthritis of the knee. *Journal of Rheumatology* 31 (4): 775–82.

De Jong OR, Hopman-Rock M, Tak EC (2004) An implementation study of two evidence-based exercise and health education programmes for older adults with osteoarthritis of the knee and hip. *Health Education Research* 19 (3): 316–25.

De Leeuw JM, Villar RN (1998) Obesity and quality of life after primary total knee replacement. *Knee* 5 (2): 119–23.

Deal CL, Schnitzer TJ, Lipstein E et al. (1991) Treatment of arthritis with topical capsaicin: a double-blind trial. *Clinical Therapeutics* 13 (3): 383–95.

Degreef I, De SL (2006) Predictors of outcome in surgical treatment for basal joint osteoarthritis of the thumb. *Clinical Rheumatology* 25 (2): 140–2.

Department of Health (2005) *Self care – a real choice: self care support: a practical option.* London: Department of Health.

Department of Work and Pensions (2005) *Opportunity age:meeting the challenges of aging in the 21st century Volume 1.* London: HM Government.

Dequeker J (1998) Improvement in gastrointestinal tolerability of the selective cyclooxygenase (COX)-2 inhibitor, meloxicam, compared with piroxicam: results of the Safety and Efficacy Large-scale Evaluation of COX-inhibiting Therapies (SELECT) trial in osteoarthritis. *British Journal of Rheumatology* 37 (9): 946–51.

Deyle GD, Allison SC, Matekel RL et al. (2005) Physical therapy treatment effectiveness for osteoarthritis of the knee: a randomized comparison of supervised clinical exercise and manual therapy procedures versus a home exercise program. *Physical Therapy* 85 (12): 1301–17.

Deyle GD, Henderson NE, Matekel RL (2000) Effectiveness of manual physical therapy and exercise in osteoarthritis of the knee. A randomized, controlled trial. *Annals of Internal Medicine* 132 (3): 173–81.

Dickens W, Lewith GT (1989) A single-blind, controlled and randomised clinical trial to evaluate the effect of acupuncture in the treatment of trapezio-metacarpal osteoarthritis. *Complementary Medical Research* 3 (2): 5–8.

Doherty M (1995) *Color Atlas and text of osteoarthritis.* USA: Mosby.

Doherty M, Mazieres B, Le BM (2003) EULAR recommendations for the treatment of osteoarthritis of the knee in general practice. Bristol-Myers Squibb and Laboratoires UPSA.

Dolin SJ, Williams AC, Ashford N et al. (2003) Factors affecting medical decision-making in patients with osteoarthritis of the hip: allocation of surgical priority. *Disability & Rehabilitation* 25 (14): 771–7.

Dominkus M, Nicolakis M, Kotz R et al. (1996) Comparison of tissue and plasma levels of ibuprofen after oral and topical administration. *Arzneimittel-Forschung* 46 (12): 1138–43.

Donovan JL, Blake DR (2000) Qualitative study of interpretation of reassurance among patients attending rheumatology clinics: 'just a touch of arthritis, doctor?'. *British Medical Journal* 320 (7234): 541–4.

Donovan JL, Blake DR, Fleming WG (1989) The patient is not a blank sheet: lay beliefs and their relevance to patient education. *British Journal of Rheumatology* 28 (1): 58–61.

Downe-Wamboldt B (1991) Coping and life satisfaction in elderly women with osteoarthritis. *Journal of Advanced Nursing* 16 (11): 1328–35.

Dracoglu D, Aydin R, Baskent A et al. (2005) Effects of kinesthesia and balance exercises in knee osteoarthritis. *JCR: Journal of Clinical Rheumatology* 11 (6): 303–10.

Dreinhofer KE, Dieppe P, Sturmer T et al. (2006) Indications for total hip replacement: comparison of assessments of orthopaedic surgeons and referring physicians. *Annals of the Rheumatic Diseases* 65 (10): 1346–50.

Duncan R, Peat G, Thomas E et al. (2007) Symptoms and radiographic osteoarthritis: not as discordant as they are made out to be? *Annals of the Rheumatic Diseases* 66 (1): 86–91.

Duncan RC, Hay EM, Saklatvala J et al. (2006) Prevalence of radiographic osteoarthritis – it all depends on your point of view. *Rheumatology* 45 (6): 757–60.

Dziedzic K, Thomas E, Hill S et al. (2007) The impact of musculoskeletal hand problems in older adults: findings from the North Staffordshire Osteoarthritis Project (NorStOP). *Rheumatology* 46 (6): 963–7.

Elson DW, Brenkel IJ (2006) Predicting pain after total knee arthroplasty. *Journal of Arthroplasty* 21 (7): 1047–53.

Elwyn G, Edwards A, Kinnersley P (1999) Shared decision-making in primary care: the neglected second half of the consultation. *British Journal of General Practice* 49 (443): 477–82.

Escobar A, Quintana JM, Bilbao A et al. (2007) Effect of patient characteristics on reported outcomes after total knee replacement. *Rheumatology* 46 (1): 112–9.

Evcik D, Kavuncu V, Yeter A et al. (2007) The efficacy of balneotherapy and mud-pack therapy in patients with knee osteoarthritis. *Joint, Bone, Spine: Revue du Rhumatisme* 74 (1): 60–5.

Evcik D, Sonel B (2002) Effectiveness of a home-based exercise therapy and walking program on osteoarthritis of the knee. *Rheumatology International* 22 (3): 103–6.

Eyigor S, Hepguler S, Capaci K (2004) A comparison of muscle training methods in patients with knee osteoarthritis. *Clinical Rheumatology* 23 (2): 109–15.

Felson DT, Lawrence RC, Dieppe PA et al. (2000) Osteoarthritis: new insights. Part 1: the disease and its risk factors. *Annals of Internal Medicine* 133 (8): 635–46.

Ferreira VM, Sherman AM (2007) The relationship of optimism, pain and social support to well-being in older adults with osteoarthritis. *Aging & Mental Health* 11 (1): 89–98.

Fielden JM, Cumming JM, Horne JG et al. (2005) Waiting for hip arthroplasty: economic costs and health outcomes. *Journal of Arthroplasty* 20: 990–7.

Fink MG, Wipperman B, Gehrke A (2001) Non-specific effects of traditional Chinese acupuncture in osteoarthritis of the hip. *Complementary Therapies in Medicine* 9 (2): 82–9.

Fioravanti A, Valenti M, Altobelli E et al. (2003) Clinical efficacy and cost-effectiveness evidence of spa therapy in osteoarthritis. The results of "Naiade" Italian Project. *Panminerva Medica* 45 (3): 211–7.

Flanagan J, Casale FF, Thomas TL et al. (1988) Intra-articular injection for pain relief in patients awaiting hip replacement. *Annals of the Royal College of Surgeons of England* 70 (3): 156–7.

Fleischmann R, Sheldon E, Maldonado CJ et al. (2006) Lumiracoxib is effective in the treatment of osteoarthritis of the knee: a prospective randomized 13-week study versus placebo and celecoxib. *Clinical Rheumatology* 25 (1): 42–53.

Focht BC, Rejeski WJ, Ambrosius WT et al. (2005) Exercise, self-efficacy, and mobility performance in overweight and obese older adults with knee osteoarthritis. *Arthritis & Rheumatism* 53 (5): 659–65.

Foley A, Halbert J, Hewitt T et al. (2003) Does hydrotherapy improve strength and physical function in patients with osteoarthritis – a randomised controlled trial comparing a gym based and a hydrotherapy based strengthening programme. *Annals of the Rheumatic Diseases* 62 (12): 1162–7.

Fransen M, McConnell S, Bell M (2002) Therapeutic exercise for people with osteoarthritis of the hip or knee. A systematic review. *Journal of Rheumatology* 29 (8): 1737–45.

Fransen M, Nairn L, Winstanley J et al. (2007) Physical activity for osteoarthritis management: a randomized controlled clinical trial evaluating hydrotherapy or tai chi classes. *Arthritis & Rheumatism* 57 (3): 407–14.

Fries JF, Bruce B (2003) Rates of serious gastrointestinal events from low dose use of acetylsalicylic acid, acetaminophen, and ibuprofen in patients with osteoarthritis and rheumatoid arthritis. *Journal of Rheumatology* 30 (10): 2226–33.

Fuchs S, Monikes R, Wohlmeiner A et al. (2006) Intra-articular hyaluronic acid compared with corticoid injections for the treatment of rhizarthrosis. *Osteoarthritis & Cartilage* 14 (1): 82–8.

Gana TJ, Pascual ML, Fleming RR (2006) Extended-release tramadol in the treatment of osteoarthritis: a multicenter, randomized, double-blind, placebo-controlled clinical trial. *Current Medical Research & Opinion* 22 (7): 1391–401.

Garfinkel MS, Schumacher HR Jr., Husain A et al. (1994) Evaluation of a yoga based regimen for treatment of osteoarthritis of the hands. *Journal of Rheumatology* 21 (12): 2341–3.

Gaw AC, Chang LW, Shaw L (1975) Efficacy of acupuncture on osteoarthritic pain. A controlled, double-blind study. *New England Journal of Medicine* 293 (8): 375–8.

Gay MC, Philippot P, Luminet O (2002) Differential effectiveness of psychological interventions for reducing osteoarthritis pain: a comparison of Erikson hypnosis and Jacobson relaxation. *European Journal of Pain* 6 (1): 1–16.

General Medical Council (2006) *Good medical practice.* London: General Medical Council.

Gibson JNA, White MD, Chapman VM et al. (1992) Arthroscopic lavage and debridement for osteoarthritis of the knee. *Journal of Bone & Joint Surgery – British Volume* 74 (4): 534–7.

Gignac MA, Davis AM, Hawker G et al. (2006) 'What do you expect? You're just getting older': a comparison of perceived osteoarthritis-related and aging-related health experiences in middle- and older-age adults. *Arthritis & Rheumatism* 55 (6): 905–12.

Gill GS, Mills D, Joshi AB (2003) Mortality following primary total knee arthroplasty. *Journal of Bone & Joint Surgery – American Volume* 85 (3): 432–5.

Golden HE, Moskowitz RW, Minic M (2004) Analgesic efficacy and safety of nonprescription doses of naproxen sodium compared with acetaminophen in the treatment of osteoarthritis of the knee. *American Journal of Therapeutics* 11 (2): 85–94.

Gottesdiener K, Schnitzer T, Fisher C et al. (2002) Results of a randomized, dose-ranging trial of etoricoxib in patients with osteoarthritis. *Rheumatology* 41 (9): 1052–61.

Goutallier D, Van DS, Manicom O et al. (2006) Influence of lower-limb torsion on long-term outcomes of tibial valgus osteotomy for medial compartment knee osteoarthritis. *Journal of Bone & Joint Surgery – American Volume* 88 (11): 2439–47.

Grace D, Rogers J, Skeith K et al. (1999) Topical diclofenac versus placebo: a double blind, randomized clinical trial in patients with osteoarthritis of the knee. *Journal of Rheumatology* 26 (12): 2659–63.

Green J, McKenna F, Redfern EJ et al. (1993) Home exercises are as effective as outpatient hydrotherapy for osteoarthritis of the hip. *British Journal of Rheumatology* 32 (9): 812–5.

Grifka JK (2004) Efficacy and tolerability of lumiracoxib versus placebo in patients with osteoarthritis of the hand. *Clinical & Experimental Rheumatology* 22 (5): 589–96.

Hampson SE, Glasgow RE, Zeiss AM (1994) Personal models of osteoarthritis and their relation to self-management activities and quality of life. *Journal of Behavioral Medicine* 17 (2): 143–58.

Hampson SE, Glasgow RE, Zeiss AM (1996) Coping with osteoarthritis by older adults. *Arthritis Care & Research* 9 (2): 133–41.

Hampson SE, Glasgow RE, Zeiss AM et al. (1993) Self-management of osteoarthritis. *Arthritis Care & Research* 6 (1): 17–22.

Harrysson OLA, Robertsson O, Nayfeh JF (2004) Higher cumulative revision rate of knee arthroplasties in younger patients with osteoarthritis. *Clinical Orthopaedics & Related Research* 421: 162–8.

Haslam R (2001) A comparison of acupuncture with advice and exercises on the symptomatic treatment of osteoarthritis of the hip – a randomised controlled trial. *Acupuncture in Medicine* 19 (1): 19–26.

Hawel R (2003) Comparison of the efficacy and tolerability of dexibuprofen and celecoxib in the treatment of osteoarthritis of the hip. *International Journal of Clinical Pharmacology & Therapeutics* 41 (4): 153–64.

Hawker GA, Wright JG, Coyte PC et al. (2001) Determining the need for hip and knee arthroplasty: the role of clinical severity and patients' preferences. *Medical Care* 39 (3): 206–16.

Hawkey C (1998) Gastrointestinal tolerability of meloxicam compared to diclofenac in osteoarthritis patients. International MELISSA Study Group. Meloxicam Large-scale International Study Safety Assessment. *British Journal of Rheumatology* 37 (9): 937–45.

Hawkey C, Svoboda P (2004) Gastroduodenal safety and tolerability of lumiracoxib compared with ibuprofen and celecoxib in patients with osteoarthritis. *Journal of Rheumatology* 31 (9): 1804–10.

Hay EM, Foster NE, Thomas E (2006) Effectiveness of community physiotherapy and enhanced pharmacy review for knee pain in people aged over 55 presenting to primary care: pragmatic randomised trial. *British Medical Journal* 333 (7576): 995.

Henderson EB, Smith EC, Pegley F et al. (1994) Intra-articular injections of 750 kD hyaluronan in the treatment of osteoarthritis: a randomised single centre double-blind placebo-controlled trial of 91 patients demonstrating lack of efficacy. *Annals of the Rheumatic Diseases* 53 (8): 529–34.

Herrero-Beaumont G, Ivorra JA, Del Carmen TM et al. (2007) Glucosamine sulfate in the treatment of knee osteoarthritis symptoms: a randomized, double-blind, placebo-controlled study using acetaminophen as a side comparator. *Arthritis & Rheumatism* 56 (2): 555–67.

Heuts PH, de Bie R, Drietelaar M et al. (2005) Self-management in osteoarthritis of hip or knee: a randomized clinical trial in a primary healthcare setting. *Journal of Rheumatology* 32 (3): 543–9.

Heyneman CA, Lawless-Liday C, Wall GC (2000) Oral versus topical NSAIDs in rheumatic diseases: a comparison. *Drugs* 60 (3): 555–74.

Hill J, Bird H (2007) Patient knowledge and misconceptions of osteoarthritis assessed by a validated self-completed knowledge questionnaire (PKQ-OA). *Rheumatology* 46 (5): 796–800.

Hinman RS, Bennell KL, Crossley KM (2003a) Immediate effects of adhesive tape on pain and disability in individuals with knee osteoarthritis. *Rheumatology* 42 (7): 865–9.

Hinman RS, Crossley KM, McConnell J et al. (2003b) Efficacy of knee tape in the management of osteoarthritis of the knee: blinded randomised controlled trial. *British Medical Journal* 327 (7407): 135.

Hinman RS, Heywood SE, Day AR (2007) Aquatic physical therapy for hip and knee osteoarthritis: results of a single-blind randomized controlled trial. *Physical Therapy* 87 (1): 32–43.

Hoeksma HL, Dekker J, Ronday HK et al. (2004) Comparison of manual therapy and exercise therapy in osteoarthritis of the hip: a randomized clinical trial. *Arthritis & Rheumatism* 51 (5): 722–9.

Hosie J (1997) Efficacy and tolerability of meloxicam versus piroxicam in patients with osteoarthritis of the hip or knee. A six-month double-blind study. *Clinical Drug Investigation* 13 (4): 175–84.

Hosie J, Distel M, Bluhmki E (1996) Meloxicam in osteoarthritis: a 6-month, double-blind comparison with diclofenac sodium. *British Journal of Rheumatology* 35 (suppl 1): 39–43.

Huang M, Lin Y, Lee C et al. (2005) Use of ultrasound to increase effectiveness of isokinetic exercise for knee osteoarthritis. *Archives of Physical Medicine & Rehabilitation* 86 (8): 1545–10.

Huang MH, Chen CH, Chen TW et al. (2000) The effects of weight reduction on the rehabilitation of patients with knee osteoarthritis and obesity. *Arthritis Care & Research* 13 (6): 398–405.

Huang MH, Lin YS, Yang RC (2003) A comparison of various therapeutic exercises on the functional status of patients with knee osteoarthritis. *Seminars in Arthritis & Rheumatism* 32 (6): 398–406.

Huang YC, Harbst K, Kotajarvi B et al. (2006) Effects of ankle-foot orthoses on ankle and foot kinematics in patients with ankle osteoarthritis. *Archives of Physical Medicine & Rehabilitation* 87 (5): 710–6.

Hubbard MJ (1996) Articular debridement versus washout for degeneration of the medial femoral condyle. A five-year study. *Journal of Bone & Joint Surgery – British Volume* 78 (2): 217–9.

Hughes SL, Seymour RB, Campbell R et al. (2004) Impact of the fit and strong intervention on older adults with osteoarthritis. *Gerontologist* 44 (2): 217–28.

Hughes SL, Seymour RB, Campbell RT et al. (2006) Long-term impact of Fit and Strong! on older adults with osteoarthritis. *Gerontologist* 46 (6): 801–14.

Hulme J, Robinson V, DeBie R et al. (2002) Electromagnetic fields for the treatment of osteoarthritis. *Cochrane Database of Systematic Reviews* (1): CD003523.

Hurley MV, Scott DL (1998) Improvements in quadriceps sensorimotor function and disability of patients with knee osteoarthritis following a clinically practicable exercise regime. *British Journal of Rheumatology* 37 (11): 1181–7.

Hurley MV, Walsh NE, Mitchell HL et al. (2007) Clinical effectiveness of a rehabilitation program integrating exercise, self-management, and active coping strategies for chronic knee pain: a cluster randomized trial. *Arthritis & Rheumatism* 57 (7): 1211–9.

Iannotti JP, Norris TR (2003) Influence of preoperative factors on outcome of shoulder arthroplasty for glenohumeral osteoarthritis. *Journal of Bone & Joint Surgery – American Volume* 85 (2): 251–8.

Ike RW, Arnold WJ, Rothschild EW et al. (1992) Tidal irrigation versus conservative medical management in patients with osteoarthritis of the knee: a prospective randomized study. *Journal of Rheumatology* 19 (5): 772–9.

Imamura K, Gair R, McKee M et al. (1996) Appropriateness of total hip replacement in the United Kingdom. *World Hospitals & Health Services* 32 (2): 10–4.

Irani MS (1980) Clinical and upper gastrointestinal effects of sulindac, indomethacin and paracetamol plus dextropropoxyphene in patients with osteoarthritis. *European Journal of Rheumatology & Inflammation* 3 (3): 222–31.

Jain SA, Roach RT, Travlos J (2003) Changes in body mass index following primary elective total hip arthroplasty: Correlation with outcome at 2 years. *Acta Orthopaedica Belgica* 69 (5): 421–5.

Jennings MB, Alfieri DM (1997) A controlled comparison of etodolac and naproxen in osteoarthritis of the foot. *Lower Extremity* 4 (1): 43–8.

Jensen EM, Ginsberg F (1994) Tramadol versus dextropropoxyphene in the treatment of osteoarthritis: a short term double-blind study. *Drug Investigation* 8 (4): 211–8.

Jinks C, Jordan K, Ong BN et al. (2004) A brief screening tool for knee pain in primary care (KNEST) 2. Results from a survey in the general population aged 50 and over. *Rheumatology* 43 (1): 55–61.

Jinks C, Ong BN, Richardson J (2007) A mixed methods study to investigate needs assessment for knee pain and disability: population and individual perspectives. *BMC Musculoskeletal Disorders* 8: 59.

Johnsen SP, Sorensen HT, Pedersen AB et al. (2006) Patient-related predictors of implant failure after primary total hip replacement in the initial, short- and long-term: a nationwide Danish follow-up study including 36,984 patients. *Journal of Bone & Joint Surgery – British Volume* 88 (10): 1303–8.

Jones CA, Voaklander DC, Johnston DW et al. (2001) The effect of age on pain, function, and quality of life after total hip and knee arthroplasty. *Archives of Internal Medicine* 161 (3): 454–60.

Jordan K, Clarke AM, Symmons DP et al. (2007) Measuring disease prevalence: a comparison of musculoskeletal disease using four general practice consultation databases. *British Journal of General Practice* 57 (534): 7–14.

Jordan K, Jinks C, Croft P (2006) A prospective study of the consulting behaviour of older people with knee pain. *British Journal of General Practice* 56 (525): 269–76.

Jubb RW, Piva S, Beinat L et al. (2003) A one-year, randomised, placebo (saline) controlled clinical trial of 500–730 kDa sodium hyaluronate (Hyalgan) on the radiological change in osteoarthritis of the knee. *International Journal of Clinical Practice* 57 (6): 467–74.

Juni P, Dieppe P, Donovan J et al. (2003) Population requirement for primary knee replacement surgery: a cross-sectional study. *Rheumatology* 42 (4): 516–21.

Junnila SYT (1982) Acupuncture superior to piroxicam (TM) in the treatment of osteoarthrosis. *American Journal of Acupuncture* 10 (4): 341–6.

Kahan A, Lleu PL, Salin L (2003) Prospective randomized study comparing the medicoeconomic benefits of Hylan GF-20 vs. conventional treatment in knee osteoarthritis. *Joint, Bone, Spine: Revue du Rhumatisme* 70 (4): 276–81.

Kalunian KC, Moreland LW, Klashman DJ (2000) Visually-guided irrigation in patients with early knee osteoarthritis: a multicenter randomized, controlled trial. *Osteoarthritis & Cartilage* 8 (6): 412–8.

Karlsson J, Sjogren LS, Lohmander LS (2002) Comparison of two hyaluronan drugs and placebo in patients with knee osteoarthritis. A controlled, randomized, double-blind, parallel-design multicentre study. *Rheumatology* 41 (11): 1240–8.

Keefe FJ, Blumenthal J (2004) Effects of spouse-assisted coping skills training and exercise training in patients with osteoarthritic knee pain: a randomized controlled study. *Pain* 110 (3): 539–49.

Kennedy LG, Newman JH, Ackroyd CE et al. (2003) When should we do knee replacements? *Knee* 10 (2): 161–6.

Kettunen JA, Kujala UM (2004) Exercise therapy for people with rheumatoid arthritis and osteoarthritis. *Scandinavian Journal of Medicine & Science in Sports* 14 (3): 138–42.

King's Fund (2005) *Social care needs and outcomes: a background paper for the Wanless Review.* London: King's Fund.

Kitchen S (2002) *Electrotherapy: evidence-based practice.* Oxford: Elsevier Health Sciences, p211.

Kivitz AJ, Moskowitz RW, Woods E (2001) Comparative efficacy and safety of celecoxib and naproxen in the treatment of osteoarthritis of the hip. *Journal of International Medical Research* 29 (6): 467–79.

Kjaersgaard AP, Nafei A, Skov O et al. (1990) Codeine plus paracetamol versus paracetamol in longer-term treatment of chronic pain due to osteoarthritis of the hip. A randomised, double-blind, multi-centre study. *Pain* 43 (3): 309–18.

Klaber Moffett JA, Richardson PH, Frost H et al. (1996) A placebo controlled double blind trial to evaluate the effectiveness of pulsed short wave therapy for osteoarthritic hip and knee pain. *Pain* 67 (1): 121–7.

Kuptniratsaikul V, Tosayanonda O, Nilganuwong S et al. (2002) The efficacy of a muscle exercise program to improve functional performance of the knee in patients with osteoarthritis. *Journal of the Medical Association of Thailand* 85 (1): 33–40.

Laborde JM, Powers MJ (1985) Life satisfaction, health control orientation, and illness-related factors in persons with osteoarthritis. *Research in Nursing & Health* 8 (2): 183–90.

Lai KC, Chu KM, Hui WM et al. (2005) Celecoxib compared with lansoprazole and naproxen to prevent gastrointestinal ulcer complications. *American Journal of Medicine* 118 (11): 1271–8.

Lastowiecka E, Bugajska J, Najmiec A et al. (2006) Occupational work and quality of life in osteoarthritis patients. *Rheumatology International* 27 (2): 131–9.

Lau EM, Symmons DP, Croft P (1996) The epidemiology of hip osteoarthritis and rheumatoid arthritis in the Orient. *Clinical Orthopaedics & Related Research* (323): 81–90.

Lefler C, Armstrong WJ (2004) Exercise in the treatment of osteoarthritis in the hands of the elderly. *Clinical Kinesiology* 58 (2): 1–6.

Lehmann R (2005) Efficacy and tolerability of lumiracoxib 100 mg once daily in knee osteoarthritis: a 13-week, randomized, double-blind study vs. placebo and celecoxib. *Current Medical Research & Opinion* 21 (4): 517–26.

Leung AT, Malmstrom K (2002) Efficacy and tolerability profile of etoricoxib in patients with osteoarthritis: A randomized, double-blind, placebo and active-comparator controlled 12-week efficacy trial. *Current Medical Research & Opinion* 18 (2): 49–58.

Levy E, Ferme A, Perocheau D et al. (1993) Socioeconomic costs of osteoarthritis in France. *Revue du Rhumatisme (French edition)* 60 (6 Pt 2): 63S–7S.

Lim BW (2002) A comparative study of open and closed kinetic chain exercise regimes in patients with knee osteoarthritis. *Physiotherapy Singapore* 5 (2): 34–40.

Lin J, Zhang W, Jones A et al. (2004) Efficacy of topical non-steroidal anti-inflammatory drugs in the treatment of osteoarthritis: meta-analysis of randomised controlled trials. *British Medical Journal* 329 (7461): 324.

Linden B, Distel M, Bluhmki E (1996) A double-blind study to compare the efficacy and safety of meloxicam 15 mg with piroxicam 20 mg in patients with osteoarthritis of the hip. *British Journal of Rheumatology* 35 (suppl 1): 35–8.

Lingard EA, Katz JN, Wright EA et al. (2004) Predicting the outcome of total knee arthroplasty. *Journal of Bone & Joint Surgery – American Volume* 86–A (10): 2179–86.

Lund B (1998) A double-blind, randomized, placebo-controlled study of efficacy and tolerance of meloxicam treatment in patients with osteoarthritis of the knee. *Scandinavian Journal of Rheumatology* 27 (1): 32–7.

MacDonald CW, Whitman JM, Cleland JA et al. (2006) Clinical outcomes following manual physical therapy and exercise for hip osteoarthritis: A case series. *Journal of Orthopaedic & Sports Physical Therapy* 36 (8): 588–99.

Maetzel A, Krahn M, Naglie G (2003) The cost effectiveness of rofecoxib and celecoxib in patients with osteoarthritis or rheumatoid arthritis. *Arthritis Care & Research* 49 (3): 283–92.

Maillefert JF, Hudry C (2001) Laterally elevated wedged insoles in the treatment of medial knee osteoarthritis: a prospective randomized controlled study. *Osteoarthritis & Cartilage* 9 (8): 738–45.

Maisiak R, Austin J, Heck L (1996) Health outcomes of two telephone interventions for patients with rheumatoid arthritis or osteoarthritis. *Arthritis & Rheumatism* 39 (8): 1391–9.

Mancuso CA, Ranawat CS, Esdaile JM et al. (1996) Indications for total hip and total knee arthroplasties. Results of orthopaedic surveys. *Journal of Arthroplasty* 11 (1): 34–46.

Mangione KK, McCully K (1999) The effects of high-intensity and low-intensity cycle ergometry in older adults with knee osteoarthritis. *Journals of Gerontology Series A – Biological Sciences & Medical Sciences* 54 (4): M184–M190.

Mann WC, Hurren D, Tomita M (1995) Assistive devices used by home-based elderly persons with arthritis. *American Journal of Occupational Therapy* 49 (8): 810–20.

March L, Irwig L, Schwarz J et al. (1994) N of 1 trials comparing a non-steroidal anti-inflammatory drug with paracetamol in osteoarthritis. *British Medical Journal* 309 (6961): 1041–5.

Martin D (1996) Interferential therapy for pain control. In: Kitchen S, Bazin S, editors. *Clayton's electrotherapy 10E.* London: WB Saunders, p 306–315.

Martin JG, Rodriguez LP, Mora CD et al. (1998) Liquid nitrogen cryotherapy effect on gait and pain in subjects with osteoarthritis of the knee. *Europa Medicophysica* 34 (1): 17–24.

Maurer BT, Stern AG, Kinossian B et al. (1999) Osteoarthritis of the knee: isokinetic quadriceps exercise versus an educational intervention. *Archives of Physical Medicine & Rehabilitation* 80 (10): 1293–9.

Mazieres B, Hucher M, Zaim M et al. (2007) Effect of chondroitin sulphate in symptomatic knee osteoarthritis: a multicentre, randomised, double-blind, placebo-controlled study. *Annals of the Rheumatic Diseases* 66 (5): 639–45.

McCaffrey R, Freeman E (2003) Effect of music on chronic osteoarthritis pain in older people. *Journal of Advanced Nursing* 44 (5): 517–24.

McCarthy CJ, Callaghan MJ, Oldham JA (2006) Pulsed electromagnetic energy treatment offers no clinical benefit in reducing the pain of knee osteoarthritis: a systematic review. *BMC Musculoskeletal Disorders* 7: 51.

McCarthy CJ, Mills PM, Pullen R et al. (2004a) Supplementation of a home-based exercise programme with a class-based programme for people with osteoarthritis of the knees: a randomised controlled trial and health economic analysis. *Health Technology Assessment* 8 (46): iii–x, 1.

McCarthy CJ, Mills PM, Pullen R et al. (2004b) Supplementing a home exercise programme with a class-based exercise programme is more effective than home exercise alone in the treatment of knee osteoarthritis. *Rheumatology* 43 (7): 880–6.

McCleane G (2000) The analgesic efficacy of topical capsaicin is enhanced by glyceryl trinitrate in painful osteoarthritis: a randomized, double blind, placebo controlled study. *European Journal of Pain* 4 (4): 355–60.

McIndoe AK, Young K (1995) A comparison of acupuncture with intra-articular steroid injection as analgesia for osteoarthritis of the hip. *Acupuncture in Medicine* 13 (2): 67–70.

McIntyre RL, Irani MS, Piris J (1981) Histological study of the effects of three anti-inflammatory preparations on the gastric mucosa. *Journal of Clinical Pathology* 34 (8): 836–42.

McKell D, Stewart A (1994) A cost-minimisation analysis comparing topical versus systemic NSAIDs in the treatment of mild osteoarthritis of the superficial joints. *British Journal of Medical Economics* 7 (2): 137–46.

McKenna F (2001) Celecoxib versus diclofenac in the management of osteoarthritis of the knee. *Scandinavian Journal of Rheumatology* 30 (1): 11–8.

Meding JB, Anderson AR, Faris PM et al. (2000) Is the preoperative radiograph useful in predicting the outcome of a total hip replacement? *Clinical Orthopaedics & Related Research* 376: 156–60.

Meenagh GK, Patton J, Kynes C et al. (2004) A randomised controlled trial of intra-articular corticosteroid injection of the carpometacarpal joint of the thumb in osteoarthritis. *Annals of the Rheumatic Diseases* 63 (10): 1260–3.

Merchan ECR, Galindo E (1993) Arthroscope-guided surgery versus nonoperative treatment for limited degenerative osteoarthritis of the femorotibial joint in patients over 50 years of age: a prospective comparative study. *Arthroscopy* 9 (6): 663–7.

Messieh M (1999) Preoperative risk factors associated with symptomatic pulmonary embolism after total knee arthroplasty. *Orthopedics* 22 (12): 1147–9.

Messier SP, Loeser RF, Miller GD et al. (2004) Exercise and dietary weight loss in overweight and obese older adults with knee osteoarthritis: the Arthritis, Diet, and Activity Promotion Trial. *Arthritis & Rheumatism* 50 (5): 1501–10.

Messier SP, Royer TD, Craven TE et al. (2000) Long-term exercise and its effect on balance in older, osteoarthritic adults: results from the Fitness, Arthritis, and Seniors Trial (FAST). *Journal of the American Geriatrics Society* 48 (2): 131–8.

Messier SP, Thompson CD, Ettinger WH, Jr. (1997) Effects of long-term aerobic or weight training regimens on gait in an older, osteoarthritic population. *Journal of Applied Biomechanics* 13 (2): 205–25.

Miceli-Richard C, Le BM, Schmidely N et al. (2004) Paracetamol in osteoarthritis of the knee. *Annals of the Rheumatic Diseases* 63 (8): 923–30.

Miller GD, Nicklas BJ, Davis C et al. (2006) Intensive weight loss program improves physical function in older obese adults with knee osteoarthritis. *Obesity* 14 (7): 1219–30.

Miller GD, Rejeski WJ, Williamson JD et al. (2003) The Arthritis, Diet and Activity Promotion Trial (ADAPT): design, rationale, and baseline results. *Controlled Clinical Trials* 24 (4): 462–80.

Minor MA (1999) Exercise in the treatment of osteoarthritis. *Rheumatic Diseases Clinics of North America* 25 (2): 397–415, viii.

Minor MA, Hewett JE, Webel RR et al. (1989) Efficacy of physical conditioning exercise in patients with rheumatoid arthritis and osteoarthritis. *Arthritis & Rheumatism* 32 (11): 1396–405.

Mitchell H, Cunningham TJ, Mathews JD et al. (1984) Further look at dextropropoxyphene with or without paracetamol in the treatment of arthritis. *Medical Journal of Australia* 140 (4): 224–5.

Moseley JB, O'Malley K, Petersen NJ et al. (2002) A controlled trial of arthroscopic surgery for osteoarthritis of the knee. *New England Journal of Medicine* 347 (2): 81–8.

Moss P, Sluka K, Wright A (2007) The initial effects of knee joint mobilization on osteoarthritic hyperalgesia. *Manual Therapy* 12 (2): 109–18.

Murray CJ, Lopez AD (1996) Evidence-based health policy – lessons from the Global Burden of Disease Study. *Science* 274 (5288): 740–3.

National Collaborating Centre for Chronic Conditions (2006) *Osteoarthritis: methodology pack*. London: National Collaborating Centre for Chronic Conditions.

National Institute for Health and Clinical Excellence (2001) Technology appraisal no 27. Guidance on the use of cyclooxygenase (Cox) II selective inhibitors, celecoxib, rofecoxib, meloxicam and etoclolae for osteoarthritis and rhematoid arthritis. London: NICE.

National Institute for Health and Clinical Excellence (2006a) *Guidelines Manual.* London: NICE.

National Institute for Health and Clinical Excellence (2006b) *Obesity: the prevention, identification, assessment and management of overweight and obesity in adults and children.* London: NICE.

National Institute for Health and Clinical Excellence (2007) *Depression: management of depression in primary and secondary care.* London: NICE.

Naylor CD, Williams JI (1996) Primary hip and knee replacement surgery: Ontario criteria for case selection and surgical priority. *Quality in Health Care* 5 (1): 20–30.

Niethard FU, Gold MS, Solomon GS et al. (2005) Efficacy of topical diclofenac diethylamine gel in osteoarthritis of the knee. *Journal of Rheumatology* 32 (12): 2384–92.

Nigg BM, Emery C, Hiemstra LA (2006) Unstable shoe construction and reduction of pain in osteoarthritis patients. *Medicine & Science in Sports & Exercise* 38 (10): 1701–8.

Nikles CJ, Yelland M, Glasziou PP et al. (2005) Do individualized medication effectiveness tests (N-of-1 trials) change clinical decisions about which drugs to use for osteoarthritis and chronic pain? *American Journal of Therapeutics* 12 (1): 92–7.

Nilsdotter AK, Aurell Y, Siosteen AK et al. (2001) Radiographic stage of osteoarthritis or sex of the patient does not predict one year outcome after total hip arthroplasty. *Annals of the Rheumatic Diseases* 60 (3): 228–32.

Nunez M, Nunez E, Segur JM et al. (2006) The effect of an educational program to improve health-related quality of life in patients with osteoarthritis on waiting list for total knee replacement: a randomized study. *Osteoarthritis & Cartilage* 14 (3): 279–85.

Ones K, Tetik S, Tetik C et al. (2006) The effects of heat on osteoarthritis of the knee. *Pain Clinic* 18 (1): 67–75.

Osiri M, Brosseau L, McGowan J et al. (2000) Transcutaneous electrical nerve stimulation for knee osteoarthritis. *Cochrane Database of Systematic Reviews*

Ostergaard M, Stoltenberg M, Gideon P et al. (1996) Changes in synovial membrane and joint effusion volumes after intraarticular methylprednisolone. *Journal of Rheumatology* 23: 1151–61.

Paker N, Tekdos D, Kesiktas N et al. (2006) Comparison of the therapeutic efficacy of TENS versus intra-articular hyaluronic acid injection in patients with knee osteoarthritis: a prospective randomized study. *Advances in Therapy* 23 (2): 342–53.

Pariser D, O'Hanlon A, Espinoza L (2005) Effects of telephone intervention on arthritis self-efficacy, depression, pain, and fatigue in older adults with arthritis. *Journal of Geriatric Physical Therapy* 28 (3): 67–73.

Parr G, Darekar B, Fletcher A et al. (1989) Joint pain and quality of life; results of a randomised trial. *British Journal of Clinical Pharmacology* 27 (2): 235–42.

Patrick DL, Ramsey SD, Spencer AC et al. (2001) Economic evaluation of aquatic exercise for persons with osteoarthritis. *Medical Care* 39 (5): 413–24.

Peacock M, Rapier C (1993) The topical NSAID felbinac is a cost effective alternative to oral NSAIDs for the treatment of rheumatic conditions. *British Journal of Medical Economics* 6: 135–42.

Peat G, Thomas E, Duncan R et al. (2006) Clinical classification criteria for knee osteoarthritis: performance in the general population and primary care. *Annals of the Rheumatic Diseases* 65: 1363–7.

Peat G, McCarney R, Croft P (2001) Knee pain and osteoarthritis in older adults: a review of community burden and current use of primary health care. *Annals of the Rheumatic Diseases* 60 (2): 91–7.

Peloquin L, Bravo G, Gauthier P et al. (1999) Effects of a cross-training exercise program in persons with osteoarthritis of the knee. A randomized controlled trial. *JCR: Journal of Clinical Rheumatology* 5 (3): 126–36.

Penninx BW, Messier SP, Rejeski WJ et al. (2001) Physical exercise and the prevention of disability in activities of daily living in older persons with osteoarthritis. *Archives of Internal Medicine* 161 (19): 2309–16.

Penninx BW, Rejeski WJ, Pandya J et al. (2002) Exercise and depressive symptoms: a comparison of aerobic and resistance exercise effects on emotional and physical function in older persons with high and low depressive symptomatology. *Journals of Gerontology Series B – Psychological Sciences & Social Sciences* 57 (2): 124–32.

Perlman AI, Sabina A, Williams AL et al. (2006) Massage therapy for osteoarthritis of the knee: a randomized controlled trial. *Archives of Internal Medicine* 166 (22): 2533–8.

Perpignano G (1994) Double-blind comparison of the efficacy and safety of etodolac SR 600 mg u.i.d. and of tenoxicam 20 mg u.i.d. in elderly patients with osteoarthritis of the hip and of the knee. *International Journal of Clinical Pharmacology Research* 14 (5–6): 203–16.

Peters TJ, Saunders C, Dieppe P et al. (2005) Factors associated with change in pain and disability over time: a community-based prospective observational study of hip and knee osteoarthritis. *British Journal of General Practice* 55: 205–11.

Petrella RJ, Petrella M (2006) A prospective, randomized, double-blind, placebo controlled study to evaluate the efficacy of intraarticular hyaluronic acid for osteoarthritis of the knee. *Journal of Rheumatology* 33 (5): 951–6.

Pham T, Maillefert JF, Hudry C et al. (2004) Laterally elevated wedged insoles in the treatment of medial knee osteoarthritis. A two-year prospective randomized controlled study. *Osteoarthritis & Cartilage* 12 (1): 46–55.

Pincus T (2004) Patient Preference for Placebo, Acetaminophen (paracetamol) or Celecoxib Efficacy Studies (PACES): two randomised, double blind, placebo controlled, crossover clinical trials in patients with knee or hip osteoarthritis. *Annals of the Rheumatic Diseases* 63 (8): 931–9.

Pipitone N, Scott DL (2001) Magnetic pulse treatment for knee osteoarthritis: a randomised, double-blind, placebo-controlled study. *Current Medical Research & Opinion* 17 (3): 190–6.

Quilty B, Tucker M, Campbell R et al. (2003) Physiotherapy, including quadriceps exercises and patellar taping, for knee osteoarthritis with predominant patello-femoral joint involvement: randomized controlled trial. *Journal of Rheumatology* 30 (6): 1311–7.

Quintana JM, Arostegui I, Azkarate J et al. (2000) Evaluation of explicit criteria for total hip joint replacement. *Journal of Clinical Epidemiology* 53 (12): 1200–8.

Qvistgaard E, Christensen R, Torp PS et al. (2006) Intra-articular treatment of hip osteoarthritis: a randomized trial of hyaluronic acid, corticosteroid, and isotonic saline. *Osteoarthritis & Cartilage* 14 (2): 163–70.

Rai J, Pal SK, Gul A et al. (2004) Efficacy of chondroitin sulfate and glucosamine sulfate in the progression of symptomatic knee osteoarthritis: a randomized, placebo-controlled, double blind study. *Bulletin, Postgraduate Institute of Medical Education & Research* 38 (1): 18–22.

Ramos-Remus C, Salcedo-Rocha AL, Prieto-Parra RE et al. (2000) How important is patient education? *Baillieres Best Practice in Clinical Rheumatology* 14 (4): 689–703.

Ravaud P, Moulinier L, Giraudeau B et al. (1999) Effects of joint lavage and steroid injection in patients with osteoarthritis of the knee: results of a multicenter, randomized, controlled trial. *Arthritis & Rheumatism* 42 (3): 475–82.

Raynauld JP, Torrance GW, Band PA et al. (2002) A prospective, randomized, pragmatic, health outcomes trial evaluating the incorporation of hylan G-F 20 into the treatment paradigm for patients with knee osteoarthritis (Part 1 of 2): clinical results. *Osteoarthritis & Cartilage* 10 (7): 506–17.

Reichenbach S, Sterchi R, Scherer M et al. (2007) Meta-analysis: chondroitin for osteoarthritis of the knee or hip. *Annals of Internal Medicine* 146 (8): 580–90.

Rejeski WJ, Craven T, Ettinger WH Jr. et al. (1996) Self-efficacy and pain in disability with osteoarthritis of the knee. *Journals of Gerontology Series B – Psychological Sciences & Social Sciences* 51 (1): 24–9.

Rejeski WJ, Focht BC, Messier SP et al. (2002) Obese, older adults with knee osteoarthritis: weight loss, exercise, and quality of life. *Health Psychology* 21 (5): 419–26.

Rejeski WJ, Martin KA, Miller ME et al. (1998) Perceived importance and satisfaction with physical function in patients with knee osteoarthritis. *Annals of Behavioral Medicine* 20 (2): 141–8.

Richards JD (2005) A comparison of knee braces during walking for the treatment of osteoarthritis of the medial compartment of the knee. *Journal of Bone & Joint Surgery – British Volume* 87 (7): 937–9.

Robinson VA, Brosseau L, Peterson J et al. (2001) Therapeutic ultrasound for osteoarthritis of the knee. *Cochrane Database of Systematic Reviews* (3)

Roddy E, Zhang W, Doherty M (2005) Aerobic walking or strengthening exercise for osteoarthritis of the knee? A systematic review. *Annals of the Rheumatic Diseases* 64 (4): 544–8.

Roder C, Staub LP, Eggli S et al. (2007) Influence of preoperative functional status on outcome after total hip arthroplasty. *Journal of Bone & Joint Surgery – American Volume* 89 (1): 11–7.

Rogind H (1997) Comparison of etodolac and piroxicam in patients with osteoarthritis of the hip or knee: a prospective, randomised, double-blind, controlled multicentre study. *Clinical Drug Investigation* 13 (2): 66–75.

Rolf C, Engstrom B, Beauchard C et al. (1999) Intra-articular absorption and distribution of ketoprofen after topical plaster application and oral intake in 100 patients undergoing knee arthroscopy. *Rheumatology* 38 (6): 564–7.

Rothacker D, Difigilo C, Lee I (1994) A clinical trial of topical 10% trolamine salicylate in osteoarthritis. *Current Therapeutic Research, Clinical & Experimental* 55 (5): 584–97.

Rothacker D, Lee I, Littlejohn III TW (1998) Effectiveness of a single topical application of 10% trolamine salicylate cream in the symptomatic treatment of osteoarthritis. *JCR: Journal of Clinical Rheumatology* 4 (1): 6–12.

Sadr AO, Bellocco R, Eriksson K et al. (2006) The impact of tobacco use and body mass index on the length of stay in hospital and the risk of post-operative complications among patients undergoing total hip replacement. *Journal of Bone & Joint Surgery – British Volume* 88 (10): 1316–20.

Salaffi F, Cavalieri F, Nolli M et al. (1991) Analysis of disability in knee osteoarthritis. Relationship with age and psychological variables but not with radiographic score. *Journal of Rheumatology* 18 (10): 1581–6.

Salim M (1996) Transcutaneous electrical nerve stimulation (TENS) in chronic pain. *Alternative Therapies in Clinical Practice* 3 (4): 33–5.

Sanda M, Collins SH, Mahady J (1983) Three-month multicenter study of etodolac (Ultradol(TM)) in patients with osteoarthritis of the hip. *Current Therapeutic Research, Clinical & Experimental* 33 (5): 782–92.

Sanders C, Donovan J, Dieppe P (2002) The significance and consequences of having painful and disabled joints in older age: co-existing accounts of normal and disrupted biographies. *Sociology of Health and Illness* 24 (2): 227–53.

Sanders C, Donovan JL, Dieppe PA (2004) Unmet need for joint replacement: a qualitative investigation of barriers to treatment among individuals with severe pain and disability of the hip and knee. *Rheumatology* 43 (3): 353–7.

Schaefer M, DeLattre M, Gao X et al. (2005) Assessing the cost-effectiveness of COX-2 specific inhibitors for arthritis in the Veterans Health Administration. *Current Medical Research & Opinion* 21 (1): 47–60.

Scheiman JM, Yeomans ND, Talley NJ et al. (2006) Prevention of ulcers by esomeprazole in at-risk patients using non-selective NSAIDs and COX-2 inhibitors. *American Journal of Gastroenterology* 101 (4): 701–10.

Schmalzried TP, Silva M, de la Rosa MA et al. (2005) Optimizing patient selection and outcomes with total hip resurfacing. *Clinical Orthopaedics & Related Research* 441: 200–4.

Schnitzer TJ, Burmester GR, Mysler E (2004) Comparison of lumiracoxib with naproxen and ibuprofen in the Therapeutic Arthritis Research and Gastrointestinal Event Trial (TARGET), reduction in ulcer complications: randomised controlled trial. *Lancet* 364 (9435): 665–74.

Schnitzer TJ, Morton C, Coker S (1994) Topical capsaicin therapy for osteoarthritis pain: achieving a maintenance regimen. *Seminars in Arthritis & Rheumatism* 23 (suppl 3): 34–40.

Scott S (1996) Shortwave diathermy. In: Kitchen S, Bazin S, editors. *Clayton's electrotherapy 10E*. London: WB Saunders Company Limited, p154–78.

Scott WA (1969) The relief of pain with an antidepressant in arthritis. *Practitioner* 202 (212): 802–7.

Segal L, Day SE, Chapman AB et al. (2004) Can we reduce disease burden from osteoarthritis? *Medical Journal of Australia* 180 (5 suppl): 1–7.

Sevick MA, Bradham DD, Muender M et al. (2000) Cost-effectiveness of aerobic and resistance exercise in seniors with knee osteoarthritis. *Medicine & Science in Sports & Exercise* 32 (9): 1534–40.

Shackel NA, Day RO, Kellett B et al. (1997) Copper-salicylate gel for pain relief in osteoarthritis: a randomised controlled trial. *Medical Journal of Australia* 167 (3): 134–6.

Sheldon EB (2005) Efficacy and tolerability of lumiracoxib in the treatment of osteoarthritis of the knee: a 13-week, randomized, double-blind comparison with celecoxib and placebo. *Clincal Therapeutics* 27 (1): 64–77.

Singh G, Fort JG, Goldstein JL et al. (2006) Celecoxib versus naproxen and diclofenac in osteoarthritis patients: SUCCESS-I Study. *American Journal of Medicine* 119 (3): 255–66.

Smugar SS, Schnitzer TJ, Weaver AL (2006) Rofecoxib 12.5 mg, rofecoxib 25 mg, and celecoxib 200 mg in the treatment of symptomatic osteoarthritis: results of two similarly designed studies. *Current Medical Research & Opinion* 22 (7): 1353–67.

Sobel DS (1995) Rethinking medicine: improving health outcomes with cost-effective psychosocial interventions. *Psychosomatic Medicine* 57 (3): 234–44.

Solomon DH, Chibnik LB, Losina E et al. (2006) Development of a preliminary index that predicts adverse events after total knee replacement. *Arthritis & Rheumatism* 54 (5): 1536–42.

Sowers JR, White WB (2005) The effects of cyclooxygenase-2 inhibitors and nonsteroidal anti-inflammatory therapy on 24-hour blood pressure in patients with hypertension, osteoarthritis, and type 2 diabetes mellitus. *Archives of Internal Medicine* 165 (2): 161–8.

Spicer DD, Pomeroy DL, Badenhausen WE et al. (2001) Body mass index as a predictor of outcome in total knee replacement. *International Orthopaedics* 25 (4): 246–9.

Spiegel BM, Targownik L, Dulai GS et al. (2003) The cost-effectiveness of cyclooxygenase-2 selective inhibitors in the management of chronic arthritis. *Annals of Internal Medicine* 138 (10): 795–806.

Stahl S, Karsh ZI, Ratzon N et al. (2005) Comparison of intraarticular injection of depot corticosteroid and hyaluronic acid for treatment of degenerative trapeziometacarpal joints. *JCR: Journal of Clinical Rheumatology* 11 (6): 299–302.

Stamm TA, Machold KP, Smolen JS (2002) Joint protection and home hand exercises improve hand function in patients with hand osteoarthritis: a randomized controlled trial. *Arthritis & Rheumatism* 47 (1): 44–9.

Stener VE, Kruse SC, Jung K (2004) Comparison between electro-acupuncture and hydrotherapy, both in combination with patient education and patient education alone, on the symptomatic treatment of osteoarthritis of the hip. *Clinical Journal of Pain* 20 (3): 179–85.

Stewart M, Brown JB, Weston WW (2003) *Patient-centered medicine: transforming the clinical method.* 2nd edition. USA: Radcliffe Medical Press.

Suarez-Otero R (2002) Efficacy and safety of diclofenac-cholestyramine and celecoxib in osteoarthritis. *Proceedings of the Western Pharmacology Society* 45: 26–8.

Superio-Cabuslay E, Ward MM, Lorig KR (1996) Patient education interventions in osteoarthritis and rheumatoid arthritis: a meta-analytic comparison with nonsteroidal anti-inflammatory drug treatment. *Arthritis Care & Research* 9 (4): 292–301.

Sutton D, Gignac MAM, Cott C (2002) Medical and everyday assistive device use among older adults with arthritis. *Canadian Journal on Aging* 21 (4): 535–48.

Tak ES (2005) The effects of an exercise program for older adults with osteoarthritis of the hip. *Journal of Rheumatology* 32 (6): 1106–13.

Tak SH, Laffrey SC (2003) Life satisfaction and its correlates in older women with osteoarthritis. *Orthopaedic Nursing* 22 (3): 182–9.

Tallon D, Chard J, Dieppe P (2000) Exploring the priorities of patients with osteoarthritis of the knee. *Arthritis Care & Research* 13 (5): 312–9.

Tannenbaum H, Berenbaum F, Reginster JY et al. (2004) Lumiracoxib is effective in the treatment of osteoarthritis of the knee: a 13 week, randomised, double blind study versus placebo and celecoxib. *Annals of the Rheumatic Diseases* 63 (11): 1419–26.

Tascioglu F, Armagan O, Tabak Y et al. (2004) Low power laser treatment in patients with knee osteoarthritis. *Swiss Medical Weekly* 134 (17–18): 254–8.

Tavakoli M (2003) Modelling therapeutic strategies in the treatment of osteoarthritis: an economic evaluation of meloxicam versus diclofenac and piroxicam. *Pharmacoeconomics* 21 (6): 443–54.

Temple AR, Benson GD, Zinsenheim JR et al. (2006) Multicenter, randomized, double-blind, active-controlled, parallel-group trial of the long-term (6–12 months) safety of acetaminophen in adult patients with osteoarthritis. *Clinical Therapeutics* 28 (2): 222–35.

ter Haar G (1999) Therapeutic ultrasound. *European Journal of Ultrasound* 9: 3–9.

Thamsborg G, Florescu A, Oturai P et al. (2005) Treatment of knee osteoarthritis with pulsed electromagnetic fields: a randomized, double-blind, placebo-controlled study. *Osteoarthritis & Cartilage* 13 (7): 575–81.

Thomas KS, Miller P, Doherty M et al. (2005) Cost effectiveness of a two-year home exercise program for the treatment of knee pain. *Arthritis & Rheumatism* 53 (3): 388–94.

Thorstensson CA, Roos EM, Petersson IF et al. (2005) Six-week high-intensity exercise program for middle-aged patients with knee osteoarthritis: a randomized controlled trial. *BMC Musculoskeletal Disorders* 6 (27)

Tillu A, Roberts C, Tillu S (2001) Unilateral versus bilateral acupuncture on knee function in advanced osteoarthritis of the knee – a prospective randomised trial. *Acupuncture in Medicine* 19 (1): 15–8.

Tillu A, Tillu S, Vowler S (2002) Effect of acupuncture on knee function in advanced osteoarthritis of the knee: a prospective, non-randomised controlled study. *Acupuncture in Medicine* 20 (1): 19–21.

Toda Y (2001) The effect of energy restriction, walking, and exercise on lower extremity lean body mass in obese women with osteoarthritis of the knee. *Journal of Orthopaedic Science* 6 (2): 148–54.

Toda Y, Tsukimura N, Kato A (2004a) The effects of different elevations of laterally wedged insoles with subtalar strapping on medial compartment osteoarthritis of the knee. *Archives of Physical Medicine & Rehabilitation* 85 (4): 673–7.

Toda Y, Tsukimura N (2004b) A comparative study on the effect of the insole materials with subtalar strapping in patients with medial compartment osteoarthritis of the knee. *Modern Rheumatology* 14 (6): 459–65.

Toda Y, Tsukimura N (2004c) A six-month follow up of a randomized trial comparing the efficacy of a lateral-wedge insole with subtalar strapping and an in-shoe lateral-wedge insole in patients with varus deformity osteoarthritis of the knee. *Arthritis & Rheumatism* 50 (10): 3129–36.

Toda Y, Tsukimura N (2006) A 2-year follow-up of a study to compare the efficacy of lateral wedged insoles with subtalar strapping and in-shoe lateral wedged insoles in patients with varus deformity osteoarthritis of the knee. *Osteoarthritis & Cartilage* 14 (3): 231–7.

Toda Y, Tsukimura N, Segal N (2005) An optimal duration of daily wear for an insole with subtalar strapping in patients with varus deformity osteoarthritis of the knee. *Osteoarthritis & Cartilage* 13 (4): 353–60.

Torrance GW, Raynauld JP, Walker V et al. (2002) A prospective, randomized, pragmatic, health outcomes trial evaluating the incorporation of hylan G-F 20 into the treatment paradigm for patients with knee osteoarthritis (Part 2 of 2): economic results. *Osteoarthritis & Cartilage* 10 (7): 518–27.

Towheed T, Maxwell L, Judd M et al. (2006a) Acetaminophen for osteoarthritis. *Cochrane Database of Systematic Reviews* (1): CD004257.

Towheed TE (2006b) Pennsaid therapy for osteoarthritis of the knee: a systematic review and metaanalysis of randomized controlled trials. *Journal of Rheumatology* 33 (3): 567–73.

Towheed TE, Maxwell L, Anastassiades TP et al. (2005) Glucosamine therapy for treating osteoarthritis. *Cochrane Database of Systematic Reviews*

Trnavsky K, Fischer M, Vogtle JU et al. (2004) Efficacy and safety of 5% ibuprofen cream treatment in knee osteoarthritis. Results of a randomized, double-blind, placebo-controlled study. *Journal of Rheumatology* 31 (3): 565–72.

Tubach F, Dougados M, Falissard B et al. (2006) Feeling good rather than feeling better matters more to patients. *Arthritis & Rheumatism* 55 (4): 526–30.

Tucker M, Brantingham JW, Myburg C (2003) Relative effectiveness of a non-steroidal anti-inflammatory medication (Meloxicam) versus manipulation in the treatment of osteoarthritis of the knee. *European Journal of Chiropractic* 50 (3): 163–83.

Tuzun EH, Aytar A, Eker L et al. (2004) Effectiveness of two different physical therapy programmes in the treatment of knee osteoarthritis. *Pain Clinic* 16 (4): 379–87.

Urwin M, Symmons D, Allison T et al. (1998) Estimating the burden of musculoskeletal disorders in the community: the comparative prevalence of symptoms at different anatomical sites, and the relation to social deprivation. *Annals of the Rheumatic Diseases* 57 (11): 649–55.

Vaile JH, Davis P (1998) Topical NSAIDs for musculoskeletal conditions. A review of the literature. *Drugs* 56 (5): 783–99.

van Baar ME, Dekker J, Oostendorp RA et al. (2001) Effectiveness of exercise in patients with osteoarthritis of hip or knee: nine months' follow up. *Annals of the Rheumatic Diseases* 60 (12): 1123–30.

van Baar ME, Dekker J, Oostendorp RA et al. (1998) The effectiveness of exercise therapy in patients with osteoarthritis of the hip or knee: a randomized clinical trial. *Journal of Rheumatology* 25 (12): 2432–9.

van der Esch M, Heijmans M, Dekker J (2003) Factors contributing to possession and use of walking aids among persons with rheumatoid arthritis and osteoarthritis. *Arthritis & Rheumatism* 49 (6): 838–42.

Veitiene D, Tamulaitiene M (2005) Comparison of self-management methods for osteoarthritis and rheumatoid arthritis. *Journal of Rehabilitation Medicine* 37 (1): 58–60.

Ververeli PA, Sutton DC, Hearn SL et al. (1995) Continuous passive motion after total knee arthroplasty: analysis of cost and benefits. *Clinical Orthopaedics & Related Research* 321: 208–15.

Victor CR, Ross F, Axford J (2004) Capturing lay perspectives in a randomized control trial of a health promotion intervention for people with osteoarthritis of the knee. *Journal of Evaluation in Clinical Practice* 10 (1): 63–70.

Victor CR, Triggs ER (2005) Lack of benefit of a primary care-based nurse-led education programme for people with osteoarthritis of the knee. *Clinical Rheumatology* 24 (4): 358–64.

Viney RC, King MT, Savage EJ et al. (2004) Use of the TTU is questionable. *Medical Journal of Australia* 181 (6): 338–9.

Waddell D, Rein A, Panarites C et al. (2001) Cost implications of introducing an alternative treatment for patients with osteoarthritis of the knee in a managed care setting. *American Journal of Managed Care* 7 (10): 981–91.

Wajon A, Ada L (2005) No difference between two splint and exercise regimens for people with osteoarthritis of the thumb: a randomised controlled trial. *Australian Journal of Physiotherapy* 51 (4): 245–9.

Walsh D (1997) *TENS Clinical applications and related theory.* New York: Churchill Livingstone.

Wang T, Belza B, Elaine TF et al. (2007) Effects of aquatic exercise on flexibility, strength and aerobic fitness in adults with osteoarthritis of the hip or knee. *Journal of Advanced Nursing* 57 (2): 141–52.

Wegman AC, van der Windt DA, De HM et al. (2003) Switching from NSAIDs to paracetamol: a series of n of 1 trials for individual patients with osteoarthritis. *Annals of the Rheumatic Diseases* 62 (12): 1156–61.

Weinberger M, Tierney WM, Booher P (1989) Common problems experienced by adults with osteoarthritis. *Arthritis Care & Research* 2 (3): 94–100.

Weiss S L (2000) Prospective analysis of splinting the first carpometacarpal joint: an objective, subjective, and radiographic assessment. *Journal of Hand Therapy* 13 (3): 218–26.

Weiss S L (2004) Splinting the degenerative basal joint: custom-made or prefabricated neoprene? *Journal of Hand Therapy* 17 (4): 401–6.

White A, Foster NE, Cummings M et al. (2007) Acupuncture treatment for chronic knee pain: a systematic review. *Rheumatology* 46 (3): 384–90.

Wielandt T, McKenna K, Tooth L et al. (2006) Factors that predict the post-discharge use of recommended assistive technology (AT). *Disability and Rehabilitation: Assistive Technology* 1 (1–2): 29–40.

Wiesenhutter CW, Boice JA (2005) Evaluation of the comparative efficacy of etoricoxib and ibuprofen for treatment of patients with osteoarthritis: a randomized, double-blind, placebo-controlled trial. *Mayo Clinic Proceedings* 80 (4): 470–9.

Wilder FV, Barrett JP, Farina EJ (2006) Joint-specific prevalence of osteoarthritis of the hand. *Osteoarthritis & Cartilage* 14 (9): 953–7.

Wilkie R, Peat G, Thomas E et al. (2007) Factors associated with restricted mobility outside the home in community-dwelling adults aged 50 years and older with knee pain: an example of use of an international classification of functioning to investigate participation restriction. *Arthritis Care & Research* 57 (8): 1381–9.

Wilkie R, Peat G, Thomas E, et al. (2006) *The potential determinants of restricted mobility outside the home in community-dwelling older adults with knee pain.*; 4 May 2006,

Williams GW, Ettlinger RE, Ruderman EM et al. (2000) Treatment of osteoarthritis with a once-daily dosing regimen of celecoxib: A randomized, controlled trial. *JCR: Journal of Clinical Rheumatology* 6 (2): 65–74.

Williams GW, Hubbard RC, Yu SS et al. (2001) Comparison of once-daily and twice-daily administration of celecoxib for the treatment of osteoarthritis of the knee. *Clincal Therapeutics* 23 (2): 213–27.

Williams PI, Hosie J (1989) Etodolac therapy for osteoarthritis: a double-blind, placebo-controlled trial. *Current Medical Research & Opinion* 11 (7): 463–70.

Witt CM, Brinkhaus B, Reinhold T et al. (2006a) Efficacy, effectiveness, safety and costs of acupuncture for chronic pain – results of a large research initiative. *Acupuncture in Medicine* 24 (suppl): S33–S39.

Witt CM, Jena S, Brinkhaus B et al. (2006b) Acupuncture in patients with osteoarthritis of the knee or hip: a randomized, controlled trial with an additional nonrandomized arm. *Arthritis & Rheumatism* 54 (11): 3485–93.

Woolf AD, Pfleger B (2003) Burden of major musculoskeletal conditions. *Bulletin of the World Health Organization* 81 (9): 646–56.

World Health Organization (2003) *The burden of musculoskeletal conditions at the start of the new millenium: report of a WHO scientific group.*

Wyatt FB, Milam S, Manske RC et al. (2001) The effects of aquatic and traditional exercise programs on persons with knee osteoarthritis. *Journal of Strength & Conditioning Research* 15 (3): 337–40.

Yelland MJ, Nikles CJ, McNairn N et al. (2007) Celecoxib compared with sustained-release paracetamol for osteoarthritis: a series of N-of-1 trials. *Rheumatology* 46 (1): 135–40.

Yen ZS, Lai MS, Wang CT et al. (2004) Cost-effectiveness of treatment strategies for osteoarthritis of the knee in Taiwan. *Journal of Rheumatology* 31: 1797–803.

Yocum D (2000) Safety and efficacy of meloxicam in the treatment of osteoarthritis: a 12-week, double-blind, multiple-dose, placebo-controlled trial. *Archives of Internal Medicine* 160 (19): 2947–54.

Yurtkuran M, Alp A, Konur S et al. (2007) Laser acupuncture in knee osteoarthritis: a double-blind, randomized controlled study. *Photomedicine and Laser Surgery* 25 (1): 14–20.

Yurtkuran M, Kocagil T (1999) TENS, electroacupuncture and ice massage: comparison of treatment for osteoarthritis of the knee. *American Journal of Acupuncture* 27 (3–4): 133–40.

Zacher J (2003) A comparison of the therapeutic efficacy and tolerability of etoricoxib and diclofenac in patients with osteoarthritis. *Current Medical Research & Opinion* 19 (8): 725–36.

Zhang W, Moskowitz RW, Nuki G et al. (2007) OARSI recommendations for the management of hip and knee osteoarthritis, Part I: critical appraisal of existing treatment guidelines and systematic review of current research evidence. *Osteoarthritis & Cartilage* 15 (9): 981–1000.

Zhao SZ, McMillen JI, Markenson JA et al. (1999) Evaluation of the functional status aspects of health-related quality of life of patients with osteoarthritis treated with celecoxib. *Pharmacotherapy* 19 (11): 1269–78.